CURRENT CONCEPTS IN COLONIC DISORDERS

Edited by **Godfrey Lule**

Current Concepts in Colonic Disorders
Edited by Godfrey Lule

Published by InTech
Janeza Trdine 9, 51000 Rijeka, Croatia

Publishing Process Manager Marina Jozipovic

Technical Editor Teodora Smiljanic

Cover Designer InTech Design Team

Additional hard copies can be obtained from orders@intechopen.com

Current Concepts in Colonic Disorders, Edited by Godfrey Lule
p. cm.
ISBN 978-953-307-957-8

For EU product safety concerns:
IN TECH d.o.o., Prolaz Marije Krucifikse Kozulić 3, 51000 Rijeka, Croatia,
info@intechopen.com or visit our website at intechopen.com.

Meet the editor

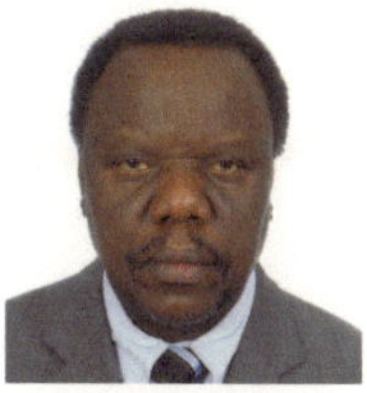

Professor Godfrey Lule was born in Kampala, Uganda, and studied medicine at Makerere University, Kampala graduating with the MBChB degree in 1976. He specialized in internal medicine at the University of Nairobi. He studied at the University of London and The London School of Tropical Medicine and Health obtaining the postgraduate Diploma in Tropical Medicine and the MSc. in infectious disease at the University of London. In 2008, he received the Fellowship of the Royal College of Physician (Edinburgh). He has published over 50 original articles in peer reviewed journals and has contributed chapters to textbooks especially covering the fields of gastroenterology and HIV disease. In 2000, he edited the first edition of "Guidelines to Antiretroviral Therapy in Kenya" followed by "Guidelines to management of opportunistic infections in Kenya". He currently works as a Professor of Medicine in the Department of Medicine, University of Nairobi medical school and is a practicing consultant physician, gastroenterologist and infectious disease specialist.

Contents

Preface

The primary objective of the first edition of this book of colonic disorders is to try to fill the gap in the fields of gastroenterology that have not been properly covered in the past.

Gastrointestinal diseases are the leading causes of morbidity and mortality in clinical practice with diarrhea and abdominal pain accounting for over 50% of the symptoms that patients present to their doctors. It is therefore not surprising that many of the chapters in this book are on diarrhea and acute or chronic abdominal pain.

The chapters have been written by world renown experts in their respective fields, all of which are related to gastroenterology.

Dr. Saulius Paskauskas has covered the area of adult intussusceptions, Prof. Azevedo et al write about prospective uses of genetic engineering, while dysbiosis of intestinal microbiota in irritable bowel syndrome has been very well covered by Dr. Anna Lyra and Dr. Sampo Lahtinen.

Other interesting titles like perforated appendicitis, travelers' diarrhea and management of various gastrointestinal conditions are some of the topics presented in simple and accessible language with well labeled illustrations where appropriate.

Advances in the pathophysiology and treatment of postoperative ileus has been covered by Dr. Tropskaya and Dr. Popova, with evidence based on experiments carried out in animal models, while Prof. Yvette Tache et al ably handle modulation of visceral pain by stress implication and modulation. The later is a must read for all professionals as it utilizes simple theories to explain some of the recurrent symptomatologies that patients present with.

This book will form useful reading for the inquisitive undergraduate medical student who wants to read more about the pathophysiology of various gastrointestinal diseases such as intussusceptions but also offers detail to the specialists out to explain causes and management of various conditions such as acute and chronic diarrhea.

Most of the chapters have an introduction and objective, epidemiology, clinical presentation and investigation sections, with outlines on management and conclusions at the end. They have been presented in this way to make them easy to understand and for quick reference by the reader while in the clinic or classroom in these days of pressure for answers and maximum time constraint.

To the reader, we hope that this book will offer you the right knowledge that would favorably modify your approach to problems of the gastrointestinal tract in the future.

Godfrey Lule FRCP (E)
Consultant Physician & Gastroenterologist/
Infectious Disease Specialist
Professor of Medicine, Department of Medicine,
University of Nairobi,
Kenya

Part 1

Intussusception

1

Adult Intussusception

Saulius Paskauskas and Dainius Pavalkis
Lithuanian University of Health Sciences
Kaunas
Lithuania

1. Introduction

Intussusception is defined as the invagination of one segment of the gastrointestinal tract and its mesentery (intussusceptum) into the lumen of an adjacent distal segment of the gastrointestinal tract (intussuscipiens). Sliding within the bowel is propelled by intestinal peristalsis and may lead to intestinal obstruction and ischemia.

Adult intussusception is a rare condition wich can occur in any site of gastrointestinal tract from stomach to rectum. It represents only about 5% of all intussusceptions (Agha, 1986) and causes 1-5% of all cases of intestinal obstructions (Begos et al., 1997; Eisen et al., 1999). Intussusception accounts for 0.003–0.02% of all hospital admissions (Weilbaecher et al., 1971). The mean age for intussusception in adults is 50 years, and and the male-to-female ratio is 1:1.3 (Rathore et. al., 2006). The child to adult ratio is more than 20:1. The condition is found in less than 1 in 1300 abdominal operations and 1 in 100 patients operated for intestinal obstruction. Intussusception in adults occurs less frequently in the colon than in the small bowel (Zubaidi et al., 2006; Wang et al., 2007).

Mortality for adult intussusceptions increases from 8.7% for the benign lesions to 52.4% for the malignant variety (Azar & Berger, 1997)

2. Etiology of adult intussusception

Unlike children where most cases are idiopathic, intussusception in adults has an identifiable etiology in 80- 90% of cases. The etiology of intussusception of the stomach, small bowel and the colon is quite different (Table 1).

50-75% of adult small bowel intussusception are due to benign pathology. The most common lesions are adhesions and Meckel's diverticulum. Other lesions include lymphoid hyperplasia, lipomas, leiomyomas, hemangiomas and idiopathic causes are more likely to occur in the small intestine than in the colon. Other conditions that predispose to small bowel intussusception include anorexia nervosa and malabsorption. The increased flaccidity of the bowel wall facilitates invagination. Unregulated anticoagulant therapy may cause submucosal hemorrhages that can lead to intussusception (Wang et al., 2007). Malignant causes of small bowel intussusception include primary leiomyosarcomas, malignant gastrointestinal stromal tumors, carcinoid tumors, neuroendocrine tumors and lymphomas. Less commonly, malignant tumors may act as lead points with metastatic disease being the most common, especially melanomas.

60-75% of large bowel intussuception are caused by malignant neoplasm. The most common malignant cause is primary adenocarcinoma and the most common nonmalignant cause is lipoma (Barussaud et al., 2006). Independent predictors of malignancy include: patients age, site of intussusception (more often colonic than enteric) and presence of anemia (hemoglobin <12g/dl) (Goh et al., 2006).

Benign or malignant neoplasms cause two thirds of these cases with a lead point; the remaining cases are caused by infections, postoperative adhesions, Crohn's granulomas, intestinal ulcers (Yersinia), and congenital abnormalities such as Meckel's diverticulum (Barussaud et al., 2006).

Lesion	**Stomach**	**Small Bowel**	**Large Bowel**
Benign	Adenoma Leiomyoma Lipoma Hamartoma Inflammatory polyps	Lipoma Leiomyoma Haemangioma Neurofibroma Adenomatous polyp Meckel diverticulum Intestinal duplication Inflammatory lesions Trauma GIST Postpoperative adhesions Lymphoid hyperplasia Adenitis Coeliac disease Henoch-Schonlein purpura Roux-en-Y anastomoses Peutz-Jeghers syndrome Tuberculosis Tropical sprue Giardiasis	Lipoma Adenomatous polyp Postpoperative adhesion Leiomyoma GIST Endometriosis (appendiceal) Previous anastomosis Crohn's disease Mucocele of apendix
Malignant	**Primary:** Adenocarcinoma Leiomyosarcoma	**Primary:** Lymphoma Malignant duodenal ulcers Malignant GIST **Secondary:** Metastatic melanoma Adenocarcinoma metastasis (lung or breast) Osteosarcoma Lymphoma	**Primary:** Adenocarcinoma Leiomyosarcoma Malignant GIST **Secondary:** Metastatic melanoma Lymphoma
Idiopathic		Motility disorder	Motility disorder

Table 1. Lesions associated with adult intussusception. GIST - gastrointestinal stromal tumor

Non neoplastic processes constitute 15–25% of cases, while idiopathic or primary intussusceptions account for only about 10%. Idiopathic causes of adult intussusception are more likely to occur in the small intestine than in the colon (Wang et al., 2007).

Some etiological differences were observed in primary adult intussusception between Western developed world and central, western Africa. This geographic variation in pathology has been attributed to the fiber content of the diet (which affects fecal load), dietary habits (large amount of beans and rice after several days without eating producing excess colonic peristalsis), and chemicals in the gut from parasites (ascaris toxins are smooth muscle stimulants) or food, and genetics (mobile right colon with a long mesentery) (VanderKolk et al., 1996).

3. Patophysiology of intussusception

The most common locations in the gastrointestinal tract where an intussusception can take place are the junctions between freely moving segments and retroperitoneally or adhesionally fixed segments. Stimulation of the gastrointestinal tract by a food bolus produces an area of constriction above the bolus and relaxation below. Any intraluminal lesion in the gastrointestinal tract or irritant within the lumen, which alters the normal peristaltic pattern, is able to initiate intussusception. The duodenum, stomach, and esophagus are rarely involved in intussusception because they are less redundant and less mobile within the abdomen (Cera, 2008). A historical cause of both antegrade and retrograde small bowel intussusception in adults is the use of long cantor tubes (Shub et al., 1978). Antegrade intussusception in this situation occurs as telescoping of the bowel over the tube especially when it is fixed in place with tape at the nose. Retrograde intussusception occurs during or after the tube is removed, especially if removed quickly and with force (Cera, 2008).

3.1 Antegrade intussusception

Antegrade intussusception occurs when any mucosal, intramural or extrinsic lead point acts as a focal area of traction in the proximal segment of the gastrointestinal tract and is pulled forward by progressive smooth muscle contractions into the distal segment (Cera, 2008). The result of this process is invagination of the involved wall and telescoping of one gastrointestinal tract segment over the adjacent segment with its mesenteric fold as result of overzealous or impaired peristalsis, further obstructing the free passage of intestinal contents and, more severely, compromising the mesenteric vascular flow of the intussuscepted segment (Figure 1). This occurrence may be transient, and therefore asymptomatic if reduction occurs spontaneously. However, more commonly, the intussusception persists because of the continued peristaltic contractions, which can lead to gastrointestinal tract obstruction accounting for the majority of the presenting symptoms. If left untreated, the mesentery involved in the intussusception may become stretched and compressed leading to vascular insufficiency, strangulation, and necrosis of the associated bowel. These events, in turn, may lead to perforation, peritonitis, and death.

In the non neoplastic cases, when lead point is absent, intussusception may be caused by functional disturbances without bowel wall abnormality, such as in coeliac disease. In these cases the loss of normal tone in the small bowel owing to the toxic effect of gluten causes flaccid, dilated bowel loops that are more prone to non obstructing intussusception.

Individuals with pelvic floor abnormalities such as nonrelaxing puborectalis and rectocele may develop rectoanal intussusception in the setting of chronic straining (Weiss & McLemore, 2008).
The origin of intussusception after gastric bypass is different from that of intussusception provoked by other causes. It is likely to be related to motility disorders in the divided small bowel, especially in the Roux limb. This rare condition may cause obstruction and lead to bowel necrosis if not recognized and treated promptly (Daellenbach & Suter, 2011).
Rectoanal intussusception is the functional disorder telescoping of the rectal wall during defecation.
Two predominant hypotheses exist regarding the etiology of rectoanal intussusception:

1. Rectoanal intussusception as a primary disorder. Some theorize that rectoanal intussusception may be the initial stage of a dynamic continuum of anomalies initiated by repetitive traumatic injury from intussusception, which may lead to solitary rectal ulcer and eventual full thickness rectal prolapse (Hwang et. al., 2006).
2. Rectoanal intussusception as a secondary phenomenon. Individuals with pelvic floor abnormalities such as nonrelaxing puborectalis and rectocele may develop rectoanal intussusception in the setting of chronic straining. Rectoanal intussusception may also develop in patients with paradoxical contraction and other spastic anal sphincter disorders (Weiss & McLemore, 2008).

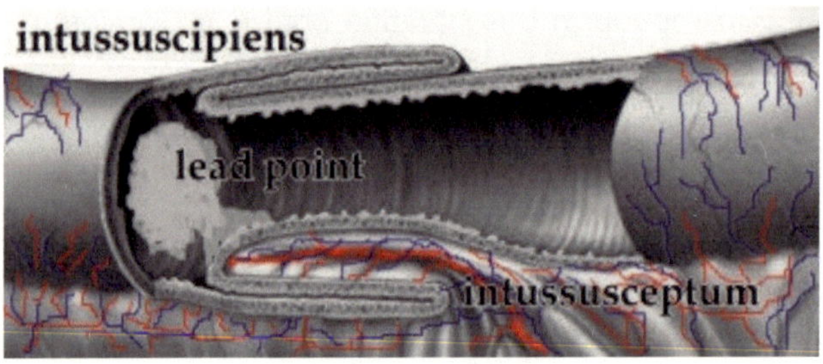

Fig. 1. Intussusception of the bowel with the lead point in the lumen.

3.1 Retrograde intussusception

Retrograde intussusception is especially rare. Altered peristalsis in focal areas of the bowel wall can lead to dysrhythmic contractions and can cause retrograde intussusception. In addition, altered peristalsis may occur as a result of functional deficits such as neuronal intestinal dysplasia where bowel dysmotility is caused by aberrant neuronal development.
The exact mechanism precipitating of an antegrade and retrograde intussusception is still unknown.

4. Classification of intussusception

There are no accepted classification of adult intussusception. We recommend to classify the intussusception according to:

1. The anatomical location of the intussusception (gastric, small bowel or colon):
- gastroenteric,
- enteroenteric,
- appendiceal,
- appendiceal-ileocolic,
- ileocolic,
- colocolic,
- rectoanal,
- stomal.
2. Cause:
2.1 neoplastic
- benign,
- malignant;
2.2 nonneoplastic
2.3 idiopathic
3. Lead point:
- intussusception with lead point;
- intussusception without lead point,
4. Direction:
- antegrade,
- retrograde.
5. Clinical course:
- acute
- chronic,
- persistent,
- recurrent
- transient.
6. Bowel obstruction:
- with lumen obstruction,
- without lumen obstruction.
7. Vascular insufficiency:
- with disturbance of the blood stream,
- without disturbance of the blood stream.

5. Clinical presentation of adult intussusception

Adult intussusceptions pose a further challenge as they are often presented with nonspecific symptoms and run a chronic indolent course. The spectrum of clinical presentation depends on the site of the intussusception, the timing of clinical presentation, and the predilection for spontaneous reduction.

The clinical presentation of adult intussusception may be presented with a variety of acute (duration less 4 days), subacute (duration 4-14days), and chronic (duration more than 14 days) or intermittent symptoms. Most patients manifest subacute (about 24%) or chronic (about 50-73%) symptoms (Barussaud et al., 2006). Duration of symptoms is longer in benign lesions as compared with malignant lesions and is longer in enteric lesions as compared with colonic lesions. The classic pediatric presentation triad of abdominal pain, palpable abdominal mass and bloody discharge from the rectum are seen only in 10% of cases. In adults, intussusception typically manifests as an acute or chronic obstruction and the presentation of adult intussusception is similar to that of small and large bowel obstruction.

Unlike intussusception in children, an acute abdomen is very occasionally present in adults. The most common symptom in the acute presentation is abdominal pain (71-100%), associated or not with an intestinal obstructive syndrome, which occurs in 78 to 100% of patients (Erkan et al., 2005; Barussaud et al., 2006; Paskauskas et al., 2010). Intermittent abdominal pain and vomiting (40-60% of the cases) and/or nausea are the major symptoms of subacute or chronic adult intussusception. Bleeding per rectum occurs in 8-27% of the cases (Table 2). This wide range is usually based on the site of the intussusception, with colonic ones bleeding more frequently than the ileal varieties. Other findings as fever, constipation or diarrhoea, tenesmus are rare in presentation of patients with intussusception.

Clinical symptoms of obstructive defecation are typical for rectoanal intussusception. One of the most common frustrations in patients with symptomatic rectoanal intussusception is the sensation of incomplete evacuation. These individuals will also frequently describe a sensation of obstruction and pressure toward the sacrum, which may increase with straining. Fecal incontinence is also a common symptom associated with rectoanal intussusception (Weiss & McLemore, 2008).

5.1 Physical and laboratorial findings of intussusception

Adult intussusception has no specific physical findings. Common physical findings include abdominal distention, hypoactive or absent bowel sounds, ocult blood test. Palpable abdominal mass or mass protruding through the anus are rare (Ahn et al., 2009; Paskauskas et al., 2010). In those with colonic lesions, up to one half can demonstrate a mass compared with 14% of those with enteric lesions. If the presentation is late in the course of the condition, signs of bowel ischemia such as pain out of proportion to examination or generalized peritonitis may result with corresponding signs of shock such as hypotension and tachycardia.

By digital examination the rectocele, anismus can be helpful to suspicion of the rectoanal intussusception (Weiss & McLemore, 2008). The longer the intussusception, the more closely the clinical examination correlated with defecography (Karlbom et al., 2004). Blood egzamination gives up to 40% evaluated leukocyte level (Table 2), with left shift on differential until 38%(Ahn et al., 2009). Anaemia is strong by associated with carcinoma as lead point of intussusception (Goh et al., 2006).

6. Diagnostic tools for adult intussusception

Preoperative diagnosis is a challenge because of rarity of adult intussusception, longstanding, intermittent, nonspecific symptoms and physical findings, and signs on imaging. Despite of the evalution of the radiological procedures, intussusception is diagnosed preoperatively from 14 to 75% of the cases. The most important factors in arriving at the correct diagnosis are an awareness of the possibility of this condition existing in any patient with symptoms, suggesting prior episodes of partial intestinal obstruction, and the vigorous approach towards complete radiographic examination in such patients (Cotlar & Cohn, 1961).

Clinical presentation	
Abdominal pain	71–100 %
Nausea	35-59 %
Vomiting	31-59 %
Loss of weight	4-33 %
Episodes of diarrhoea	9-28%
Hematochezia, rectal bleeding	8-27%
Constipation	13-26%
Fever	4-25%
Tenesmus	3 %
Physical findings	
Abdominal distension	23-54%
Palpable abdominal mass	8-33%
Mass protruding through the anus	2-8 %
Laboratorial blood tests	
Anaemia (hemoglobin <12 g/dl)	43%
Leukocytosis	40%

Table 2. Common clinical, physical and laboratorial findings of adult patients with intussusception.

Non-invasive radiologic imaging techniques can be of significant help in identifying an intussusception, but most cases are diagnosed at emergency operation, after abdomen exploration and excision of the intussuscepted segment of the gastrointestinal tract.

6.1 Plain abdominal film

Plain abdominal films are typically the first diagnostic tool in acute abdomen and usually demonstrate signs of acute intestinal obstruction (air-fluid levels) and may provide information regarding to the site of obstruction (Eisen et al., 1999). Sensitivity of this diagnostic tool regarding to intussusception is only about 25% (Yakan et al., 2009).

6.2 Barium enema

Barium enema examination is cheap, quite easy to carry out, and seems to be useful method with an accuracy rates from 20 to 45% for the diagnosis of intussusceptions, but remains limited to the ileocolic or colonic lesions (Barussaud et al., 2006; Goh et al., 2006). Barium enema with barium reflux in the lumen of the space between the intussusceptum and intussuscipiens can help to identify the site and cause (Figure 2) of the intussusception, particularly in more chronic cases. Signs of intussusception include a spiral, "coil spring" or "stacked coin" appearance with narrowed central canal (Eisen et al., 1999). These signs result from the retrograde filling of the contrast between the walls of the invaginated bowel loop. The narrowed central canal is the edematous, obstructing intussusceptum (Goh et al., 2006).

Contrast studies are obviously contraindicated if there is a possibility of bowel perforation or ischemia.

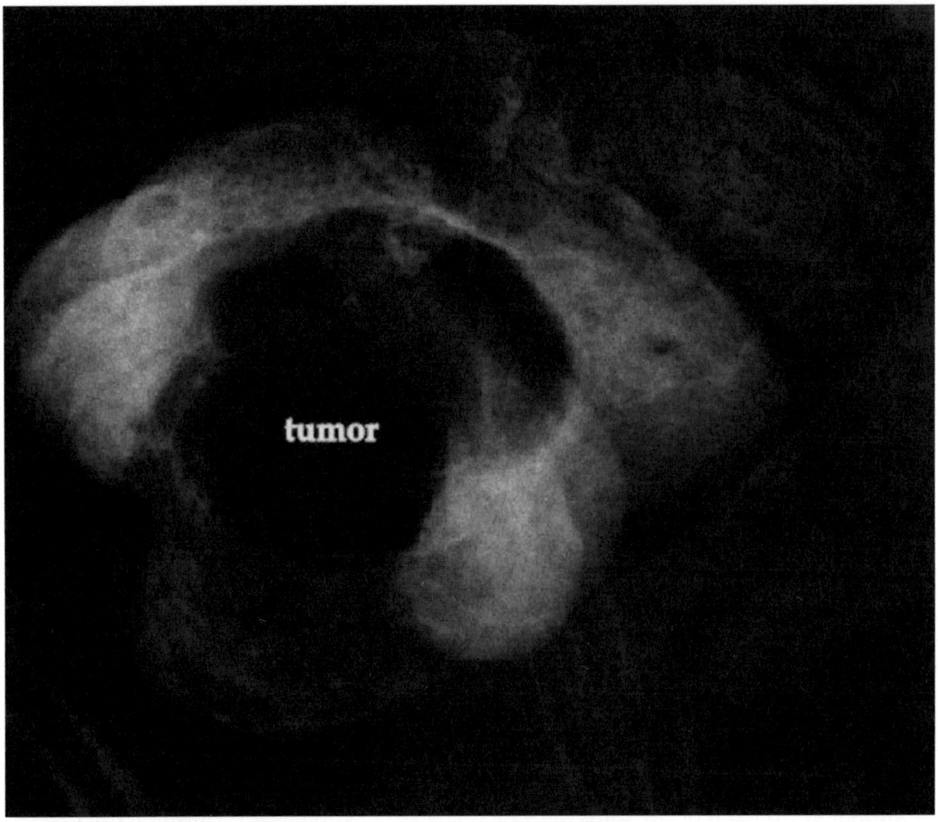

Fig. 2. Colonic intussusception with tumor as lead point in the bowel lumen (figure from Paskauskas et al., 2010).

6.3 Ultrasonography

Ultrasonography is considered to be a useful tool for the diagnosis of suspected intussusception (Figures 3, 4), when the characteristic a „target and doughnut sign" (an even thickened hypoechoic outer and a central hyperechoic core on transverse view), a „crescent-in-doughnut sign" (an even outer hypoechoic rim with a central hyperechoic crescent) or a „multiple concentric rings sign" (a mass with multiple alternating hypoechoic and hyperechoic concentric rings (Figures 5, 6)), and other views are shown (Figures 3, 4). It is quick and cost-effective and shows, when done by an experienced physician, similar sensitivity and specificity like a CT scan (Martin-Lorenzo et al., 2004). Ultrasonography is a more available and generalized technique than CT, enabling it to be used more often with emergency and acute symptoms and thus being available at times of abdominal crisis in intermittent processes. Sonography allows a study on all planes and in real time, which is important as intussusception is often a dynamic phenomenon. The most characteristic, in fact most specific, sonographic aspect of intestinal invagination is obtained on a cross-section and depends on the area of the invagination in which it is performed, its length and the existence or not of a lesion that acts as a head (Martin-Lorenzo et al., 2004). If color flow Doppler is used, the presence of bowel necrosis may be demonstrated by showing compromised blood flow to the intussusceptum. The major disadvantage of ultrasound is masking by gas-filled loops of bowel, and operator dependency.

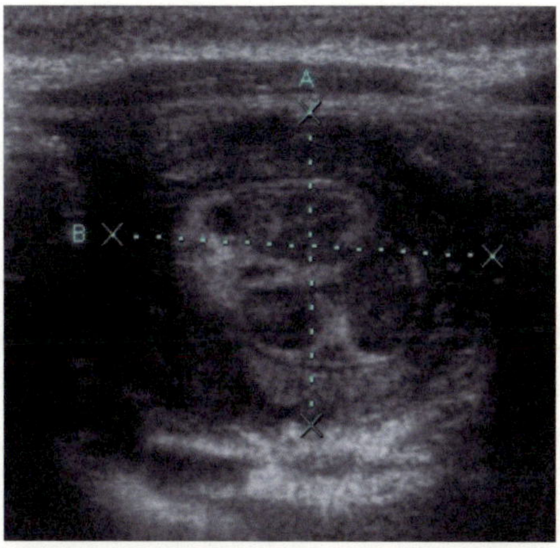

Fig. 3.

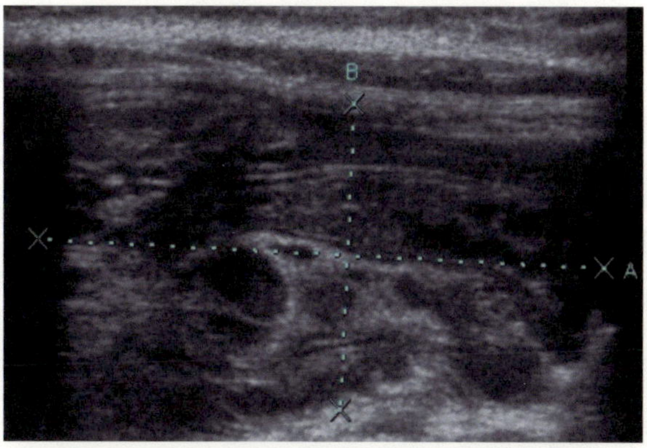

Fig. 4.

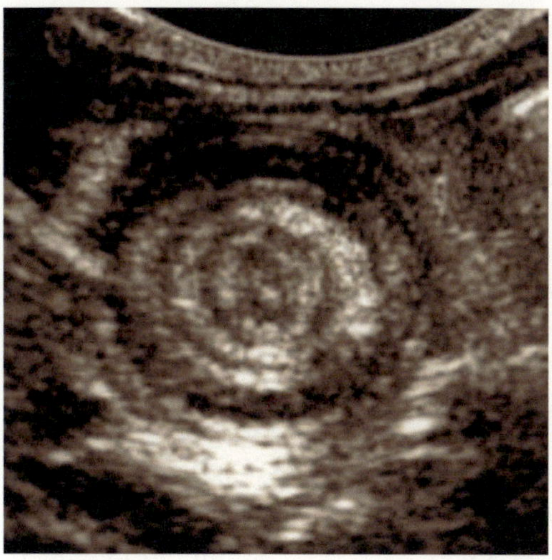

Fig. 5.

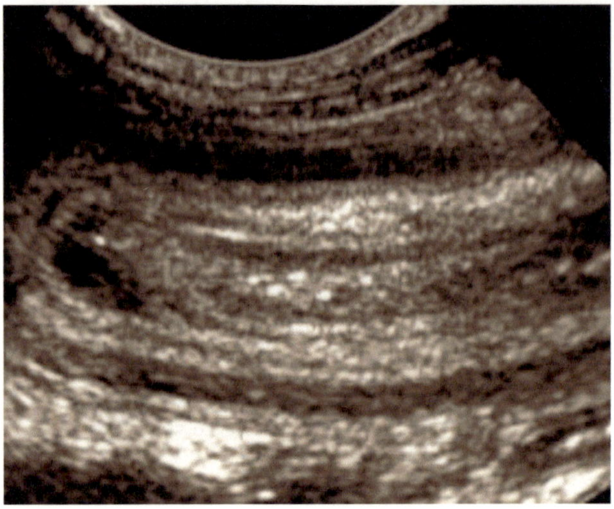

Fig. 6.

Fig. 3 - Fig. 6. Ultrasonography views of an intussusception (figures are provided from Radiology department of Lithuanian University of Health Sciences).
Figures 3 and 5 show a transverse view of the intussuscepted bowel. Figure 4 and 6 represent longitudinal view of the intussuscepted bowel. In figures 3 and 4 the lines A and B mark the intussuscepted bowel lumen. In figure 5 alternating hyperechoic and hypoechoic concentric rings are present within the lumen of a distended loop of bowel, giving the typical "target" sign. In figure 6 multiple layers of bowel wall are shown within the lumen of the intussuscipiens.

6.4 Computed tomography

In recent years, CT has become the first imaging method performed, after plain abdominal films, in the evaluation of patients with non-specific abdominal complaints. Intussusception is well diagnosed on multi-slice spiral computed tomography with a diagnostic accuracy near 100%. Abdominal CT is the most useful diagnostic tool not only for detecting an intussusception, but also helps in identifying the underlying cause (Huang & Warshauer, 2003). CT demonstrates the collapsed intussusceptum lying within the opacified lumen of the distal intussuscipiens (Figures 7, 8). The CT appearance of an intussusception is often a complex target-shaped or sausage-shaped in-homogeneous soft tissue mass with an eccentric area of fat density contained within, which represents the mesenteric fat (Yakan et al., 2009). Later, a layering effect occurs as a result of longitudinal compression and venous congestion in the intussusceptum (Bar-Ziv & Solomon, 1991). Multislice CT facilitates the assessment of vascular supply to the affected bowel loop in cases of intussusception where impending ischemia is suspected (Gayer et al., 2002). Especially in cases in which a malignancy is suspected, CT can be useful for diagnosing the surrounding area (Martin-Lorenzo et al., 2004). In comparison to ultrasonography CT has the limitations of less accessibility and a static and initially only single-plane exploration, apart from involving a dose of radiation and generally requiring the administration of oral and intravenous contrast material, which delays the study and may entail adverse effects.

Abdominal CT scanning is the preferred noninvasive radiologic modality for diagnosing intussusception from colonic lipomas (Taylor & Wolff, 1987). The CT characteristics of lipoma include a spherical or ovoid shape; smooth, sharply demarcated margins with a thin fibrous septa and homogeneous fatty density with CT values between -40 and -120 Hounsfield units (Chiang et Lin, 2008). If prominent fibrous septa and nodularity are evident, the most imperative differential diagnosis is a well-differentiated liposarcoma, despite the few reports of gastrointestinal liposarcomas in the literature (Pereira et al., 2005).

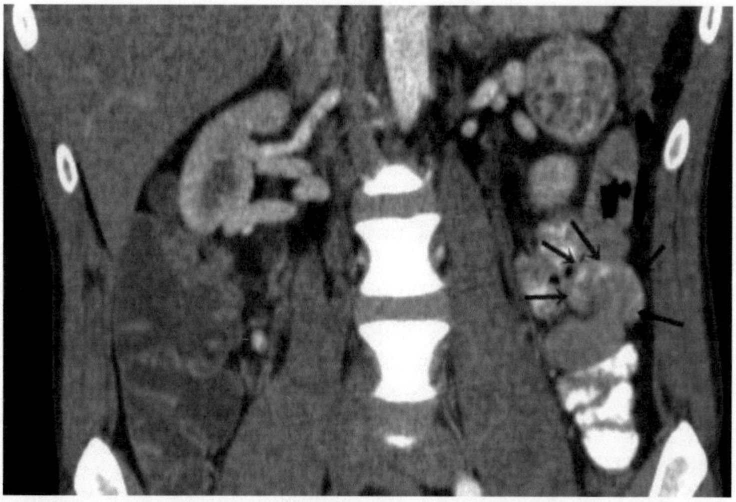

Fig. 7. Coronaric view of small bowel intussusception (marked with arrows) and tumor of the left kidney. (Figure is provided from Radiology department of Lithuanian University of Health Sciences).

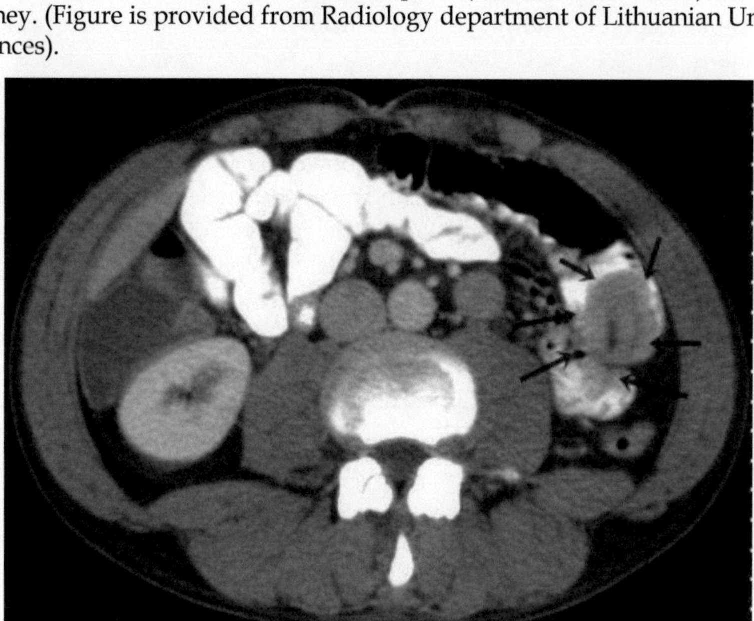

Fig. 8. Axial view of small bowel intussusception (marked with arrows). (Figure is provided from Radiology department of Lithuanian University of Health Sciences).

6.5 Magnetic resonance imaging

The general imaging characteristics of adult intussusception on MRI are similar to those on CT. Unlike CT, MR examination, is not technically limited by the presence of previously administered barium (Tamburrini et al., 2004).

6.6 Capsule endoscopy

Intussusception during capsule endoscopy is an accidental finding (Culliford et al., 2005).

6.7 Colonoscopy

Colonoscopy is also a useful tool for evaluating intussusception, especially when the present ing symptoms indicate a large bowel obstruction, but have limitations in small bowel egzamination. Colonoscopy plays a role in the evaluation of large bowel obstruction caused by intussusception by defining benign from malignant causes. It can be used as part of the preoperative assessment or, if the intussusception is found intraoperatively as it most commonly occurs, can be performed intraoperatively to facilitate appropriate surgical management (Cera, 2008). It may not be advisable to perform endoscopic biopsy or polypectomy in those individuals with long-term symptoms because of the high risk of perforation, which is more likely to happen in the phase of chronic tissue ischemia, and perhaps necrosis because of vascular compromise in intussusception (Erkan et al., 2005).

6.8 Defecography

Defecography is the gold standard for the diagnosis of the rectoanal intussusception. Dynamic pelvic magnetic resonance imaging and transperineal ultrasound are attractive alternatives to defecography; however, their sensitivity is poor in comparison to the gold standard at this time.

6.9 Laparoscopy

Laparoscopy, although not an imaging study, is obviously an excellent evaluation tool when intussusception is suspected in a patient with bowel obstruction. It allows for identification of the location, the nature of the lead point, and the presence of compromised bowel. It aids in the choice of an appropriate location for the incision that would minimize length (Barussaud et al., 2006).

Laparoscopic operation may be applicable as a less-invasive method, but not in acute bowel obstruction.

The sensitivities of the different radiological methods are abdominal ultrasounds (35%), upper gastrointestinal barium study (33%), abdominal computed tomography (58-100%), barium enema (73%), and colonoscopy (66%) (Huang et al., 2003; Erkan et al., 2005; Barussaud et al., 2006; Yakan et al., 2009).

7. Differential diagnosis

Because the symptoms are similar to other causes of intestinal obstruction and acute abdomen an intussusception in adults must be suspected in the differential diagnosis of these conditions.

8. Treatment

Many therapeutic interventions have been tried for the treatment of adult intussusception, which vary from conservative treatment to various surgical procedures. Treatment is almost always surgical in adults when compared to children and invariably leads to resection of the involved bowel segment with subsequent primary anastomosis. The choice of using a laparoscopic or open approach depends on the clinical condition of the patient, the location and extent of intussusception, the possibility of underlying disease, and the availability of surgeons with sufficient laparoscopic expertise. Emergency operations are necessary in about 35-60% of all adult patients with intussusception. For all patients who present with signs of perforation, shock, or peritonitis, immediate laparotomy is necessary. In the absence of these signs, the majority of adult patients are brought to the operating room with the preoperative diagnosis of bowel obstruction and an intussusception seen at the time of exploration. Unlike children, preoperative reduction with barium or air should not be recommended in adults as a definitive treatment (Huang et al., 2003). Overall, the type of surgical intervention depend on the cause of intussusception (benign or malignant), patients age, functional status, medical history and intraoperative findings (a gangrenous bowel or a perforation with peritonitis; location and length of intussuscepted segment) (Paskauskas et. al., 2010). The main problem is to distinguish the benign and the malignant lesions preoperatively (Nagorney et al., 1981; Chiang & Lin, 2008). Patients with malignant disease may undergo major surgery, including resection of the involved segment and regional lymph nodes, while patients with benign lesions may undergo simple resection (Figure 9). In most cases, the histological diagnosis is arrived at only after the excision of the tumor. Intraoperative histopathology is important examination for selected doubtful cases of adult intussusception, which can also assist in guiding the exact diagnosis and optimize surgical treatment planning (Jiang et al., 2007; Paskauskas et al., 2010).

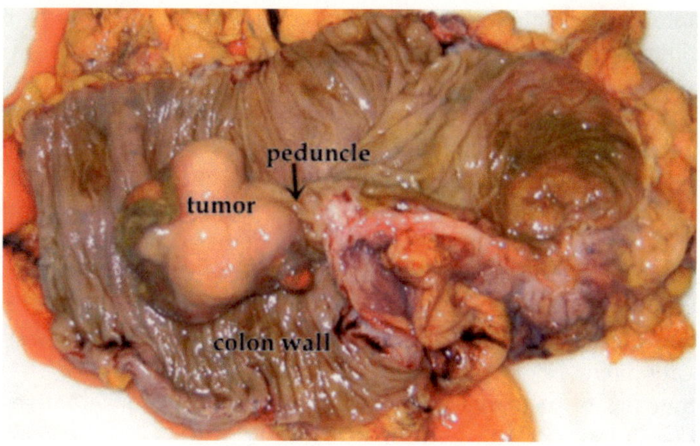

Fig. 9. Pedunculated colonic lipoma in lumen of resected specimen.

Recently, minimally invasive techniques such as endoscopic procedure, laparoscopic small and large bowel resections, have been applied to the treatment of small or large bowel obstruction and intussusception. The minilaparotomy approaches have many advantages over conventional laparotomy.

In specific situations, of both the large and small intestine intussusceptions of benign etiology an adhesolysis, appendectomy, enterotomy, polypectomy, or diverticulectomy is the sufficient treatment after reduction providing the bowel is viable (Erkan et al., 2005; Wang et al., 2007), but a polypectomy through a limited colotomy or enterotomy is done through an oedematous bowel, with an increased theoretic risk of leak (Barussaud et al., 2006).

Gastroduodenal and coloanal intussusceptions are extremely rare and may require innovative surgical techniques (Yalarmathi et al., 2005).

The optimal management of adult intussusception still remains controversial, but in any case it should be cut out.

8.1 Conservative treatment

In selected patients, when intermittent intussusception is associated with celiac disease, Crohn's disease and malabsorption syndrome as a result of abnormal intestinal contractions, these transient ones can be managed conservatively in the absence of any severe abdominal symptoms (Catalano, 1997).

8.2 Surgical treatment of large bowel intussusception

In adults, large bowel intussusception almost always requires surgical therapy (laparoscopy or laparatomy).

Two-thirds of colonic intussusceptions are resulted from malignant processes, therefore not diagnosed benign lesions before operation must be interpreted as cancer and should be treated by surgical oncological principles (Azar &Berger, 1997; Wang et al., 2007; Chiang & Lin, 2008). In most cases of adult colonic intussusception, primary resection without reduction should be performed due to the theoretical risks of perforation and the seeding of colonic microorganisms or tumor to the peritoneal cavity and venous embolization in regions of ulcerated bowel mucosa, after exposing and handling the ischemic, friable, and edematous bowel tissue (Nagorney et al., 1981).

An oncologic en bloc resection, after evaluation of the abdomen in search of distant metastases, is the surgical treatment of choice in cases of large bowel intussusception (Figure 10), if the intraoperative condition of the patient is stable (Erkan et al., 2005; Franz et al., 2010), particularly in those over 60 years of age due to a higher risk of malignancy.

En bloc resection eliminates the possibility of recurrence, is beneficial in patients at risk for short gut, and avoids enterotomy or anastomosis in edematous or compromised bowel. The reductions of intussuception also increase the risk of anastomotic complications (the bowel wall may be weakened during manipulation) and the potential for bowel perforation. For this reason, some authors advocate en bloc resections of all intussusception in adults regardless of location (enteric or colonic) or cause (benign or malignant).

Management strategies of rectoanal intussusception including conservative measures such as biofeedback and surgical procedures including mucosal proctectomy (Delorme), rectopexy, and stapled transanal rectal resection (STARR) procedures have varied degrees of efficacy (Weiss & McLemore, 2008). Overall, treatment of this pathology is multidisciplinary.

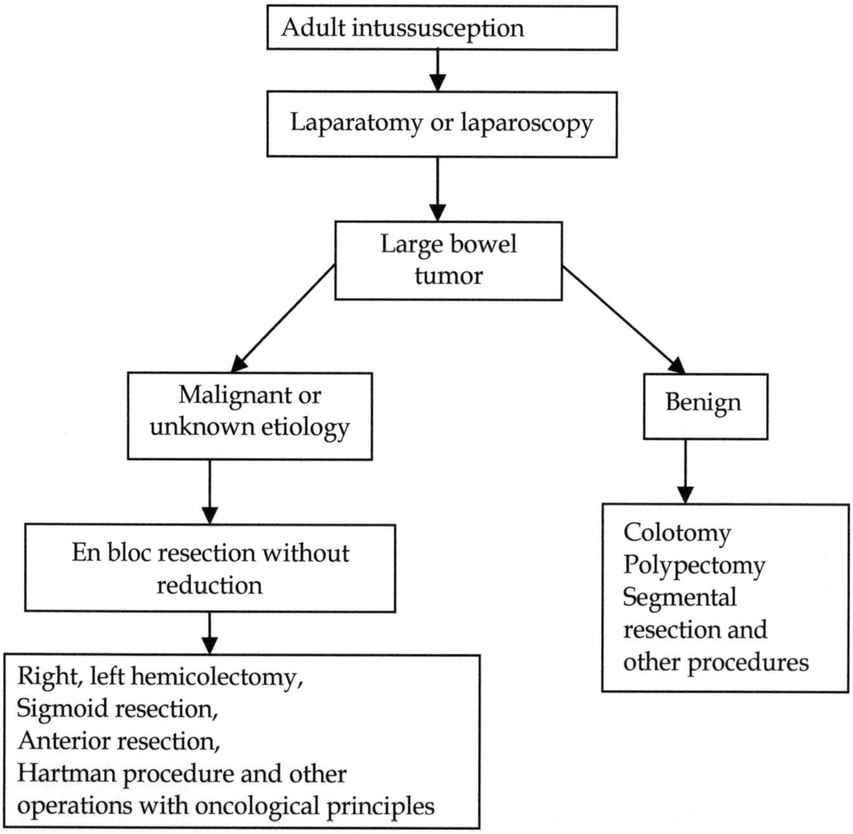

Fig. 10. Algorithm of surgical treatment of adult large bowel intussusception with tumor.

8.3 Surgical treatment of small bowel intussusception

Surgical treatment of small bowel intussusception is limited by remaining bowel length (Figure 11). In small bowel intussusception, initial reduction first of enteric lesions, before resection should be carried out in cases if the pre-operative diagnosis of benign etiology is confirmed, the bowel is viable or it entails resecting massive lengths of small bowel with the risk of short gut syndrome as a sequela (Takeuchi et al., 2003; Erkan et al., 2005; Khan et al., 2008; Franz et al., 2010).

Some authors reported the need for en bloc resection without reduction even in small bowel intussusception because of the inability to differentiate benign from malignant etiology preoperatively or intraoperatively (Wang et al., 2007). Reductions of these intussusceptions with subsequent enterotomy, biopsy, and excision of the etiologic lesion necessitate an enterotomy in edematous and previously ischemic bowel. The reduction of an intussusception secondary to a malignant lead point is potentially detrimental, as there is the theoretic risk of intraluminal or intraperitoneal seeding of the cancer, but oncologic resection is limited by the length of the remaining bowel. On the other hand, many malignancies causing enteric intussusception are metastatic implants in which the benefit of a formal oncologic resection is questionable and extent of resection does not impact overall survival and prognosis.

Benign enteric lesions that are not associated with adhesions require resection to prevent recurrent intussusception. The exception to this concept is postoperative adhesions, which are felt to be safe to reduce without resection as long as the bowel is viable (Azar & Berger, 1997). Because the leading tumors of intussusception in the small intestine are benign in frequency, laparoscopic operation may be applicable as a less-invasive method in not urgent situations.

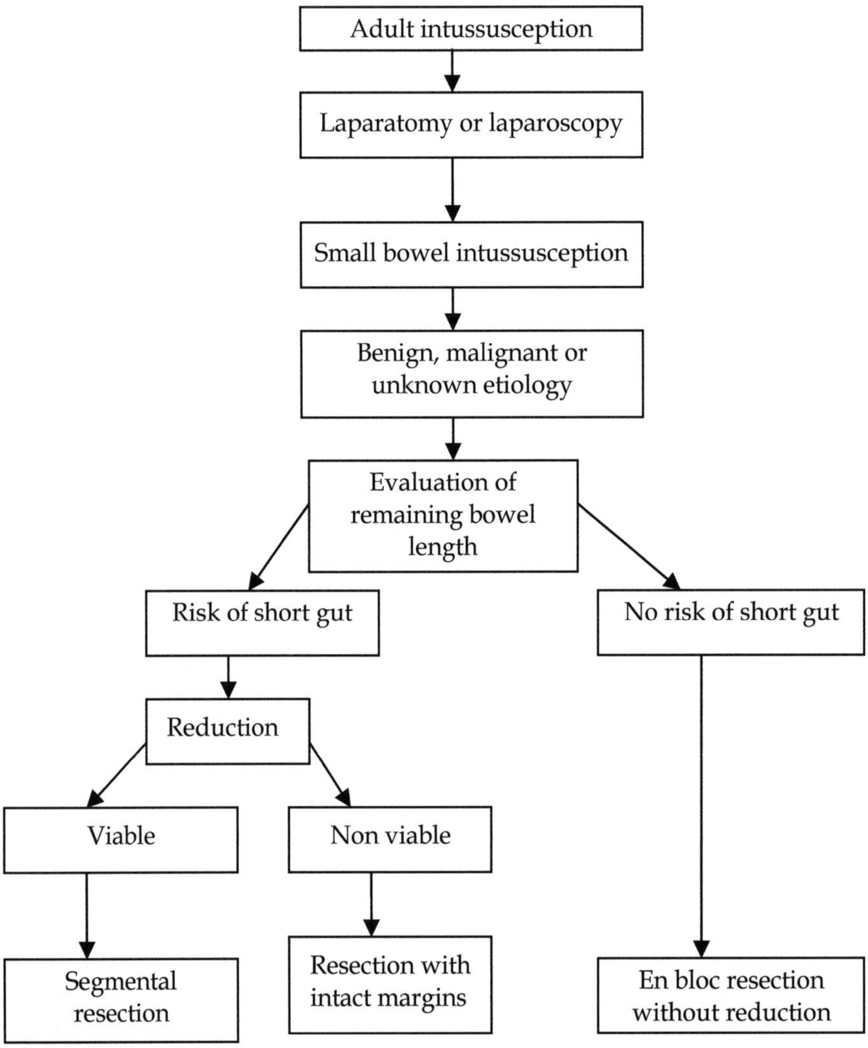

Fig. 11. Algorithm of treatment of adult small bowel intussusception.

9. Prognosis and complications of intussusception

Intussusceptions themselves have a good prognosis and depend on the cause. Mortality for adult intussusceptions increases from 8.7% for the benign lesions to 52.4% for the malignant cause. Intussusception-associated infant mortality rate account up to 2.3 per 1 000 000 live births (Parashar et al., 2000). Risk of mortality depends on bowel obstruction, complications, urgent operation, associated malignancy, but not on intussusceptions themselves. In children, if left untreated, intussusception can cause severe complications, which are directly related to the amount of time that passes from when the intussusception occurred until it is treated. Most patients who are treated within the first 24 hours recover completely. Further delay increases the risk of complications, which include bowel ischemia, necrosis and perforation, infection, and death (untreated 2-5 days). Mortality with treatment is 1-3%. Recurrence of an adult intussusception after surgical treatment is rare condition (Barussaud et al., 2006). In children, recurrence is observed in 3-11% of cases. Most recurrences involve intussusceptions that were reduced with contrast enema.

10. Differences between adult and pediatric intussusception

The adult intussusception is distinct from pediatric intussusception in various aspects. Intussusception is most commonly encountered in children and has been reported to be the most common abdominal emergency in early childhood and the second most common cause of intestinal obstruction after pyloric stenosis. It typically occurs from age 6 to 18 months and occurs more commonly in boys than girls. After 2 years of age, the incidence of intussusception declines. Only 30% of all cases of intussusception occur in children older than 2 years. Formation of the intussusceptum occurs differently in the pediatric and adult population. Factors involved in causation include anatomic features of the developing gastrointestinal tract and infectious influences.

The presentation of pediatric intussusception often is acute with sudden onset of intermittent colicky pain, vomiting, and bloody mucoid stools, and the presence of a palpable mass. In contrast, the adult entity may present with acute, subacute, or chronic non-specific symptoms. In the adult population, intussusception presents a preoperative diagnostic challenge and the rate of a preoperative correct diagnosis in the pediatric group is higher (Demirkan et al., 2009).

The decreased rigidity in the wall of the pediatric cecum (secondary to delayed development of the teniae coli) naturally allows for easy intussusception of the thickened muscle of the ileocecal valve which, in children, tends to be more anteriorly located and therefore more mobile and prone to prolapse.

Infections in the pediatric population, most commonly adenovirus and rotavirus, are thought to cause hypertrophy of Peyer's patches, increased bowel motility during diarrhoea resulting in an intussusceptum (Cera, 2008). In children, intussusception is idiopathic in 90% of cases and results in the common scenario of ileocolic intussusception (Demirkan et al., 2009). In contrast to children, adult intussusception is a rare disorder and is usually not idiopathic. In less than 10% of pediatric cases, a lead point or underlying cause may be found. These non idiopathic causes may be due to congenital gastrointestinal tract abnormalities, such as Meckel's diverticulum and intestinal duplication, or due to the presence of neoplastic lead points such as polyps, hamartomas, or lipomas. With increasing age, the non idiopathic causes tend to become more prevalent. Malignant causes of intestinal intussusception in pediatrics include lymphomas, carcinoma as associated with juvenile polyposis syndrome, and leiomyosarcoma (Cera, 2008). The diagnosis and management in the pediatric population is relatively standardized with nonoperative reduction attempted first. In children, abdominal ultrasound and air or contrast studies are the most useful

(Demirkan et al., 2009). Ultrasound is quick and cost-effective when done by an experienced radiologist with sensitivity and specificity approaching 100%. Ultrasound is less useful in adults because massive air in distended bowel loops and obesity limit image quality. Pneumatic or hydrostatic (air contrast enemas) reduction of the intussusception is sufficient to treat the condition in 80% of the patients. In contrast, almost 90% of the cases of intussusception in adults are secondary to a benign or malignant lesion. Due to a significant risk of associated malignancy, radiologic decompression is not addressed preoperatively in adults. More than 90% of adult cases of intussusception require surgical treatment.

11. Conclusion

Adult intussusception is a rare condition wich can occur in any site of gastrointestinal tract from stomach to rectum. Because of the rarity of adult intussusception and because of the nonspecific symptoms and physical finding, and signs on imaging, preoperative diagnosis is difficult. In adults, the treatment of intussusception is almost always surgical, emploing resectional approach. Intussusception themselves have a good prognosis, but this depend on the primary disease causing intussusception.

12. Acknowledgements

We thank Dr. K. Zviniene and Dr. D. Mitraite for providing us with ultrasonography and computed tomography images.

13. References

Agha FP. (1986). Intussusception in adults. *AJR Am J Roentgenol.*, (Mar 1986), 146, 3, pp. 527–531. PMID:3484870

Ahn JH, Choi SC, Lee KJ & Jung YS. (2009). A Clinical Overview of a Retrospective Study About Adult Intussusceptions: Focusing on Discrepancies Among Previous Studies. *Dig Dis Sci.*, (Dec 2009), 54, 12, pp. 2643–2649. PMID:19101801

Azar T & Berger DL. (1997). Adult intussusception. *Ann Surg.*, (Aug 1997), 226, 2, pp.134–138. PMID:9296505

Bar-Ziv J & Solomon A. (1991). Computed tomography in adult intussusception. *Gastrointest Radiol.*, (Summer 1991), 16, 3, pp. 264-266. PMID:1879648

Barussaud M, Regenet N, Briennon X, de Kerviler B,. Pessaux P, Kohneh-Sharhi N, Lehur PA, Hamy A, Leborgne J, le Neel JC & Mirallie E. (2006). Clinical spectrum and surgical approach of adult intussusceptions: a multicentric study. *Int J Colorectal Dis.*, (Jun 2005), 21, 8, pp. 834–839. PMID:15951987

Begos DG, Sandor A & Modlin IM. (1997). The diagnosis and management of adult intussusception. *Am J Surg.*, (Feb 1997), 173, 2, pp. 88–89. PMID:9074370

Catalano O. (1997). Transient small bowel intussusception: CT findings in adults. *Br J Radiol.*, (Aug 1997);70, 836, pp. 805–808. PMID:9486044

Cera SM. (2008). Intestinal Intussusception. *Clin Colon Rectal Surg.*, (May 2008), 21, 2, pp.106–113. PMID:20011406

Chiang JM & Lin YS. (2008). Tumor spectrum of adult intussusception. *J Surg Oncol.*, (Nov 2008), 98, 6, pp. 444-447. PMID:18668640

Cotlar AM & Cohn I. (1961). Intussusception in adults. *Am J Surg.*, (Jan 1961), 101, pp. 114–120. PMID:13695859

Culliford A, Daly J, Diamond B, Rubin M & Green PHR. (2005). The value of wireless capsule endoscopy in patients with complicated celiac disease. *Gastrointest Endosc.*, (Jul 2005), 62, 1, pp. 55-61. PMID:15990820

Huang BY, Warshauer DM. (2003). Adult intussusception: diagnosis and clinical relevance. *Radiol Clin North Am.*, (Nov 2003), 41, 6, pp. 1137–1151. PMID: 14661662

Daellenbach L & Suter M. (2011). Jejunojejunal intussusception after Roux-en-Y gastric bypass: a review. *Obes Surg.*, .(Feb 2011), 21, 2, pp.253-263. PMID:20949329

Demirkan A, Yagmurlu A, Kepenekci I, Sulaimanov M, Gecim E & Dindar H. (2009). Intussusception in Adult and Pediatric Patients: Two Different Entities. *Surg Today*, (Sep 2009), 39, 10, pp. 861–865. PMID: 19784724

Eisen LK, Cunningham JD, Aufses AH Jr. (1999). Intussusception in adults: institutional review. *J Am Coll Surg.*, (Apr 1999), 188, 4, pp. 390-395. PMID:10195723

Erkan N, Hacıyanlı M, Yıldırım M, Sayhan H, Vardar E & Polat AF. (2005). Intussusception in adults: an unusual and challenging condition for surgeons. *Int J Colorectal Dis.*, (Sep 2005) 20, 3, pp. 452–456. PMID:15759123

Franz B, Rabl C, Neureiter D, Ofner D & Emmanuel K. (2010). Emergency surgery for enteric and colonic intussusception in adults. *Eur Surg.*, (Aug 2010), 42, 4, pp. 180–183.

Gayer G, Zissin R, Apter S, Papa M & Hertz M. (2002). Pictorial review: adult intussusception - a CT diagnosis. *Br J Radiol.*, (Feb 2002), 75, 890, pp. 185–190. PMID:11893645

Goh BK, Quah HM, Chow PK, Tan KY, Tay KH, Eu KW, Ooi LL & Wong WK. (2006). Predictive factors of malignancy in adults with intussusception. *World J Surg.*, (Jul 2006), 30, 7, pp. 1300–1304. PMID:16773257

Huang BY & Warshauer DM. (2003). Adult intussusception: diagnosis and clinical relevance. *Radiol Clin North Am* ., (Nov 2003), 41, 6, pp. 1137–1151. PMID:14661662

Hwang YH, Person B, Choi JS, Nam YS, Singh JJ, Weiss EG, Nogueras JJ & Wexner SD. (2006). Biofeedback therapy for rectal intussusception. *Tech Coloproctol.*, (Mar 2006), 10, 1, pp. 11–15. PMID:16528489

Jiang L, Jiang LS, Li FY, Ye H, Li N, Cheng NS & Zhou Y. (2007). Giant submucosal lipoma located in the descending colon: a case report and review of the literature. *World J Gastroenterol.*, (Nov 2007), 13, 42, pp. 5664-5667. PMID:17948945

Karlbom U, Graf W, Nilsson S & Pahlman L. (2004). The accuracy of clinical examination in the diagnosis of rectal intussusception. *Dis Colon Rectum.*, 2004, 47, 9, pp. 1533–1538. PMID:15486753

Khan MN, Agrawal A & Strauss P. (2008). Ileocolic Intussusception - A rare cause of acute intestinal obstruction in adults; Case report and literature review. *World J Emerg Surg.*, (Aug 2008), 4;3:26-31. PMID:18680588

Martin-Lorenzo JG, Torralba-Martinez A, Liron-Ruiz R, Flores-Pastor B, Miguel-Perelló J, Aguilar-Jimenez J & Aguayo-Albasini JL. (2004). Intestinal invagination in adults: preoperative diagnosis and management. *Int J Colorectal Dis.*, (Jan 2004), 19, 1, pp. 68–72. PMID:12838363

Nagorney DM, Sarr MG & McIlrath DC. (1981). Surgical management of intussusception in the adult. *Ann Surg.* (Feb 1981), 193, 2, pp. 230–236. PMID:7469558

Parashar UD, Holman RC, Cummings KC, Staggs NW, Curns AT, Zimmerman CM, Kaufman SF, Lewis JE, Vugia DJ, Powell KE, Glass RI. (2000). Trends in intussusception-associated hospitalizations and deaths among US infants. *Pediatrics.*(Dec 2000), 106, 6, pp. 1413-1421. PMID:11099597

Paskauskas S, Latkauskas T, Valeikaitė G, Parseliūnas A, Svagzdys S, Saladzinskas Z, Tamelis A & Pavalkis D. (2010). Colonic intussusception caused by colonic lipoma: a case report. *Medicina* (Kaunas)., 2010, 46, 7, pp. 477-481.

Pereira JM, Sirlin CB, Pinto PS & Casola G. (2005). CT and MR imaging of extrahepatic fatty masses of the abdomen and pelvis: techniques, diagnosis, differential diagnosis, and pitfalls. *Radiographics,* (Jan-Feb 2005), 25, 1, pp. 69-85. PMID:15653588

Rathore MA, Andrabi SI & Mansha M. (2006). Adult intussusception--a surgical dilemma. *J Ayub Med Coll Abbottabad.,* (Jul-Sep 2006), 18, 3, pp. 3–6. PMID:17348303

Shub HA, Rubin RJ & Salvati EP. (1978). Intussusception complicating intestinal intubation with a long Cantor tube: Report of 4 cases. *Dis Colon Rectum.,* (Mar 1978), 21, 2, pp. 130–134. PMID:648291

Takeuchi K, Tsuzuki Y, Ando T, Sekihara M, Hara T, Kori T & Kuwano H. (2003) The diagnosis and treatment of adult intussusception. *J Clin Gastroenterol.,* (Jan 2003), 36, 1, pp. 18–21. PMID:12488701

Tamburrini S, Stilo A, Bertucci B & Barresi D. (2004). Adult colocolic intussusception: demonstration by conventional MR techniques. *Abdom Imaging.,* (Jan-Feb 2004), 29, 1, pp. 42-44. PMID:15160752

Taylor B & Wolff B. (1987). Colonic lipomas. Report of two unusual cases and review of the Mayo Clinic experience, 1976–1985. *Dis Colon Rectum,* (Nov 1987), 30, 11, pp. 888–893. PMID:3677966

VanderKolk WE, Snyder CA & Figg DM. (1996). Cecal-colic adult intussusception as a cause of intestinal obstruction in Central Africa. *World J Surg.,* (Mar-Apr 1996), 20, 3, pp.341-344. PMID:8661842

Wang L-T, Wu CC, Yu JC, Hsiao CW, Hsu CC & Jao SW. (2007). Clinical entity and treatment strategies for adult intussusceptions: 20 years' experience. *Dis Colon Rectum,* (Nov 2007), 50, 11, pp. 1941–1949. PMID:17846839

Weilbaecher D, Bolin JA, Hearn D & Ogden W. (1971). Intussusception in adults. Review of 160 cases. *Am J Surg.,* (May 1971), 121, 5, pp. 531–535. PMID:5557762

Weiss EG & McLemore EC. (2008). Functional Disorders: Rectoanal Intussusception. *Clin Colon Rectal Surg.,* (May 2008), 21, 2, pp. 122–128. PMID:20011408

Yakan S, Caliskan C, Makay O, Denecli AG & Korkut MA. (2009). Intussusception in adults: clinical characteristics, diagnosis and operative strategies. *World J Gastroenterol.,* (Apr 2009), 28, 15, 16, pp. :1985-1989. PMID:19399931

Yalarmathi S & Smith RC. (2005). Adult intussusception: case reports and review of literature. *Postgrad Med J.,* 2005, 81:174–177.

Zubaidi A, Al-Saif F & Silverman R. (2006). Adult intussusception: a retrospective review. *Dis Colon Rectum.,* (Oct 2006), 49, 10, pp. 1546–1551. PMID:16990978

2

Predictors and Ultrasonographic Diagnosis of Intussusception in Children

Luca Lideo and Milan Roberto
Private Veterinary Clinic
Cartura, Padua,
Italy

1. Introduction

INTUSSUSCEPTION IS THE invagination of a portion of the intestine, called intussusceptum, into the lumen of an adjacent segment of intestine, called intussuscipiens, in the direction of the normal peristalsis or occasionally in a retrograde direction. The intussusceptum is composed of an inner or entering wall and an outer or returning wall.

The first description of intussusception appears in 1793 by Hunter. The first successful operative reduction was reported by Hutchinson in 1873. In 1876, Hirschsprung published the first of several reports on the reduction of intussusception by hydrostatic pressure. Later in 1926, Hipsley described a series of patients managed with this method of treatment.

In human medicine, intussusception is a disease primarily of infants and toddlers, although intussusception can occur at any age; only 10% to 25% of cases occur after 2 years of age.2 The peak incidence occurs between 5 and 9 months,9 and then decline. It rarely occurs younger than 2 months but may occur even in neonatal period. Although rare, intussusception has been reported in preterm infants. Males are affected approximately twice as often as females.

The small intestine is the most difficult part to examine of the gastrointestinal (GI) tract because of its length and tortuous course. The traditional investigations with small bowel enteroclysis and small bowel follow-through reveal information sparingly, and unfortunately involve radiation exposure of the patient. Although it is an organ that is spared from frequent disease, more precise and patient-friendly methods are needed. In the last three decades, new imaging techniques have been developed that have proven useful. Computerized tomography (CT), magnetic resonance imaging (MRI), wireless capsule endoscopy and double-balloon endoscopy are all relatively new additions to the diagnostic armamentarium.

Compared with these methods, transabdominal bowel sonography (TABS), has the advantage of being cheap, portable, flexible and user- and patient-friendly. There are challenges with depth penetration and intestinal air precluding optimal image quality, and the flexibility of ultrasonography (US) warrants a systematic approach by the examiner. However, the development of improved scanner technology and high-resolution transducers has provided the clinician with image data of high temporal and spatial resolution, thus making it a useful tool in the diagnosis of small intestinal diseases. When using US frequencies in the range of 7,5-14 MHz, the wall of the small intestine usually exhibits five different layers that correspond well to the histological layers.

B-mode ultrasonography has been used successfully in the diagnosis of intestinal intussusception in children. The most common sonographic pattern observed in transverse sections of the bowel is a target-like mass consisting of multiple hyperechoic and hypoechoic concentric rings around a hyperechoic center that represents the entrapped mesentery. In longitudinal sections, multiple hyperechoic and hypoechoic parallel lines are usually visible. Exploratory celiotomy followed by manual reduction or resection of the intussuscepted bowel is the usual method of treatment of intestinal intussusception in animals. In children, the primary method of treatment is hydrostatic or pneumatic reduction of the intussusception under radiologic control. However, pneumatic reduction should never be attempted where the bowel is necrotic or perforated.

Prediction of bowel viability and reducibility is of most importance if hydrostatic or pneumatic reduction of gangrenous intussuscepted bowel is to be avoided. A number of ultrasonographic criteria useful in predicting bowel reducibility have been described in children. However, the recognition of blood flow in the intussuscepted bowel using color flow Doppler ultrasonography appears to be the most valuable for predicting bowel reducibility. Radiologically controlled reduction of the intussuscepted bowel is not usually performed to treat intestinal intussusception in small animals. However, ability to predict the reducibility of the intussuscepted bowel could lead to improved prognosis and timing for surgical intervention.

The aim of this review article was to describe ultrasound technic in gastrointestinal examination, US pattern of intussusception and US predictive factors of surgery for intussusception in childrens.

2. Ultrasound of the bowel in children: How we do it

Transabdominal US is currently a well-established method for the evaluation of the small and large bowel [1]. The traditional imaging modalities of the bowel, contrast fluoroscopic studies, are facing competition from or some are being replaced by US of the bowel. Advances in US like high-resolution transducers, harmonic imaging, panoramic modality and contrast-enhanced US have overcome some of the obstacles in bowel sonography that existed in the past. Despite these facts the routine use of US of the small and large bowel in children has significant geographic variations, particularly when looking beyond the evaluation of the appendix. It appears to be more commonly integrated as part of the pediatric bowel imaging work-up in Europe and Canada than in the USA.

A very important application of US of the bowel in children is in the evaluation of inflammatory bowel disease (IBD), particularly Crohn disease. In this group of pediatric patients comparative studies of US of the bowel and ileocolonoscopy and histology have demonstrated the range of sensitivity and specificity to be 74–88% and 78–93%, respectively. It is meant to serve like a recipe and facilitate the routine performance of bowel US in the pediatric age group.

2.1 Step-by-ste approach to performing US of the bowel

A. Patient preparation

US of the bowel can be conducted without any kind of preparation. It is known that significant gaseous distention of the bowel can be an impediment to bowel US.

Lack of even very small amount of fluid in the intestine leads to completely collapsed bowel loops and reduction in peristalsis. The intake of carbonated fluid or very long duration of fasting can lead to such states. Particularly, in such cases the following preparatory step may turn out to be helpful. The oral intake of non-carbonated fluid about 30 min before the US examination may be helpful to reduce the air and also slightly distend the bowel loops. Placing the child in a right lateral decubitus position will hasten the emptying of the fluid from the stomach. A partially filled bladder will assist in the evaluation of the distal sigmoid colon and rectum.

B. Selection of US modalities

The appropriate selection of transducers and modalities will lead to optimal results of the bowel US. After initial trial of various settings a default setting for bowel US needs to be saved for further use. For ease of annotation, where possible, the following labels should also be saved in full or abbreviated: duodenum—DUO, jejunum—JEJ, ileum—IL, terminal ileum—TI, ileocecal valve—ICV, cecum—CEC, ascending colon—AC, hepatic flexure—HF, transverse colon—TC, splenic flexure—SF, descending colon—DC, sigmoid colon—SC, rectum—REC, right upper quadrant— RUQ, right lower quadrant—RLQ, left upper quadrant— LUQ, left lower quadrant—LLQ. Having these annotations allows quick and exact labeling of the image. The body markers are less suitable for exact labeling of the different parts of the bowel. High-frequency, harmonic and panoramic imaging are important US modalities for high-quality imaging of the bowel and can be used in combination or separately.

1. High-frequency imaging: This entails the use of transducers with high frequency. With the advancement of US transducer technology what we regard as high frequency is shifting, too. If 10 years ago a 7.5 MHz transducer was presented as the high-frequency transducer, nowadays many pediatric diagnostic US scanners have transducers that go higher than 15 MHz. It is important to remember the inverse relationship between frequency and penetration depth of the US wave. Thus the right choice of frequency depends on the body habitus of the patient. For practical purposes it is prudent to start with the available highest-frequency transducer for abdominal imaging and switch to lower ones, if sufficient penetration and visualization is not possible. Predominantly linear, but also convex transducers are needed.
2. Harmonic imaging: This is based on the non-linear propagation property of acoustic signal as it travels through the body. Harmonic waves are generated within the tissue and build up with depth to a point of maximal intensity before they decrease due to attenuation. On the contrary, conventional US waves are generated at the surface of the transducer and progressively decrease in intensity as they traverse the body. The harmonic waves are selectively utilized for imaging, eliminating the fundamental frequency. The latter is achieved by highpass filters or through pulse/phase inversion technique, or both. Harmonic frequencies are higher integer multiples of the transmitted frequency. Some US scanners only use the 2nd harmonic for imaging (narrow band), whereas others are capable of implementing a wider range of harmonics (wide band). There is image-quality difference between these two modalities, in general the wide band harmonics modality is of better quality. Harmonic imaging improves axial resolution due to shorter wavelength and lateral resolution through better focusing with higher frequencies. As the harmonic waves are produced beyond the body wall the defocusing effect of the body wall is reduced. The relatively small

amplitude of the harmonic waves results in artifact reduction. In addition, side lobes are less likely to occur and degrade the image. Artifact-free, clear images with higher contrast and spatial resolution are the result. The advantage and superiority of harmonic imaging compared to conventional US for the bowel has been demonstrated in both adults and children.

3. Panoramic imaging: The bowel is a long convoluted structure. The depiction of a longer segment of the bowel by conventional US is limited. To overcome this limitation and to allow documentation of a bowel loop longer the an the length of the transducer one can attempt to use a low-frequency curved-array transducer or dual display mode. These are by far less optimal than panoramic or extended field-of-view imaging. Panoramic imaging involves acquiring multiples of successive US images. With the advanced computational capabilities of US scanners ultrafast motion detection and image processing is possible in realtime. Up to a length of 60 cm can be scanned at one time. It is possible to follow the course of the bowel and make correct length measurements. Moreover, we can use smaller window to evaluate short segments within the scanned bowel.

C. Method of scanning

US of the bowel is conducted with the child in supine position. It is easier for the manual handling if the child is lying closer to the edge of the table nearer to the examiner.

1. Compression techniques: The most important technique to use is graded compression. Non-performance of this maneuver is probably the most frequent reason for suboptimal US images of the bowel. Graded compression is not a technique reserved only for appendix imaging, it is also important for the rest of the bowel. It is prudent in older children to inform them that you are going to compress the abdomen and intermittently look at their facial expression to gauge the pressure exerted. Graded compression displaces disturbing air and adjacent bowel loops, shortens the distance for visualization and isolates the bowel loop of interest. An inflamed bowel is non-compressible in contrast to a normal bowel loop. An additional less known maneuver, but one that we have successfully applied is the adjuvant use of a posterior manual compression technique in combination with the graded compression. The hand not holding the transducer is placed under the back. The back is pushed anteriorly at the same time the graded compression is done in the posterior direction. This technique compounds the effects of the graded compression. It is most useful for depicting the terminal ileum, ileocecal valves and cecum.
2. Scan planes: Each bowel segment is documented in both the transverse and longitudinal planes. Two planes are more important as it allows a better overview of the mesentery.
3. Doppler US: The bowel wall and mesentery do not normally demonstrate significant color signals on power or color Doppler. In contrast an inflamed bowel loop or mesentery can have increased color signals. Thus whenever abnormal bowel wall or mesentery is visualized color or power Doppler examination needs to done. The color Doppler is more commonly used than the power Doppler as it is less sensitive to motion, both from bowel peristalsis and patient movement. The setting of the Doppler has to be very low in order to capture small increase in hyperemia. Color Doppler US is useful for follow-up as it may be the first sign to change prior to significant reduction in bowel wall thickness. Some US scanners have the option of color panoramic modality, too.

4. US clip: The documentation of the presence, absence or relative decrease of peristalsis is done with a short clip. The respective bowel is isolated and the transducer fixed withoutmovement of the hand. An inflamed bowel shows reduced or no peristalsis compared to a normal one.
5. Measurements: If an inflamed loop is detected, two measurements need to be carried out. The bowel wall thickness is measured from the hyperechogenic mucosal to the hyperechogenic serosal interfaces. A 3-mm cut-off for normal bowel wall thickness is generally applicable. Specifically for inflammatory bowel disease in the pediatric age group a thickness for the small and large bowels of greater than 2.5 and 2.9 mm, respectively, are regarded as abnormal [7]. The length of an inflamed bowel segment is best measured using panoramic imaging. Some scanners provide the additional feature of measurement of curved distances.
6. "Itinerary": Using a linear transducer we start with the depiction of the psoas muscle and iliac vessels in the right lower quadrant in the axial plane. From this point it is easy to localize the terminal ileum in its longitudinal plane. We follow the terminal ileum to the ileocecal valves. The ileocecal junction is best viewed at a more obliquely angled view. This is followed by the evaluation of the cecum and ascending colon. These are the bowel loops located most laterally on the right. The transducer is moved along the ascending colon to the hepatic flexure and then turned to the transverse colon. It is important to carefully trace the path of the transverse colon as the stomach and proximal small bowel loops may be easily mistaken for the transverse colon. After that the transducer is moved to the left over the splenic flexure downward tracing the descending colon. This is the bowel loop normally found most laterally on the left. At the distal end of the descending colon the transducer is turned medially to trace the sigmoid colon. The sigmoid colon is depicted in its longitudinal plane over the axial section of the left psoas muscle and iliac vessels. Further tracing of the large bowel to the rectum with a linear transducer may be difficult. Prior to switching to a convex transducer we go on to evaluate the left upper quadrant, the left lower quadrant, the right upper quadrant and right lower quadrants for the duodenum, jejunum and proximal ileum. After a switch to a convex transducer we continue tracing the remaining sigmoid colon and rectum. The latter is best visualized behind a partially full bladder. It is important to remember that at each step the proper selection of US modality is necessary. Furthermore, at each step the use of graded compression, portrayal in axial and longitudinal planes, color Doppler, clips and measurements whenever appropriate is to be stressed. It is also important to document pathological changes of the mesentery around an inflamed bowel loop. Significant gaseous distention of the bowel and adipose body habitus may hinder depiction of all parts of the bowel. The ease of visualization of pathological findings in the different parts of the bowel is also variable, being more difficult in the more proximal small bowel loops than in the distal ones.

There are currently emerging advanced US modalities in bowel sonography. These new applications are starting to be used primarily in adults, but may have potential benefits in children, too. Hydrosonography is a method in which a contrast liquid with low echogenicity is administered orally or rectally for distending the bowel and improving the scan. The specific study for the small bowel is also known under the name small-intestinecontrast- enhanced US or SICUS. An isotonic polyethylene glycol (PEG) solution is commonly used. In Crohn disease hydrosonography of the small bowel was found to be comparable to ileocolonoscopy, wireless capsule endoscopy, and small-bowel sonography in the assessment of the number, site, extension, and postoperative recurrence of small-bowel lesions. In comparison to conventional US the use of oral contrast agent increased the overall sensitivity from 4% to 11%. In particular, it proved advantageous in depiction of proximal small bowel lesions, from 80% to 100%, and in the evaluation of the number and site of small bowel stenoses, increasing the detection by 11–22%. It is important to realize that when we do bowel US without any bowel preparation as described previously that we are doing so with some degree of limitation. Further advanced application includes contrastenhanced US with intravenous administration of US contrast agent for better evaluation of the blood flow to the bowel wall. US elastography or strain imagings are US applications for detecting the elasticity or stiffness of a tissue and providing a visual display. Endoscopic sonography using miniprobes is another new application.

D. Reporting findings

A prepared reporting form or a macro for dictation is helpful to standardize the reporting and provide the referring clinician with clear and consistent sonographic information. Such reporting also makes the follow-up evaluation easier. A sample of a form for reporting has been provided in Table 1. The following sample macro of a normal bowel US finding can serve as the basis for reporting the results and be modified accordingly.

REPORT: ULTRASOUND OF THE BOWEL

BOWEL LOOP:

DUO=Duodenum, JEJ=Jejunum, IL=Ileum [Pro=proximal, Ter=terminal]

CEC=Cecum, ASC=ascending colon, TRA=transverse colon, DES=descending colon, SIG sigma, REC=rectum

*Thickness = if abnormal in mm; *Length = if inflamed bowel length in cm; Extramural findings localized to the closest bowel loop(s)

REPORT:

US of the small and large bowel

HISTORY: Rule out inflammatory bowel disease

COMPARISON: None

TECHNIQUE: US study targeting only the small and large bowel loops. High-resolution US imaging combined with color Doppler.

FINDINGS: An adequate evaluation of the small and large bowel loops could be carried out. The small bowel loops duodenum, jejunum and ileum—were visualized. There was no abnormal wall thickening or pathological color Doppler finding. Specifically, the terminal ileum was depicted and traced to the ileocecal valves. The terminal ileum also has normal bowel thickness and there is no increase in color

Doppler signal. The large bowel loops—cecum, ascending colon, transverse colon, descending colon, sigmoid colon and rectum—were visualized. They did not show any evidence of abnormal wall thickening or pathological color Doppler finding. In addition, the mesenteric echogenicity was normal and there was no mesenteric thickening and hyperemia. There is normal peristalsis. No free fluid is detected.

IMPRESSION: Normal US of the small and large bowel without evidence of inflammatory bowel disease.

Status	Parameter		Bowel loop									
			DUO	JEJ	IL		COLON					
					Pro	Ter	CEC	ASC	TRA	DES	SIG	REC
Not visualized												
Visualized	**Bowel wall**	**Thickness***										
		Echogenicity										
		Stratification										
		Blood flow										
		Peristalisis										
		Ulceration										
		Disruption										
		Phlegmon /Abscess										
		Stenosis										
		Length*										
	Mesentery	**Thickening**										
		Bowel separation										
		Echogenicity										
		Blood flow										
		Fistula										
	Lymph nodes	**Enlargement**										
		Blood flow										
	Abscess											
	Bowel conglo-merate											

Table 1. Standardized form for reporting findings of US of the small and large bowel

2.2 Ultrasonographic findings

High-resolution US can demonstrate the multiple layers of the bowel wall Fig. 1. The innermost hyperechoic line corresponds to the mucosal interface with the lumen. The mucosa itself is hypoechoic and this is followed by the hyperechoic submucosa and hypoechoic muscularis. The outermost layer is hyperechoic and represents an interface echo between the surrounding structures and the serosa. We speak in US of normal stratification of the bowel wall if five layers are visible and of loss of stratification if one or more US layers are missing. The jejunum demonstrates more folds and peristalsis than the ileum. The colon displays even less peristalsis and more air-filling. If the bowel loop contains gas, only the front wall may be visible while the rear wall is concealed by the shadow cone and by the gas generated reverberation artifacts.

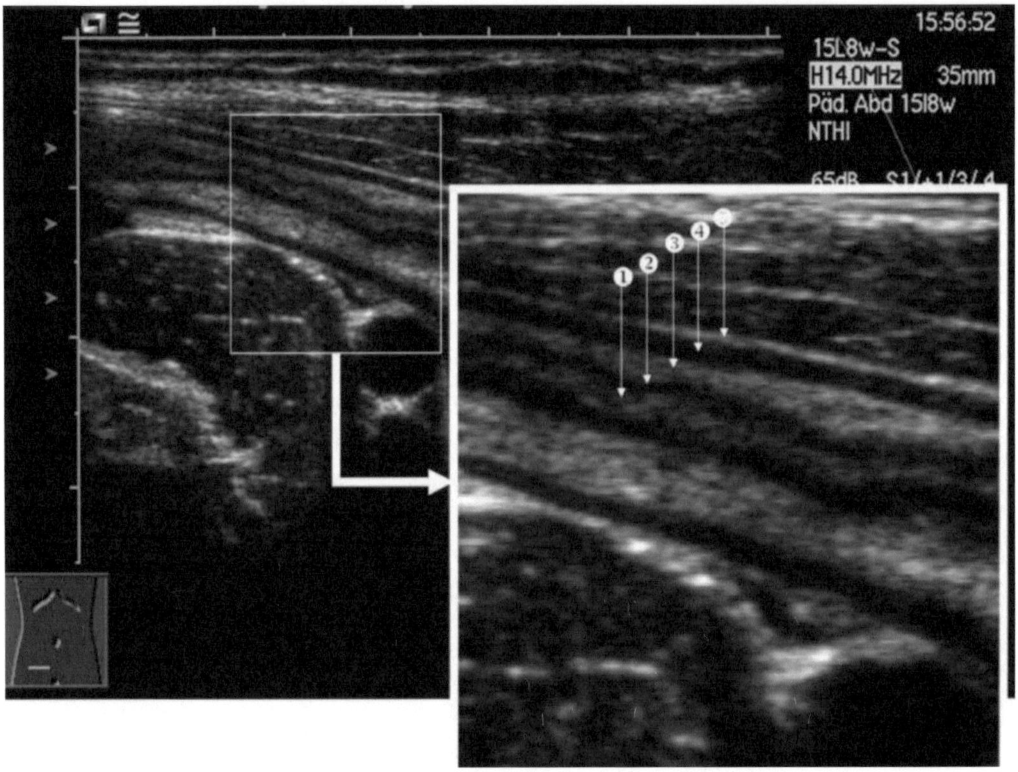

Fig. 1. The terminal ileumscanned with a linear transducer at 14 MHz. All the five layers of the bowel wall are well visualized. A magnified view with labeling of each layer is provided: ❶ HYPERechoic mucosal interface, ❷ HYPOechoic mucosa, ❸ HYPERechoic submucosa, ❹ HYPOechoic muscularis, ❺ HYPERechoic serosal interface

3. Pathophysiology of intestinal intussusception in infants and children

Intussusception is one of the most common causes of acute abdomen in infancy. The condition occurs when a segment of intestine (the intussusceptum) prolapses into a more caudal segment of intestine (the intussuscipiens). This condition usually occurs in children between 5 months to 2 years of age. In this age group most intussusceptions are idiopathic with no pathologic lead point demonstrated. More than 90% of intussusceptions are believed to be secondary to enlarged lymphoid follicles in the terminal ileum.

Intussusception is more common in boys and the condition is rare in children younger than 3 months. The peak incidence is between 5 and 9 months of age. Lead points are noted in children younger than 3 months of age or greater than 2 years of age. Lead points include such entities as Meckel's diverticulum, duplication cysts, intestinal polyps, lymphoma, and intramural hematomas. Transient intussusception is seen in patients with celiac disease (sprue). Most intussusceptions involve the ileocolic region (75%), where the ileum becomes telescoped into the colon. This is followed in decreasing frequency by ileoileocolic, ileoileal, and colocolic intussusceptions. The classic clinical triad of acute abdominal pain (colic), currant jelly stools or hematochezia, and a palpable abdominal mass is present in less than 50% of children with intussusception. Up to 20% of patients may be pain free at presentation. Additionally, in some instances lethargy or convulsion is the predominant sign or symptom. This situation results in consideration of a neurologic disorder rather than intussusception. Given the uncertainty of achieving an accurate clinical diagnosis, imaging is required in most cases to achieve an early and quick diagnosis to reduce morbidity and mortality. Delay may be life threatening because of the development of bowel necrosis and its complications.

3.1 Literature review of intestinal intussusception in infants and children

Much controversy exists in the literature related to the diagnosis and management of intussusception. Realistically speaking children with intussusception can be managed successfully in a number of different ways. It is best to use diagnostic tools that are as benign as possible, however, to avoid potential harm to these children and to lessen the discomfort to the children who are not shown to have intussusception.

The coiled spring sign is produced when the edematous mucosal folds of the returning limb of the intussusception are outlined by contrast material in the lumen of the colon. The enema examination, however, can be a very unpleasant experience for both the parent and child and is also associated with radiation.

The role of sonography in the diagnosis of intussusception is well established with a sensitivity of 98% to 100% and a specificity of 88% to 100%. It has been suggested that sonography should be the initial imaging modality and that the enema examination should only be performed for therapeutic reasons. Sonography not only aids in the diagnosis of intussusception but it also allows the identification of patients who are candidates for therapeutic reduction. Sonography may also detect other abnormalities that are overlooked by the enema examination. In addition, there is a high level of patient comfort and safety with US.

A technique of graded compression is used for the sonographic evaluation of suspected intussusception. Because deep penetration of the US beam is not necessary in small children, a linear high-resolution transducer, 5 to 10 MHz, can be used to improve the definition of the image. The abdomen and the pelvis should be scanned in both longitudinal and transverse planes. The intussusception mass is a large structure, usually greater than 5 cm. Most intussusception occurs in the subhepatic region often displacing adjacent bowel loops. Even inexperienced operators can readily identify the intussusception on sonography. An intussusception is a complex structure.

The intussuscipiens (the receiving loop) contains the folded intussusceptum (the donor loop), which has two components: the entering limb and the returning limb. The attached mesentery is dragged between the entering and returning limbs. Sonographically, the intussusception may demonstrate an outer hypoechoic region surrounding an echogenic center, referred to as a "target" or "doughnut" appearance.

The hypoechoic outer ring seen on axial scans is formed by the everted returning limb, which is the thickest component of the intussusception and the thin intussuscipiens. The echogenic center of intussusception contains the central or entering limb, which is of normal thickness and is eccentrically surrounded by hyperechoic mesentery. Another pattern of imaging that has been described is that of multiple con- centric rings. Within the bowel wall the mucosa and submucosa are echogenic, whereas the muscularis layer is hypoechoic. Multiple hypoechoic and hyperechoic layers are identified when there is little bowel edema present. This represents the mucosa, submucosa, and muscularis layers of the intussusceptum and intussuscipiens. With increasing degrees of bowel edema, the hyperechoic mucosal and submucosal echoes are obliterated in the intussusceptum resulting in fewer layers. On long axis scans the hypoechoic layers on each side of the echogenic center may result in a reniform or pseudokidney appearance. The pseudokidney sign is seen if the intussusception is curved or imaged obliquely.

Although the target and pseudokidney signs are the most common ultrasonographic signs used, they are not pathognomic because they have also been seen in normal or pathologic intestinal loops. Differential consideration for the US findings includes other causes of bowel wall thickening, such as neoplasm, edema, and hematomas. An inexperienced operator may mistake stool or psoas muscle for an intussusception.

In addition to diagnosing the intussusception US has other advantages. US may detect the presence of a lead point, which is present in approximately 5% of intussusception. Various sonographic findings have been reported to be predictive of success of hydrostatic reduction. A study shows that the sonographic presence of enlarged mesenteric lymph node in the intussusception is a prediction of hydrostatic irreducibility. Small amounts of free peritoneal fluid are seen in up to 50% of cases. The presence of trapped peritoneal fluid within an intussusception correlates significantly with ischemia and irreducibility, however, because it reflects vascular compromise of the everted limb. Additionally, the absence of flow within the intussusception on color Doppler sonography correlates with a decreased success of reduction and a higher likelihood of bowel ischemia, and presence of color flow within the intussusception correlates with higher success rate of its reduction.

There are many different techniques used to reduce intussusception described in the literature. Water-soluble contrast material, barium, air enema guided by fluoroscopy, and physiologic saline solution combined with US have all been used. The use of sonography to guide hydrostatic reduction has been predominately performed in the eastern hemisphere and is increasingly being used in Europe. The reduction rate is high (76%- 95%), with only 1 perforation in 825 cases reported. The procedure may be performed with water, saline solution, or Hartmann solution. The instilled fluid is followed as it courses through the large bowel until the intussusception is no longer visualized and the terminal ileum and distal small bowel are filled with fluid or air. There has been little experience with US-guided air enema therapy. Because air prevents the passage of the US beam, it may be difficult to visualize the ileocecal valve; therefore, small residual ileoileal intussusception can be observed. Additionally, it is difficult to detect perforation resulting in pneumoperitoneum. Sonography has been shown to be highly successful in the diagnoses and reduction of intussusception. The appropriate use of US in children with suspected intussusception obviates the necessity for diagnostic enema, and the use of enema should be limited to therapeutic purposes.

In children with intussusception or intestinal invagination, the typical finding on transabdominal bowel sonography (TABS) is a multilayered lesion with concentric circles (onion sign) in the right fossa, when seen in the transversal lane. When the mesentery is involved, this forms an echo-rich crescent open towards the ante-mesenteric side. This is called the crescent in the donut sign. When seen longitudinally, the mesentery is seen as an echo-rich layer between two multilayered structures, the sandwich sign. Using these criteria, a sensitivity of nearly 100% and a specificity around 90% have been found in prospective studies. TABS can also be used as guide in treatment procedures with hydrostatic reduction. Color Doppler examination of children with intussusception shows that absence of flow in the wall of the invaginated intestine makes reduction more difficult, but does not necessarily

mean the intestine is necrotic. In adults, TABS has proven useful as a primary diagnostic method, but since intestinal invagination is a rare cause of bowel obstruction in adults, it is often found by other means. The TABS appearance is similar to that in children, but there is often other pathology present that is the pathological lead point of the invagination.
As a result of the low number of incidents, there have been no prospective studies in the literature. Transient intestinal invaginations occur in children and adults, and mostly without symptoms. If there are no pathological lead points, the discovery is incidental, and if the intestinal segment is shorter than 3.5 cm, they are considered harmless.

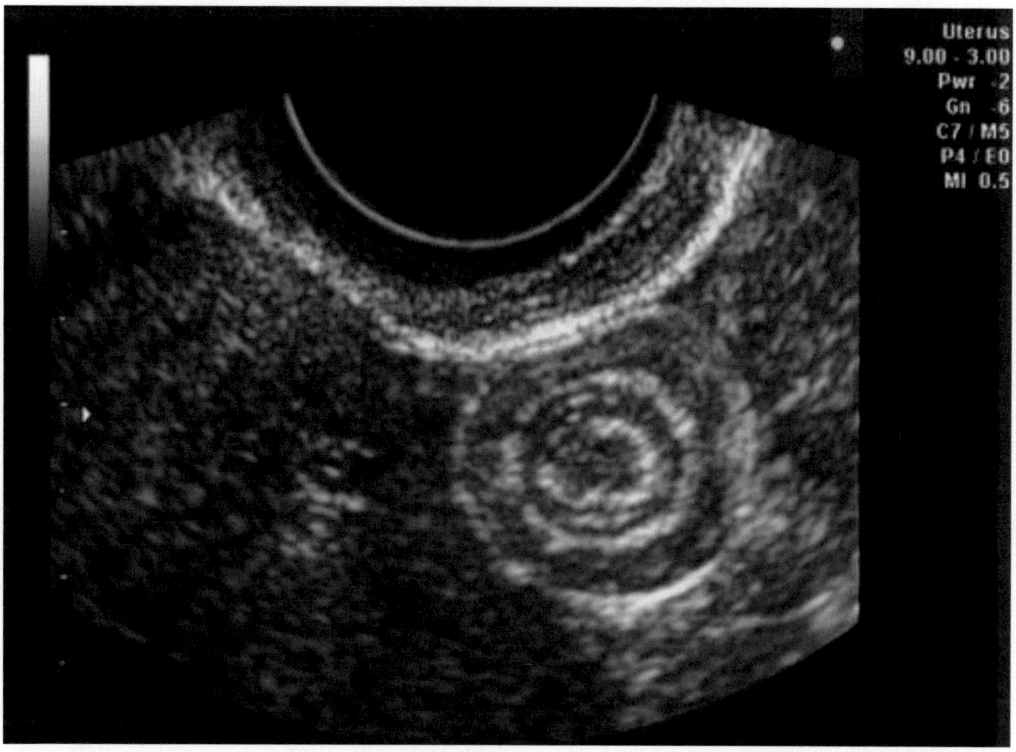

Fig. 2. Target sign noted adjacent to the uterus on a transvaginal scan.

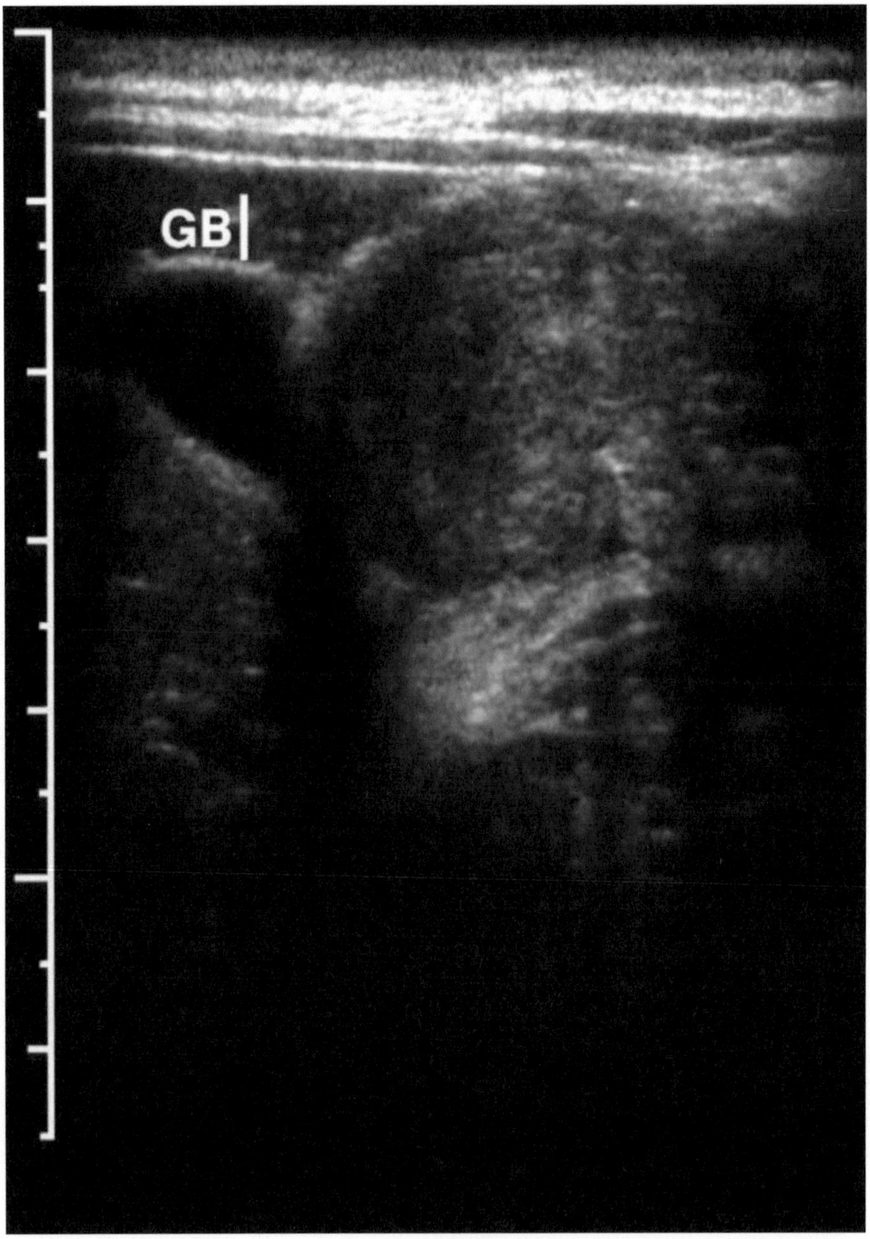

Fig. 3. Intestinal intussusception. Transverse sonographic image demonstrates a soft tissue mass in the right upper quadrant adjacent to the gallbladder (GB)

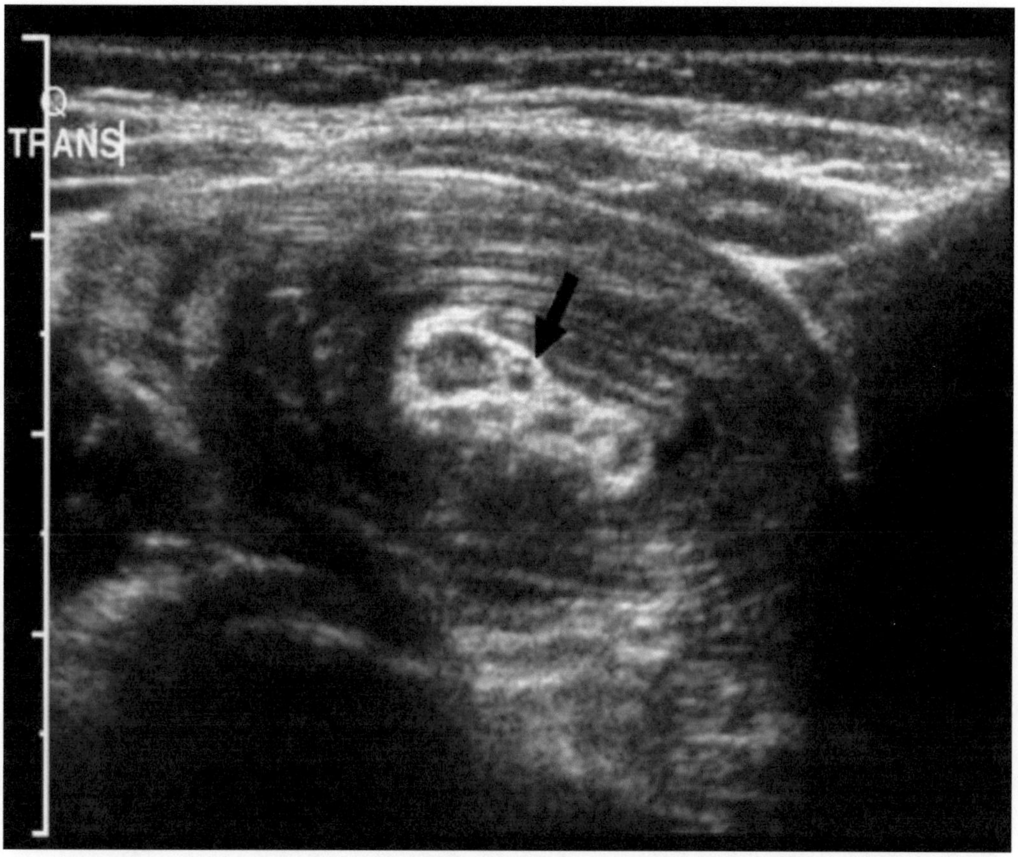

Fig. 4. Target appearance. Transverse sonographic view demonstrates the intussusception. The hypoechoic outer layer represents the intussuscipiens and the central echogenic layer represents the intussusceptum (arrow).

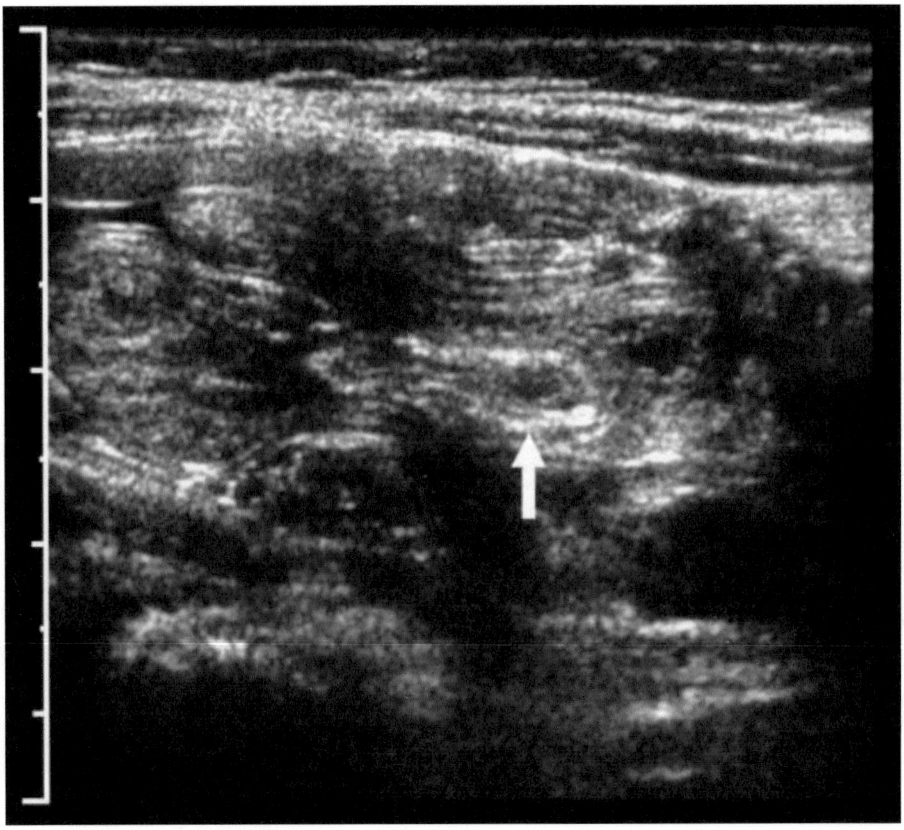

Fig. 5. Long-axis sonographic view shows an elongated appearance resulting in a pseudokidney appearance (arrow).

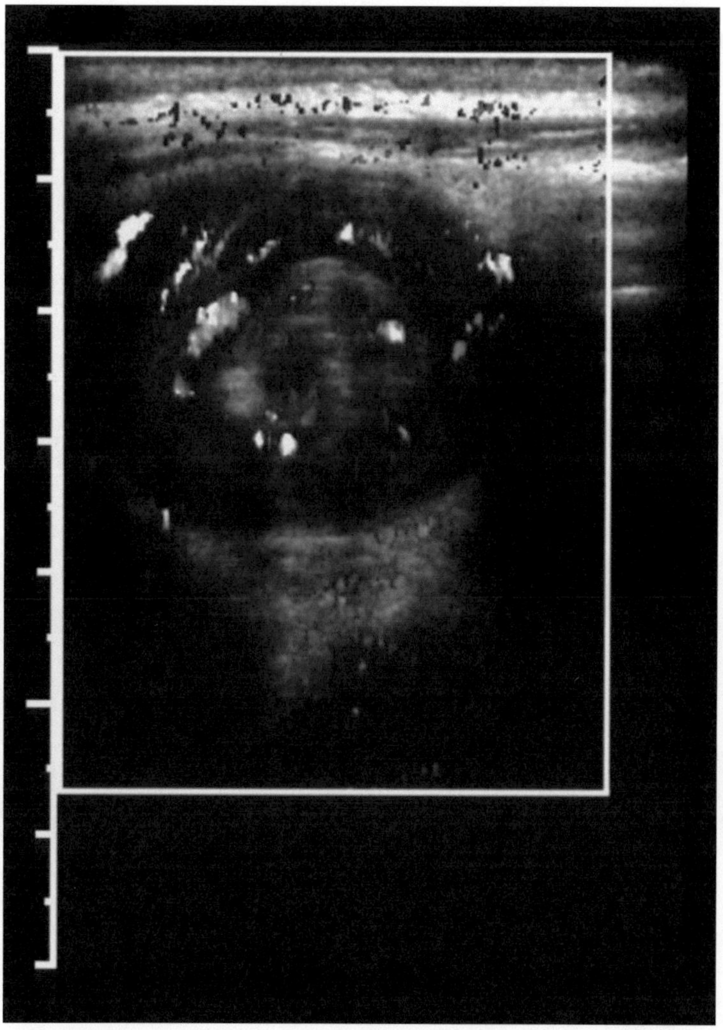

Fig. 6. Use of Doppler ultrasound to evaluate intussusception. Doppler ultrasound shows blood flow within the intussusception, suggesting its reducibility.

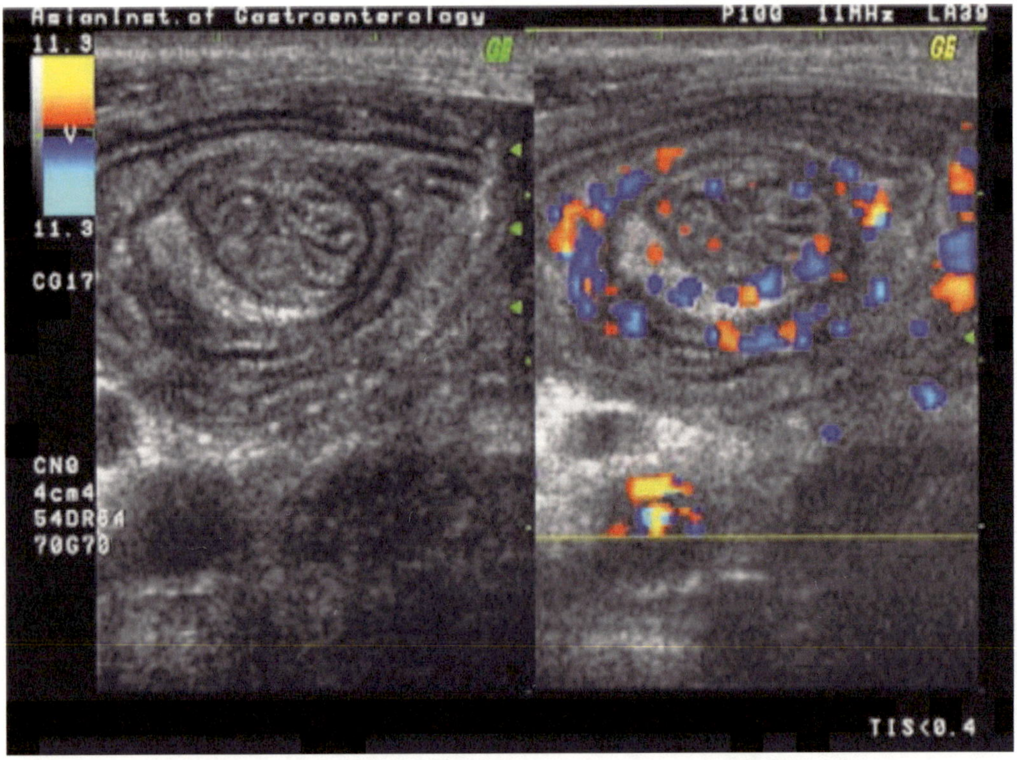

Fig. 7. Color Doppler demonstrating the vascularity of the intussusception.

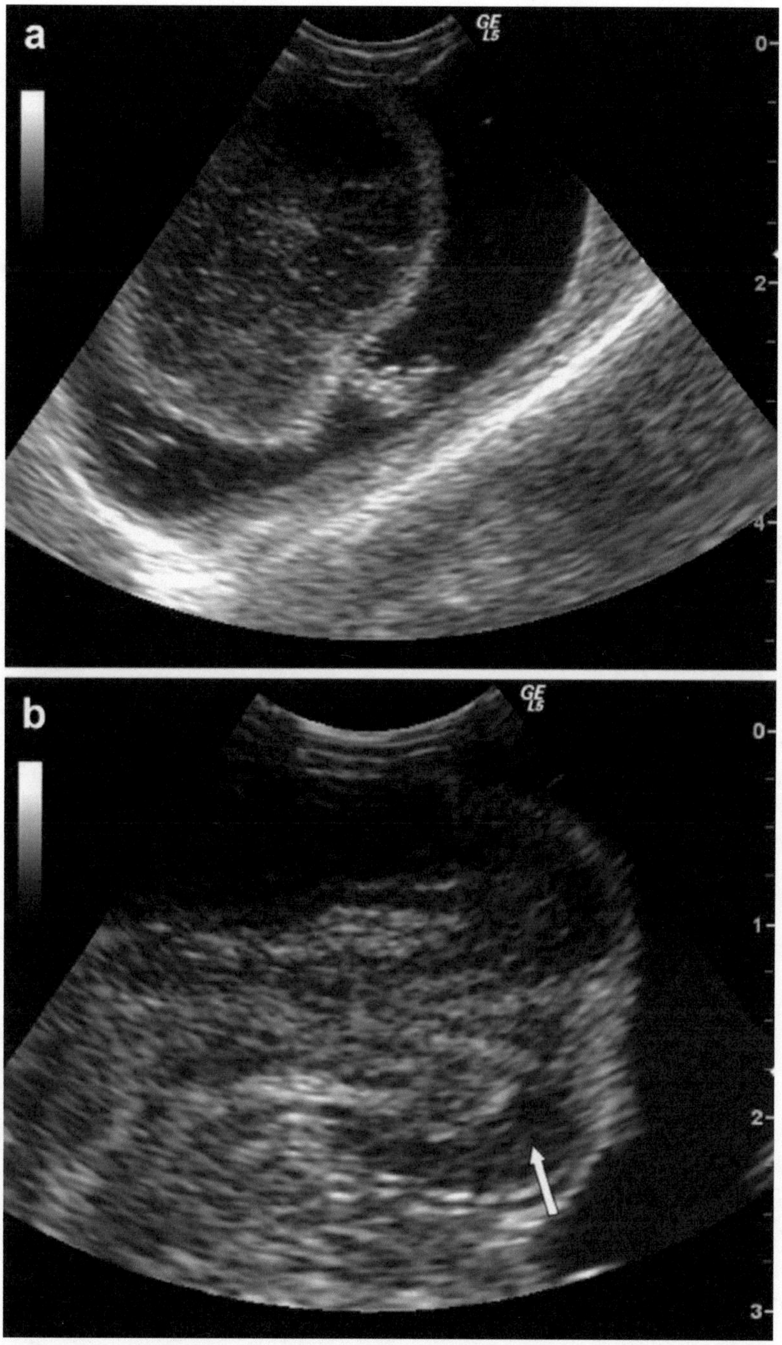

Fig. 8. US examination of the pylorogastric intussusceptions (rare case). (a) Transverse image of the pyloric region. Multiple concentric echogenic and echolucent rings were visible. (b) Longitudinal image of intussusceptions seen in (a); pylorus and proximal duodenum were displaced into the pyloric antrum and fundus; severely hypoechoic gastric mucosal layer caused by edema (arrow).

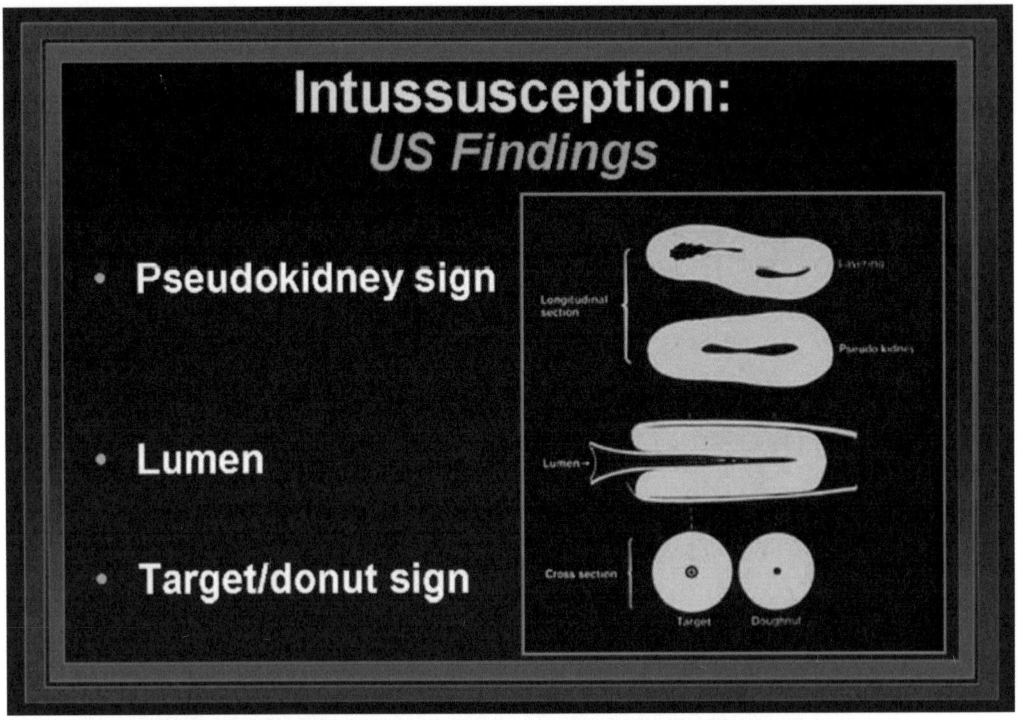

Fig. 9. Various signs of intussusception on cross-sectional imaging. Depending upon the plane through which an intussusception is imaged, various configurations may be demonstrated. On cross section, the head of the walls of the intussusception may appear as a double donut or target sign. The image on the right demonstrates the pseudokidney sign obtained by imaging the intussusception in a longitudinal plane.

4. Discussions and conclusion

Acute intussusception is the most common condition causing an acute abdomen in infants, and typical clinical manifestations include paroxysmal crying, abdominal pain, abdominal mass, and bloody stool. Intussusceptions are usually located in the ileocolic region and ileocecal junction, and these two types comprise approximately 80% of the intussusceptions in pediatric patients. Small bowel intussusceptions (SBIs) are relatively rare and accounts for <10% of the intussusceptions in pediatric patients. Clinical manifestations of SBIs are not typical, patients may present with non-specific signs and symptoms, an abdominal mass and bloody stool occur infrequently, and diagnosis may be delayed resulting in intestinal necrosis and a potential life-threatening situation.

Ultrasound is highly accurate for the diagnosis of ileocolic intussusceptions with a reported sensitivity of 98–100%, and the ultrasound detection rate for SBIs is approximately 76%. Diagnosis of an intussusception is made by the appearance of characteristic findings on ultrasound. Because some SBIs reduce spontaneously, it is controversial whether or not surgical treatment is necessary for all cases in pediatric patients. Doi et al. reported that spontaneous reduction happens in most cases of SBI in children, and only clinical observation, rather than surgical intervention, is needed and has termed these transient intussusceptions, benign SBIs. Sönmez et al consider that SBIs secondary to Henoch-Schonlein purpura can be reduced spontaneously, and conservative treatment is feasible. However, Ko et al. report that persistent SBIs are often associated with intestinal ischemia, necrosis, and perforation, and surgical intervention is warranted once diagnosed. Koh et al. consider that though spontaneous reduction can be achieved in most cases of SBIs, surgical treatment is inevitable in some patients with intestinal ischemia or a pathological lead point. Therefore, it is clinically very important to determine whether an SBI is likely to reduce spontaneously in order to avoid complications and perform surgery in a timely manner, as well as avoid surgery when not necessary. In the present study, we carried out a retrospective analysis of pediatric patients with SBIs who required surgery and in whom the intussusception resolved spontaneously in order to identify ultrasound characteristics predictive of the need for surgical management. That an intussusception diameter ≥2.1 cm, length ≥4.2 cm, and thickness of the outer rim ≥0.40 cm predict the need for surgical management in pediatric patients with SBIs. These values may be of assistance to clinicians when determining if surgery is required in pediatric patients with SBIs. Values below those determined from these data should be interpreted with caution in patients with signs and symptoms of mechanical ileus or intestinal ischemia.

Incidentally detected, small bowel intussusceptions with no identifiable pathological lead point, normal wall thickness, a length of less than 3.5 cm, normal nondilated proximal bowel and normal vascularity on color Doppler are due to physiological variations in peristalsis. These transient nonobstructive intussusceptions may be incidental findings on US due to minor transient disturbances in bowel motility with no clinical significance as they reduce spontaneously and their presence warrants only conservative (TSBI) is underestimated. If the patients had not been undergoing an US examination at that particular time, these intussusceptions would not have been detected. Nevertheless, we believe that TSBI occur in both adult and pediatric populations. Whatever be the possible etiology, their presence does not warrant intervention.

5. References

Agha FP (1986) Intussusception in adults. AJR 146:527–531

Aliotta A, Pompili M, Rapaccini GL, De Vitis I, Caputo S, Cedrone A, Grattagliano A, Gasbarrini G. Doppler ultrasonographic evaluation of blood flow in the superior mesenteric artery in celiac patients and in healthy controls in fasting conditions and after saccharose ingestion. *J Ultrasound Med* 1997; 16: 85-91;

Applegate KE. Evidence-based diagnosis of malrotation and volvulus. Pediatr Radiol. 2009 Apr;39 Suppl 2:S161-3. DOI 10.1007/s00247-009-1177-x

Applegate KE. Intussusception in children: evidence-based diagnosis and treatment. Pediatr Radiol. 2009 Apr;39 Suppl 2:S140-3 DOI 10.1007/s00247-009-1178-9

Applewhite AA, Cornell KK, Selcer BA (2001). Pylorogastric intussusceptions in the dog: a case report and literature review. *J Am Anim Hosp Assoc*;37:238e43

Applewhite AA, Cornell KK, Selcer BA. (2001) Diagnosis and treatment of intussusceptions in dogs. *Comp Cont Educ Pract Vet*; 24:110e27.

Bhisitkul DM, Listernick R, Shkolnik A, Donaldson JS, Henricks BD, Feinstein KA, Fernbach SK. Clinical application of ultrasonography in the diagnosis of intussusception. *J Pediatr* 1992; 121: 182-186

Bolondi L, Gaiani S, Brignola C, Campieri M, Rigamonti A, Zironi G, Gionchetti P, Belloli C, Miglioli M, Barbara L. Changes in splanchnic hemodynamics in inflammatory bowel disease. Non-invasive assessment by Doppler ultrasound flowmetry. *Scand J Gastroenterol* 1992; 27: 501-507

Bowerman R.A., Silver T.M., Jaffe M.H., Real-Time ultrasound diagnosis of intussusception in children, Radiol Radiology 143: 527-529, May 1982

Bozkurt T, Richter F, Lux G. Ultrasonography as a primary diagnostic tool in patients with inflammatory disease and tumors of the small intestine and large bowel. *J Clin Ultrasound* 1994; 22: 85-91

Bremner AR, Griffiths M, Argent JD et al (2006) Sonographic evaluation of inflammatory bowel disease: a prospective, blinded comparative study. Pediatr Radiol 36:947–953

Cammarota T, Sarno A, Robotti D et al (2008) Us evaluation of patients affected by IBD: how to do it, methods and findings. Eur J Radiol 69:429–437

Canani RB, de Horatio LT, Terrin G et al (2006) Combined use of noninvasive tests is useful in the initial diagnostic approach to a child with suspected inflammatory bowel disease. J Pediatr Gastroenterol Nutr 42:9–15

Carnevale E, Graziani M, Fasanelli S (1994) Post-operative ileoileal intussusception: sonographic approach. Pediatr Radiol 24:161–163

Castiglione F, Rispo A, Cozzolino A, Camera L, D'Argenio G, Tortora R, Grassia R, Bucci C, Ciacci C. Bowel sonography in adult celiac disease: diagnostic accuracy and ultrasonographic features. *Abdom Imaging* 2007; 32: 73-77

Catalano (1997) Transient small-bowel intussusception: CT findings in adults. Br J Radiol 70:805–808

Cerro P, Magrini L, Porcari P, De Angelis O. Sonographic diagnosis of intussusceptions in adults. Abdom Imaging. 2000 an-Feb;25(1):45-7. DOI: 10.1107/s002619910008

Cittadini G, Giasotto V, Garlaschi G, de Cicco E, Gallo A, Cittadini G. Transabdominal ultrasonography of the small bowel after oral administration of a non-absorbable anechoic solution: comparison with barium enteroclysis. *Clin Radiol* 2001; 56: 225-230

Claudon M, Cosgrove D, Albrecht T, Bolondi L, Bosio M, Calliada F, Correas JM, Darge K, Dietrich C, D'Onofrio M, Evans DH, Filice C, Greiner L, Jäger K, Jong N, Leen E, Lencioni R, Lindsell D, Martegani A, Meairs S, Nolsøe C, Piscaglia F, Ricci P, Seidel G, Skjoldbye B, Solbiati L, Thorelius L, Tranquart F, Weskott HP, Whittingham T. Guidelines and good clinical practice recommendations for contrast enhanced ultrasound (CEUS) - update 2008. *Ultraschall Med* 2008; 29: 28-44

Cochran AA, Higgins GL 3rd, Strout TD. Intussusception in traditional pediatric, nontraditional pediatric, and adult patients. Am J Emerg Med. 2011 Jun;29(5):523-7. Epub 2010 Apr 2.

Cohen MD, Lintott DJ (1978) Transient small bowel intussusceptions in adult celiac disease. Clin Radiol 29:529–534

Cosgrove D. Ultrasound contrast agents: an overview. *Eur J Radiol* 2006; 60: 324-330

Darge K, Anupindi S, Keener H, Rompel O. (2010) Ultrasound of the bowel in children: how we do it. *Pediatr Radiol.* Apr;40(4):528-36 DOI 10.1007/s00247-010-1550-9

Dell'Aquila P, Pietrini L, Barone M, Cela EM, Valle ND, Amoruso A, Minenna MF, Penna A, De Francesco V, Panella C, Ierardi E. Small intestinal contrast ultrasonography-based scoring system: a promising approach for the diagnosis and follow-up of celiac disease. *J Clin Gastroenterol* 2005; 39: 591-595

Del-Pozo G, Albillos JC, Tejedor D, et al. (1999) Intussusception in children: current concepts in diagnosis and enema reduction. Radiographics 19:299–319

Epifanio M, Baldisserotto M, Spolidoro JV et al (2008) Grey-scale and colour Doppler sonography in the evaluation of children with suspected bowel inflammation: correlation with colonoscopy and histological findings. Clin Radiol 63:968–978

Folvik G, Bjerke-Larssen T, Odegaard S, Hausken T, Gilja OH, Berstad A. Hydrosonography of the small intestine: comparison with radiologic barium study. *Scand J Gastroenterol* 1999; 34: 1247-1252

Fraquelli M, Colli A, Colucci A, Bardella MT, Trovato C, Pometta R, Pagliarulo M, Conte D. Accuracy of ultrasonography in predicting celiac disease. *Arch Intern Med* 2004; 164: 169-174

Gilja OH, Heimdal A, Hausken T, Gregersen H, Matre K, Berstad A, Ødegaard S. Strain during gastric contractions can be measured using Doppler ultrasonography. *Ultrasound Med Biol* 2002; 28: 1457-1465

González-Spínola J, Del Pozo G, Tejedor D, Blanco A. Intussusception: the accuracy of ultrasound-guided saline enema and the usefulness of a delayed attempt at reduction. *J Pediatr Surg* 1999; 34: 1016-1020

Hanquinet S, Anooshiravani M, Vunda A, et al. (1998) Reliability of color Doppler and power Doppler sonography in the evaluation of intussuscepted bowel viability. Pediatr Surg Int 13:360–362

Havre RF, Elde E, Gilja OH, Odegaard S, Eide GE, Matre K, Nesje LB. Freehand real-time elastography: impact of scanning parameters on image quality and in vitro intra and interobserver validations. *Ultrasound Med Biol* 2008; 34: 1638-1650

Heimdal A, Gilja OH. Strain Rate Imaging - A new tool for studying the GI tract. In: Odegaard S, Gilja OH, Gregersen H, editors. Basic and new aspects of gastrointestinal ultrasonography. Singapore: World Scientific, 2005: 243-263

Heyne R, Rickes S, Bock P, Schreiber S, Wermke W, Lochs H. Non-invasive evaluation of activity in inflammatory bowel disease by power Doppler sonography. *Z Gastroenterol* 2002; 40: 171-175

Hiorns MP (2008) Imaging of inflammatory bowel disease. How? Pediatr Radiol 38(Suppl 3):S512–S517

Hughes UM, Connolly BL, Chait PG, et al. (2000) Further report of small-bowel intussusceptions related to gastrojejunostomy tubes. Pediatr Radiol 30:614–617

Kiesling VJ, Tank ES (1989) Postoperative intussusception in children. Urology 33:387–389

Kim JH (2004) US features of transient small bowel intussusception in pediatric patients. Korean J Radiol 5(3):178–184

Kimmey MB, Martin RW, Haggitt RC, Wang KY, Franklin DW, Silverstein FE. Histologic correlates of gastrointestinal ultrasound images. *Gastroenterology* 1989; 96: 433-441

Kimmey MB, Wang KY, Haggitt RC, Mack LA, Silverstein FE. Diagnosis of inflammatory bowel disease with ultrasound. An in vitro study. *Invest Radiol* 1990; 25: 1085-1090

Knowles MC, Fishman EK, Kuhlman JE, et al. (1989) Transient Intussusception in Crohn_s disease: CT evaluation. Radiology 170:814

Kong MS, Wong HF, Lin SL, Chung JL, Lin JN. Factors related to detection of blood flow by color Doppler ultrasonography in intussusception. *J Ultrasound Med* 1997; 16: 141-144

Kornecki A, Daneman A, Navarro O, et al. (2000) Spontaneous reduction of intussusception: clinical spectrum, management and outcome. Pediatr Radiol 30:58–63

Kunihiro K, Hata J, Haruma K, Manabe N, Tanaka S, Chayama K. Sonographic detection of longitudinal ulcers in Crohn disease. *Scand J Gastroenterol* 2004; 39: 322-326

Lagalla R, Caruso G, Novara V, et al. (1994) Color Doppler ultrasonography in pediatric intussusception. Ultrasound Med 13:171–174

Lee JH, Jeong YK, Hwang JC et al (2002) Graded compression sonography with adjuvant use of a posterior manual compression technique in the sonographic diagnosis of acute appendicitis. AJR 178:863–866

Lee H, Yeon S, Lee H, et al (2005). Ultrasonographic diagnosis-pylorogastric intussusceptions in a dog. *Vet Radiol Ultrasoun*; 46:317e8.

Lideo L, Milan R.,. Feliciati A, Bonetti G.,. Baroni E (2010), Diagnosi ecografica di intussuscezione pilorogastrica in un cucciolo di chihuahua. Abstract Book XXII Congresso Nazionale Società Italiana di Ultrasonologia in Medicina e Biologia (SIUMB) e XXV Giornate Internazionali di Ultrasonologia, Turin, 77

Lideo L, Mutinelli f; Milan R (2010), Pylorogastric intussusception in a Chihuahua puppy. A case report. *Journal of Ultrasound* 13, 175e178 doi:10.1016/j.jus.2010.10.004

Lim HK, Bae SH, Lee KH, et al. (1994) Assessment of reducibility of ileocolic intussusception in children: usefulness of color Doppler sonography. Radiology 191:781–785

Ludwig D, Wiener S, Brüning A, Schwarting K, Jantschek G, Stange EF. Mesenteric blood flow is related to disease activity and risk of relapse in Crohn's disease: a prospective follow-up study. *Am J Gastroenterol* 1999; 94: 2942-2950

Lvoff N, Breiman RS, Coakley FV, et al. (2003) Distinguishing features of self-limiting adult small-bowel intussusception identified at CT. Radiology 227:68–72

Maconi G, Bianci P (eds) (2007) Ultrasound of the gastrointestinal tract. Medical Radiology. Diagnostic Imaging Series. Springer-Verlag, Heidelberg

Maconi G, Radice E, Bareggi E et al (2009) Hydrosonography of the gastrointestinal tract. AJR 193:700–708

Maconi G, Radice E, Greco S, Bezzio C, Bianchi Porro G. Transient small-bowel intussusceptions in adults: significance of ultrasonographic detection. *Clin Radiol* 2007; 62: 792-797

Martín-Lorenzo JG, Torralba-Martinez A, Lirón-Ruiz R, Flores-Pastor B, Miguel-Perelló J, Aguilar-Jimenez J, Aguayo-Albasini JL. Intestinal invagination in adults: preoperative diagnosis and management. *Int J Colorectal Dis* 2004; 19: 68-72

Mateen MA, Saleem S, Rao PC, Gangadhar V, Reddy DN. Transient small bowel intussusceptions: ultrasound findings and clinical significance Abdom Imaging. 2006 Jul-Aug;31(4):410-6. Epub 2006 Aug 30. DOI: 10.1007/s00261-006-9078-z

Mateen MA, Saleem S, Rao PC, Gangadhar V, Reddy DN. Transient small bowel intussusceptions: ultrasound findings and clinical significance. *Abdom Imaging* 2006; 31: 410-416

Milan R, Lideo L, G. Bonetti, E. Baroni 2010 Pylorogastric intussusception in a chihuahua puppy dog, *Proceeding 65° SCIVAC International Congress,* Rimini, 297

Mollitt DL, Ballantine TVN, Grosfeld J (1979) Postoperative intussusception in infancy and childhood: analysis of 119 cases. Surgery 86:402–408

Morrison SC, Stork E (1990) Documentation of spontaneous reduction of childhood intussusception by ultrasound. Pediatr Radiol 20:358–359

Navarro O, Dugougeat F, Kornecki A, Shuckett B, Alton DJ, Daneman A. The impact of imaging in the management of intussusception owing to pathologic lead points in children. A review of 43 cases Pediatr Radiol. 2000 Sep;30(9):594-603.

Neugut AI, Jacobson JS, Suh S, Mukherjee R, Arber N. The epidemiology of cancer of the small bowel. *Cancer Epidemiol Biomarkers Prev* 1998; 7: 243-251

Nylund K, Odegaard S, Hausken T et al (2009) Sonography of the small intestine. World J Gastroenterol 15:1319–1330

Nylund K, Ødegaard S, Hausken T, Folvik G, Lied GA, Viola I, Hauser H, Gilja OH. Sonography of the small intestine. World J Gastroenterol. 2009 Mar 21;15(11):1319-30. ISSN 1007-9327

Ødegaard S, Kimmey MB. Location of the muscularis mucosae on high frequency gastrointestinal ultrasound images. *Eur J Ultrasound* 1994; 1: 39-50

Pallotta N, Baccini F, Corazziari E. Small intestine contrast ultrasonography. *J Ultrasound Med* 2000; 19: 21-26

Pallotta N, Baccini F, Corazziari E. Small intestine contrast ultrasonography (SICUS) in the diagnosis of small intestine lesions. *Ultrasound Med Biol* 2001; 27: 335-341

Pallotta N, Tomei E, Viscido A, Calabrese E, Marcheggiano A, Caprilli R, Corazziari E. Small intestine contrast ultrasonography: an alternative to radiology in the assessment of small bowel disease. *Inflamm Bowel Dis* 2005;11: 146-153

Parente F, Greco S, Molteni M, Anderloni A, Sampietro GM, Danelli PG, Bianco R, Gallus S, Bianchi Porro G. Oral contrast enhanced bowel ultrasonography in the assessment of small intestine Crohn's disease. A prospective comparison with conventional ultrasound, x ray studies, and ileocolonoscopy. *Gut* 2004; 53: 1652-1657

Perko MJ, Just S. Duplex ultrasonography of superior mesenteric artery: interobserver variability. *J Ultrasound Med* 1993; 12: 259-263

Pracros JP, Tran-Mihn VA, Morin de Finfe CH, et al. (1987) Acute intestinal intussusception in children. Contribution of ultrsonography (145 cases). Ann Radiol 30:535–530

Riccabona M (2006) Modern pediatric ultrasound: potential applications and clinical significance. A review. Clin Imaging 30:77–86

Roebuck DJ, McLaren CA. Gastrointestinal intervention in children Pediatr Radiol (2011) 41:27–41 DOI 10.1007/s00247-010-1699-2

Sandrasegaran K, Kopecky KK, Rajesh A, et al. (2004) Proximal small bowel intussusceptions in adults: CT appearance and clinical significance. Abdom Imaging 29:653–657

Schmidt T, Hohl C, Haage P et al (2005) Phase-inversion tissue harmonic imaging compared to fundamental B-mode ultrasound in the evaluation of the pathology of large and small bowel. Eur Radiol 15:2021–2030

Strouse PJ, DiPietro MA, Saez F (2003) Transient small-bowel intussusception in children on CT. Pediatr Radiol 33:316–320(Epub 2003 February 26)

Swischuk LE, John SD, Swischuk PN (1994) Spontaneous reduction of intussusception: verifications with US. Radiology 192:269– 271

Tarján Z, Tóth G, Györke T, Mester A, Karlinger K, Makó EK. Ultrasound in Crohn's disease of the small bowel. *Eur J Radiol* 2000; 35: 176-182

Tranquart F, Grenier N, Eder Vet al (1999) Clinical use of ultrasound tissue harmonic imaging. Ultrasound Med Biol 25:889–894

Tröger J, Darge K (1998) SieScape - a new dimension of ultrasound imaging in pediatric radiology. Radiologe 38:417–419

Turgut AT, Cos ZU, Kısmet K et al (2008) Comparison of extended field of view and dual image ultrasound techniques for the measurement of the longitudinal dimension of enlarged thyroid glands. J Med Ultrasound 16:150–157

Van Oostayen JA, Wasser MN, van Hogezand RA, Griffioen G, Biemond I, Lamers CB, de Roos A. Doppler sonography evaluation of superior mesenteric artery flow to assess Crohn's disease activity: correlation with clinical evaluation, Crohn's disease activity index, and alpha 1-antitrypsin clearance in feces. *AJR Am J Roentgenol* 1997; 168: 429-433

Vasavada P. Ultrasound evaluation of acute abdominal emergencies in infants and children. Radiol Clin North Am. 2004 Mar;42(2):445-56

Verschelden P, Filiatrault D, Garel L, Grignon A, Perreault G, Boisvert J, Dubois J. Intussusception in children: reliability of US in diagnosis--a prospective study. *Radiology* 1992; 184: 741-744

Warshauser DM, Lee JKT (1999) Adult intussusception detected at CT or MR imaging: clinical imaging correlation. Radiology 212:853–860

Wilson SR (2000) The gastrointestinaltract. In: Rumack CM, Wilson SR, Charboneau JW, (eds). Diagnostic ultrasound, 2nd edn.St. Louis: Mosby

Ying M, Sin MH (2005) Comparison of extended field of view and dual image ultrasound techniques: accuracy and reliability of distance measurements in phantom study. Ultrasound Med Biol 31:79–83

Zhang Y., Yu-Zuo Bai, Shi-Xing Li & Shou-Jun Liu & Wei-Dong Ren & Li-Qiang Zheng (2011). Sonographic findings predictive of the need for surgical management in pediatric patients with small bowel intussusceptions, *Langenbecks Arch Surg.* 2011 Jan 28. DOI 10.1007/s00423-011-0742-6

3

Appendiceal Intussusception

Nikolaos Varsamis, Konstantinos Pouggouras, Nikolaos Salveridis, Aekaterini Theodosiou, Eftychios Lostoridis, Georgios Karageorgiou, Athanasios Mekakas and Konstantinos Christodoulidis
1st Department of Surgery, General Hospital of Kavala
Greece

1. Introduction

Diseases of the appendix constitute a problem of daily practice in the routine of the general surgeon. One should be well aware and familiar with all the spectrum of its pathology and, of course, he should be able to deal with it successfully and uneventfully. It is not a coincidence that appendectomy is the first operation a general surgeon is trained to perform. Moreover, statistics claim that appendectomy is the most common emergent general surgery procedure performed in the United States. Finally, with 250,000 appendectomies performed there every year, Addiss et al estimated in 1990 the lifetime risk of appendectomy to be 8.6% for men and 6.7% for women (Chaar et al, 2009).

Despite being such a common matter of daily medical practice, diseases of the appendix may comprise lesions that are not so usually encountered by a general surgeon. Therefore it is important and worthy to try to illuminate them and bring some useful information concerning them to the foreground.

Intussusception of the appendix is such an infrequent appendiceal lesion with an incidence of 0.01% among patients receiving an appendectomy. Although it may clinically mimic more common acute and chronic abdominal conditions, it is an important entity to recognize, since it could be discovered as a caecal mass or mistaken for a gastrointestinal neoplasm. However, diagnosis is rarely made preoperatively due to its variable and non-specific symptoms.

All the information mentioned above point out the importance of the thorough presentation concerning the clinical entity of the intussusception of the vermiform appendix that is going to be given in the following pages of this essay.

2. Appendiceal intussusception: A challenge for the general surgeon

2.1 Materials and methods

Appendiceal intussusception, despite being a rare entity, is a distinctive and by means of diagnosis challenging condition. The literature referring to appendiceal intussusception mainly consists of case report articles. Our objective is to present a thorough review of the existing literature, based on articles published in journals accessible via Medline (Pub Med database source).

A research in Pub Med/Medline was performed by our team using the key words "Appendiceal Intussusception" and MeSH ("Appendix"[Majr]) AND "Intussusception"

[Majr]. In the first instance our research resulted in 160 titles of articles, whereas in the second we found 183 ones. All of them having an abstract or full text available were reviewed and taken into consideration as a source of data for our essay. During our research we found out that in 2009 Chaar et al made a comprehensive review of the English literature concerning appendiceal intussusception and presented a series of 191 cases published, including one who was their patient. We decided to use those 191 cases as our initial material and add all the cases of appendiceal intussusception published after Chaar's review up until 2011, while we also added some articles from previous years that weren't included in his review. Finally, we gathered a total of 28 articles describing 29 new cases of appendiceal intussusception plus some cases where the appendiceal stump acted as the leading point for intussusception. Thus our material comprises 220 cases of appendiceal intussusception described in English literature from which all data that are presented below have emerged.

2.2 Definition and classification of intussusception

Intussusception represents a rare form of bowel obstruction, which is defined as the telescoping of a proximal segment of the gastrointestinal tract, called intussusceptum, into the lumen of the adjacent distal segment of the gastrointestinal tract, called intussuscipiens.
Lesions within the lumen of the bowel have a higher likelihood to cause invagination, because peristalsis drags them forward. These lesions act as "leading points" for intussusception (Kim et al, 2006).
This entity was first reported in 1674 by Barbette of Amsterdam and further presented in a detailed report in 1789 by John Hunter as "introssusception". Historically, Sir Jonathan Hutchinson was the first to operate on a child with intussusception in 1871 (Marinis et al, 2009).
The most common locations in the gastrointestinal tract where an intussusception can take place are the junctions between freely moving intestinal segments, and retroperitoneally or adhesionally fixed bowel segments. The types of intussusception have been classified according to their location into four categories :

- entero-enteric intussusception , confined to the small bowel
- colo-colic intussusception, involving only the large bowel
- ileo-colic intussusception, defined as the prolapse of the terminal ileum within the ascending colon
- ileo-caecal intussusception, where the ileo-cecal valve is the leading point of the intussusception and that is distinguished with some difficulty from the ileo-colic variant

(Marinis et al, 2009).

2.3 Basic anatomy and physiology of the appendix

The appendix is located in the right iliac fossa and usually its base is situated in a line joining the right superior iliac spine to the umbilicus in relation to the anterior abdominal wall (one third of the way from the right superior iliac spine). The vermiform appendix is a narrow, muscular diverticulum containing numerous lymphoid follicles. Its length varies from 8 to 13 cm (3 to 5 in.) and its base arises from the posteromedial surface of the caecum approximately 2,5 cm (1 in.) below the ileocolic valve. It usually has a complete peritoneal covering and it attaches to the mesentery of the small intestine by the mesoappendix. The latter contains the appendicular vessels and nerves. The teniae coli of the caecum converge to the base of the appendix and form a muscle coat. It is divided in three parts: base, body and tip of the appendix. The tip of the appendix is moving freely and may be found inside (85%) or outside the peritoneum (15%) (Anson & McVay, 1971). In the first case, the most common position of the appendix is coiled up behind the caecum (65%). In 20% of cases, it hangs down into the pelvis against the right pelvic wall. Less common sites are in front or behind the terminal part of the ileum. In the second case, it projects upward along the lateral site of the caecum or the ascending colon. In cases of intestinal malrotation or situs inversus, it may be located in the right upper quadrant or in the left iliac fossa, respectively (Snell, 2008).

The appendicular artery is a branch of the ileocolic artery, which originates from the superior mesenteric artery. In 30% of the cases, a second branch from the posterior caecal artery exists. The appendicular vein drains into the ileocolic vein and finally to the portal vein (through upper mesenteric vein). The lymph vessels drain into one or two nodes lying in the mesoappendix, into the ileocaecal nodes and eventually into the superior mesenteric nodes (Snell, 2008).

The nerve supply derives from the superior mesenteric plexus, which gives the sympathetic and parasympathetic (vagus) nerves. The visceral pain of the appendix is conducted by afferent nerve fibers that enter the spinal cord at the level of the 10th thoracic segment (Snell, 2008).

The role of the appendix as a part of the immune system remains unknown. Its physiologic function is related to the presence of lymphoid follicles in the submucosal layer of the appendix. The lymphoid follicles appear two weeks after birth and number about 200 or more between the ages of 15 and 25 years. They progressively decline and become atrophic in the elderly with fibrosis of the wall and total or partial obliteration of the lumen of the appendix (Schumpelick et al, 2000). Mucous is secreted into the lumen of appendix with a rate of 2-3 ml per day (Sbarounis, 1991).

2.4 Intussusception of the vermiform appendix

2.4.1 Historical background

In 1858 McKidd was the first who described a case of complete invagination of the appendix into the caecum of a 7 year-old boy as a post mortem finding (Gilpin, 1989; McKidd, 1858). In 1890, the first operation for appendiceal intussusception in a 13-months-old child was reported. Wright, Renshaws, Pitts and McGraw performed successful operations for appendical intussusception. In 1964, Collins concluded a 40-year study on 71,000 appendices obtained from surgical and autopsy material and reported prevalence of 0.01% for intussusception of the appendix; the prevalence of endometriosis and adenocarcinoma of the appendix were 0.05% and 0.08%, respectively (Collins, 1963; Ryu et al, 2005).

Since the first report, the literature on appendiceal intussusception has been limited to case reports and small case series. Forshall in 1953 and Bachman and Clement in 1971 wrote the largest case series, presenting 7 patients each. Some investigators attempted limited reviews of the literature. Fink et al reviewed the literature in 1964 and found that less than 118 cases had been previously reported. Finally, Chaar et al made a comprehensive review in 2009 and presented 191 cases of appendiceal intussusception described in the English literature since then (Chaar et al, 2009).

From all the above it is clear that appendiceal intussusception is an extremely rare lesion of the appendix. Despite its rarity, it is a disease encountered and described one and a half century ago, and it still remains in the centre of medical interest, since case reports and reviews continue to be published nowadays.

2.4.2 Demographics

There is an objective difficulty in presenting accurate data referring to demographics and incidence of appendiceal intussusception due to the infrequency of this condition. Most articles in the literature are limited in case reports or small case series. Moreover, results presented in these articles are often variant and controversial.

Fink et al reviewed the literature and found that less than 118 cases were reported. Their paper was published in 1964 and stated that appendiceal intussusception is predominantly a pediatric condition, with most cases observed in the first decade of life, with the average age of occurrence being 16 years old. Men seemed to be affected 4 to 5 times more frequently than women (Fink et al, 1964). Jevon et al reviewed the cases reported between 1984 and 1991 and found 12 reports of appendiceal intussusception. He concluded that this lesion occurs mostly in adults and has an equal sex distribution (Jevon et al, 1992). Finally, Chaar et al in 2009 concluded that appendiceal intussusception is more often encountered in adult women, with a predominance of occurrence in the 4th decade of life. He presented demographic data from 189 out of 191 patients mentioned. (Chaar et al, 2009).

Our team worked out with a total of 218 patients' demographic data. 189 patients came from Chaar's review and 29 patients from our research in the literature. Male patients were 82 out of 218 in total (37.6%), whereas female patients were 136 out of 218 (62.4%). Consequently, male/female ratio of patients suffering from appendiceal intussusception was approximately 1/3. Moreover, pediatric patients affected by this lesion were 52 out of 218 (23.8%), while adult patients were 166 out of 218 (76.2%). Thus, appendiceal intussusception is more commonly encountered in the age group of adults, with a frequency which is more than 2 times higher than that of the pediatric age group.

Interestingly, intussusception of the vermiform appendix happens more often in male population in the pediatric age group, while female patients are more in the age group of adults. In particular, 32 out of 52 patients (61.5%) in the pediatric age group were male, whereas 116 out of 166 patients (69.9%) in the age group of adults were female. It is clear that there is an inversion in the frequency and rate of appearance (1/3) among the two sexes in the two different age groups of pediatric and adult population. This phenomenon can be explained by the fact that appendiceal intussusception in adults is predominantly secondary to appendiceal endometriosis or mucocele, as we will more thoroughly explain in a following chapter of this essay. However, endometriosis happens only to women and mucocele of the appendix is also more often in women. Moreover, appendiceal intussusception in pediatric age group is almost always primary with elements of inflammation, thus female dominance stops to exist. Therefore, there seems to be a rational explanation for the observed inversion in the frequencies among the two sexes.

Patients' terminal ages varied from 17 days after gestation to 85 years of life, and the total average age of occurrence lied between 35 and 36 years (35.6 years). In the pediatric age group average age of presentation was 6.8 years. Finally, in the age group of adults appendiceal intussusception emerged in the average age of 45.5 years.

2.4.3 Classification

Appendiceal intussusception was first classified by Moschowitz in 1910 and later modified by McSwain in 1941. The classification is anatomically based on which part of the appendix is the intussusceptum and where the intussuscipiens is located. McSwain described 5 types as follows (**Fig. 1**):

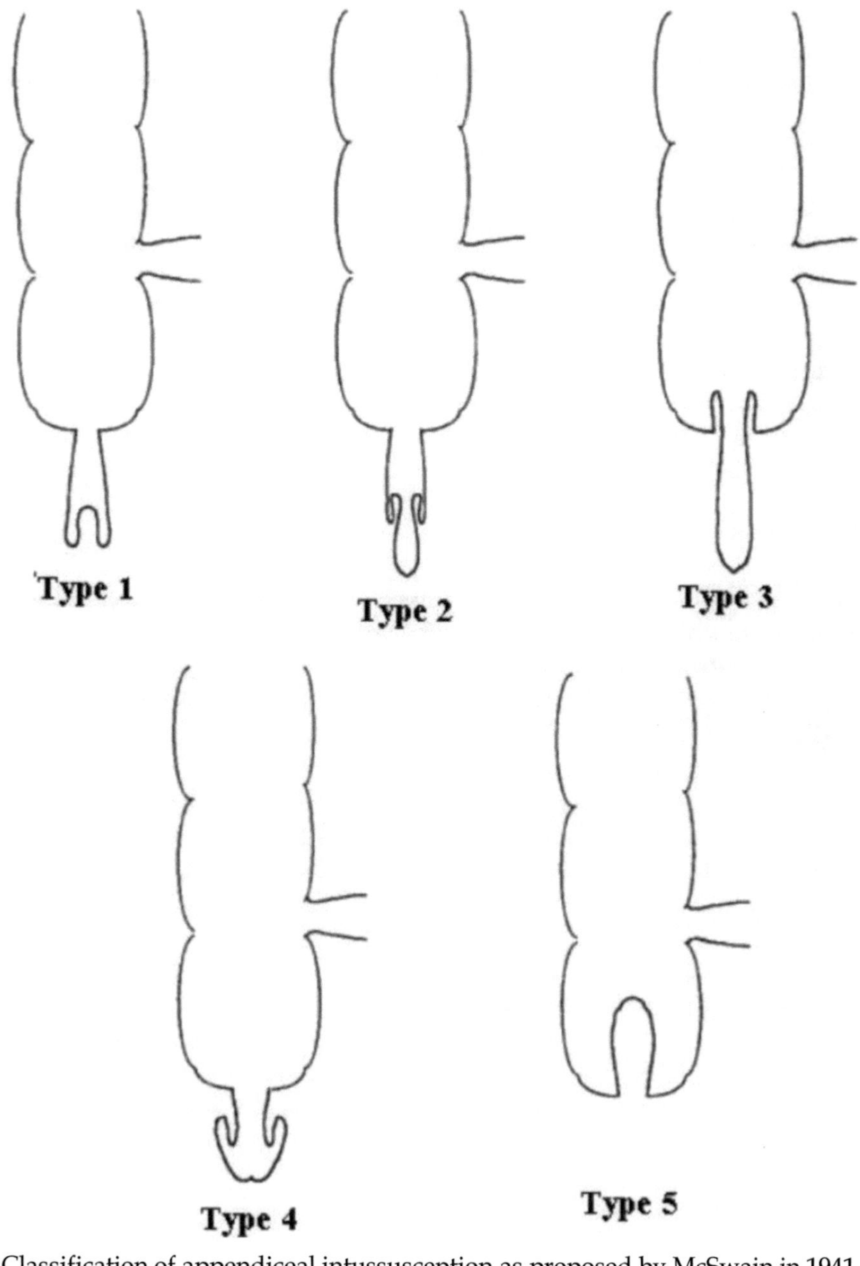

Fig. 1. Classification of appendiceal intussusception as proposed by McSwain in 1941 (Taban et al, 2006).

Type I: The tip of the appendix forms the intussusceptum and is invaginated into the proximal appendix, which is the intussuscipiens.
Type II: The invagination starts at some point along the length of the appendix. The intussuscipiens is the adjacent tissue.
Type III: The invagination starts at the junction of the appendix and caecum. The caecum is the intussuscipiens.
Type IV: This is retrograde intussusception, where the proximal appendix is invaginated into the distal appendix.
Type V: Complete invagination of the appendix into the caecum from progression of types I and II or type III. (Chaar et al, 2009).
All types of the previously described primary appendiceal intussusceptions, possibly with the exception of type IV, can initiate a secondary intussusception. The question of whether the intussuscepted appendix initiates a secondary intussusception presumably depends upon both the degree of irritation by its presence inside the caecum and the anatomy of the caecum. A fixed caecum is unlikely to intussuscept, whereas a mobile caecum with rotational anomaly may be more likely to produce intussusception (Atkinson et al, 1976). Characteristically, Dunavant and Wilson reported in 1952 the case of an intussuscepted appendix leading to complete colonic intussusception and protrusion of the inverted appendix from the anus as a mass (Dunavant & Wilson, 1952).
Langsam proposed in 1958 a simpler classification for appendiceal intussusception:
Type I begins at the tip of the appendix (the intussusceptum) which intussuscepts into its more proximal portion (the intussuscipiens).
Type II begins in the base of the appendix (intussusceptum) and the caecum is the intussuscipiens.
In **type III**, the base of the appendix is the intussusceptum received by the appendiceal tip.
Type IV refers to complete inversion of the appendix with accompanying ileocaecal intussusception, whereby the appendix remains the leading point of the intussusceptum. This can result from types I and II of appendiceal intussusception (Salehzadeh et al, 2010).
Finally, Jacobs in 1963 argued that the term "intussusception of the appendix" should be reserved only for the condition in which the appendix intussuscepts into itself, in the same way that ileum intussuscepts into ileum in the ileo-ileal type of intussusception. This condition is equivalent to retrograde appendiceal intussusception, described as type IV by McSwain, and its rarity is pointed out by the fact that Collins in 1963 in a review of 71,000 human specimens after appendectomy found that particular lesion only in one case (Collins, 1963; Jacobs, 1963).

2.4.4 Etiology and predisposing conditions

The etiology of most cases of appendiceal intussusception remains unknown; however certain predisposing conditions are thought to make intussusception more likely to happen. Pathophysiological features that determine the invagination of the appendix can be divided in two large groups: anatomical and pathological.
Anatomical conditions are represented by:

- a fetal type of caecum, with the appendix originating from its tip
- a wide appendicular lumen with the proximal lumen having a greater diameter than its distal part
- a mesoappendix that is thin, free from fat and with a narrow base

- a mobile appendicular wall capable of active peristaltism
- an appendix that is free, unfixed by peritoneal folds or adhesions.

Most workers theorize that abnormal appendiceal peristalsis secondary to local irritation is the chief pathologic predisposing factor. The most commonly accepted view, which has been suggested by Rolleston in 1898, proposes that either an intramural or an intraluminal lesion produces irritation of the normal appendiceal peristaltic activity, which leads to an attempt by the appendix to extrude the offending lesion. The appendix itself undergoes strong peristaltic contractions which may become more vigorous if the appendiceal wall is irritated. This may lead to part of its wall being pushed in, or out, acting as the leading point for an intussusception. Spasm of the muscular sphincter at the base of the appendix might also form the apex of an intussusception. It seems likely as mentioned before that a combination of anatomical, physiological and minor pathological changes interact to produce this rare condition.

Local pathological irritants such as parasites, fecaliths, foreign bodies, neoplasms (polyps, mucoceles, adenocarcinomas, carcinoid tumors), hypertrophic lymphoid follicles, mucoceles, endometrial implants and postinflammatory scars have been implicated as predisposing lesions for the development of appendiceal intussusception (Atkinson et al, 1976; Gilipin, 1989; Komine et al, 2004; Taban et al, 2006).

In our clinic we have encountered the case of a calcified appendiceal mucocele acting as the leading point for caecoclic intussusception (Varsamis et al, 2010). An intraoperative photo of the mucocle after manual reduction of the caecocolic intussusception can be seen in **Fig. 2.**

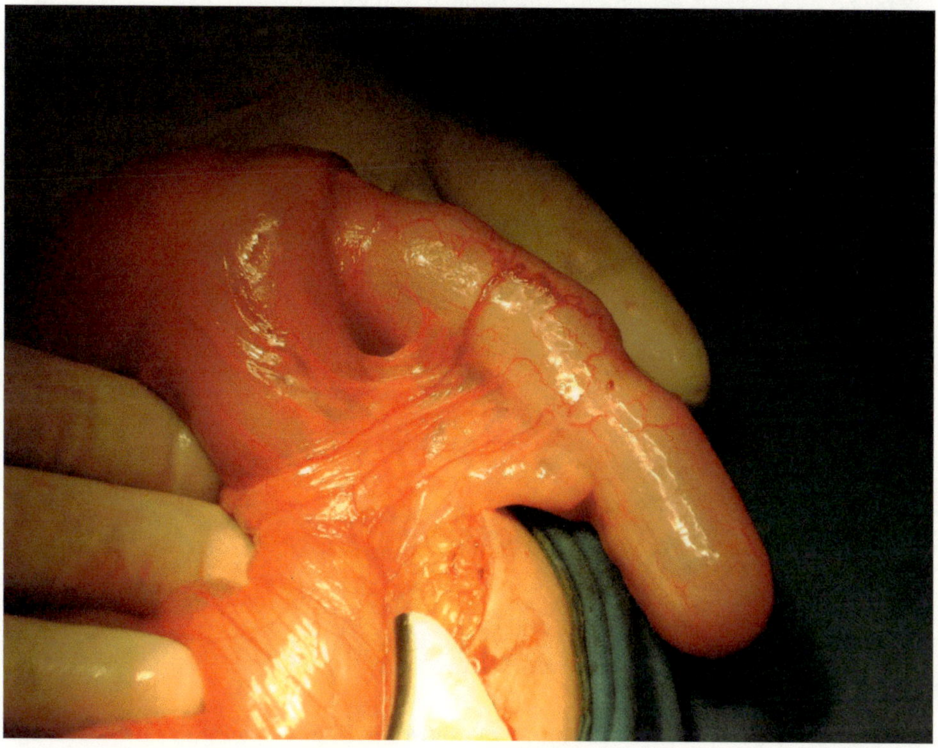

Fig. 2. Intraoperative photo of a large mucocele with its base intussuscepted into the lumen of the caecum. **Type III** of appendiceal intussusception according to McSwain's classification. (From our clinic's photo archive).

Finally, cases where the inverted appendiceal stump after appendectomy acted as the leading point for a secondary ileo-colic intussusception have been described in the literature. Those cases comprise mainly pediatric and young adult male patients, with the intussusception taking place commonly during the first few post-operative days. When the appendiceal stump is inverted into the caecum after appendectomy, conceivably a leading point for intussusception could be created. Yeager in 1947 studied methods of appendiceal stump closure and showed that an inverted stump was more intramural than intraluminal. However, swelling and inflammatory reaction caused by a foreign body at the site of an intramural stump could encroach on the caecal lumen sufficiently to be caught in normal peristalsis and lead to intussusception (Arora et al, 2008; Bridger , 1956; Hanson et al, 1967; Lipskar et al, 2008; Yeager, 1947).

2.4.5 Histopathological findings

Histopathological examination of the intussuscepted appendix and results were reported in 153 cases used by Chaar in his review. We added the histopathological findings of our 29 new cases to those previously mentioned and gathered a total of 182 results concerning cases of appendiceal intussusception.
Inflammatory lesions consistent with acute appendicitis were reported in 51 patients suffering from appendiceal intussusception. Inflammation was the most frequent histopathological finding with a percentage of occurrence estimated in 28%. The second commonest diagnosis was endometrial implants in the intussuscepted appendix, which was found in 43 female patients (23.6%). Simple mucoceles **(Fig.3)** acted as the leading points for intussusception in 29 cases (15.9%) and mucinous cystadenomas in 8 cases (4.4%). Adenomas of the intussuscepted appendix were diagnosed in 14 patients (7.7%), adenocarcinomas in 8 patients (4.4%), carcinoid tumors in 9 patients (4.9%) and histopathological findings of neuroendocrine carcinoma with a metastatic lymph node were reported in 1 patient (0.55%). Other tumors of the intussuscepted appendix comprised 1 case of papilloma (0.55%), 1 case of hamartoma (0.55%) and 1 case of juvenile polyp (0.55%).

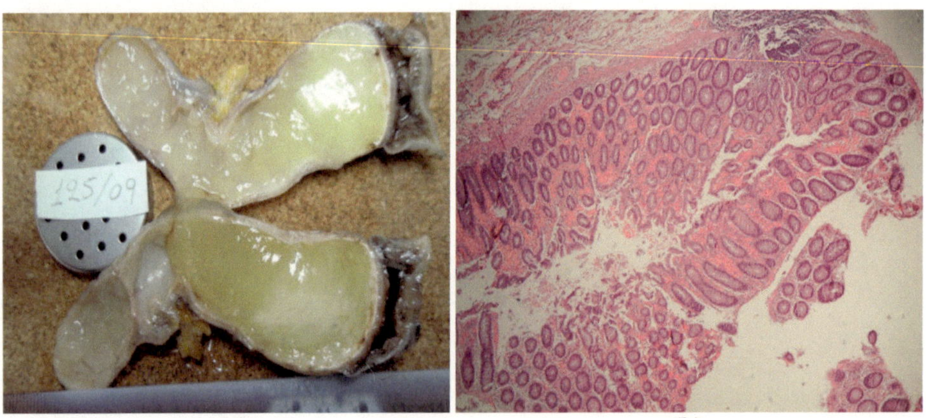

(a) (b)

Fig. 3. **(a)** Gross section of the simple mucocele shown in Figure 2, with its lumen full of yellow, gelatinous mucus. **(b)** Histopathological image of the same mucocele showing mucus producing glands in its wall, with no elements of cellular atypia (H&E Stain x 100. From our clinic's photo archive).

Moreover, 1 patient with Mucosa Associated Lymphoid Tissue (MALT) Lymphoma (0.55%) and also 1 patient (0.55%) with ileo-caecal Non-Hodgkin Lymphoma (NHL) were encountered in the literature. In total, 74 patients (40.6%) suffered from a primary benign or malignant neoplasia of the vermiform appendix which took place in the development of a secondary appendiceal intussusception.

Other less common lesions found at histopathological examination were 3 cases of appendiceal distention due to Cystic Fibrosis (1.65%), 2 cases of an inverted appendiceal stump with no elements of inflammation (1.1%), 2 cases of colonoscopically taken biopsies which revealed normal appendiceal mucosa (1.1%), 2 cases of fecalith material (1.1%), 1 case of a granuloma due to Crohn's Disease (0.55%), 1 case of microscopic melanosis coli (0.55%), 1 case with angiodyspastic foci in the appendix causing anemia (0.55%), 1 case of Schistosomiasis with occupation of the appendiceal base and several lymph nodes by Schistosome's eggs (0.55%) and 1 final case with simple lymphoid hyperplasia of the appendix (0.55%).

In the pediatric age group, 23 out of 36 patients having an histopathological examination came with the final diagnosis of appendiceal inflammation (63.9%). Inflammation was the commonest diagnosis in children because other lesions causing appendiceal intussusception like tumors normally emerge in adolescence. In the adult group of patients endometriosis of the appendix was the commonest diagnosis, with 43 reported women out of 146 patients (29.5%). Finally, simple mucocele and inflammation, both encountered in 26 out of 146 patients (17.8%), were the second commonest lesions causing appendiceal intussusception in adults.

2.4.6 Clinical presentation

Symptoms of appendiceal intussusception have classically been divided into four groups. In the first group, onset of symptoms is abrupt similarly to acute appendicitis and these cases are frequently taken to surgery with the diagnosis of acute appendicitis. At operation partial or complete intussusception of the appendix is found.

In the second group, the symptoms are consistent with intestinal intussusception. Abdominal pain and vomiting usually occur for several days. Bowel movements may be normal. Less commonly, there may be constipation, diarrhea or melena. Examination frequently reveals an abdominal mass which is recognized as an underlying intussusception. These cases have a compound intussusception and the appendiceal invagination is discovered only after the main intussusception has been reduced either by surgery or by barium enema examination.

A third group includes cases with a prolonged history of repeated intermittent severe attacks of right lower quadrant abdominal pain. Vomiting and melena may be present. The interval between the attacks is quite variable. Physical examination between attacks is unrevealing. The acute pain can be due to intermittent secondary intussusception which follows intussusception of the appendix. A patient with a history of multiple attacks of intermittent abdominal pain deserves a thorough clinical and radiological examination with the possibility of appendiceal intussusception considered in the differential diagnosis.

There is a fourth group of patients in which primary appendiceal intussusception is asymptomatic. In these cases, appendiceal intussusception is described as an incidental finding in screening colonoscopical or radiological investigation of the patient. Brewer and Wangenstein suggested in 1974 a fifth group, in which intermittent bleeding from rectum is found in otherwise asymptomatic patients (Atkinson et al, 1976).

In our material of 220 patients suffering from appendiceal intussusception the observed symptoms and signs had a variable frequency of presentation. Abdominal pain, reported in 161 out of 220 cases, turned out to be the commonest symptom with a percentage of 73.2%. It was mainly located in the right lower quadrant or periumbilically and its character was colicoid. Nausea and emesis were present in 56 out of 220 patients and followed in frequency with 25.5%. Blood per rectum or melena occurred in 47 patients and was the third commonest symptom (21.4 %). A mass could be palpated on physical examination of the abdominal wall in 38 patients (17.3%). Other symptoms or signs reported according to their frequency of existence were diarrhea in 28 cases (12.7%), constipation in 21 cases (9.5%), weight loss in 12 cases (5.5%), anorexia in 10 cases (4.5%), abdominal tenderness in 10 cases (4.5%) and bowel distention in 5 cases (2.3%). Finally, 3 patients were totally asymptomatic, representing 1.4% of cases.

2.4.7 Laboratory, radiological and colonoscopical investigation

Elaborate investigation of patients suffering from appendiceal intussusception is a very important parameter in the effort to reach a precise diagnosis. As mentioned before, in most cases patients referred with atypical and non-specific symptoms, like abdominal pain, nausea and constipation. Therefore, complete laboratory, radiological and colonoscopical examination should be performed to all the patients with obscure clinical presentation, in order to achieve a correct preoperative diagnosis.

Laboratory findings were not certain or specific according to the literature. In most cases, laboratory values and temperature were within normal limits. Leukocytosis with a polymorphonuclear white blood cell type were the commonest observed pathological findings. An elevated value of C-reactive protein (CRP) or mild pyrexia could be present in the event of co-existing inflammation. Moreover, anemia was reported in some cases where blood per rectum or melena were also observed. Finally, in two asymptomatic patients, screening blood tests revealed an increased serum γ-glutamyltranspeptidase (γGTP) in the first and an elevated serum carcinoembryonic antigen (CEA) in the second one. Both patients suffered from appendiceal intussusception due to preexisting mucoceles (Lu et al, 2009; Okuda et al, 2008).

In most cases of appendiceal intussusception, radiographical findings were normal, unless a small-bowel obstruction co-existed. "Air-fluid" levels of the small intestine could then be present in plain abdominal X-Ray films (Koumanidou et al, 2001; Varsamis et al, 2010).

Cases of appendiceal invagination were diagnosed during double-contrast barium enema examination, sometimes at asymptomatic patients. Levin *et al.* described in 1985 11 cases with characteristic radiological signs, like a "coiled-spring" sign in the caecum or nonfilling of the appendix. Radiological abnormalities included:

- no abnormality seen in the caecal region, with absence of the appendix
- oval or round bosselated intraluminal filling defects, usually in the medial wall of the caecum, with no visualization of the appendix (partial appendiceal invagination)
- intraluminal, "finger-like" filling defects within the caecum, usualy arising from its medial wall (complete appendiceal invagination)
- reduction of the filling defect out of the caecum during fluoroscopy (Bachman & Clemett, 1971; Levine et al, 1985; Taban et al, 2006).

Ultrasonography has played a role in the diagnosis of appendiceal intussusception, especially in children. A "donut" sign or a "target" lesion is virtually diagnostic of

intussusception (Holt & Samuel, 1978). Appendiceal intussusception may appear as the "multiconcentric ring" sign on transverse scans, while longitudinal sonograms may show the inverted appendix protruding into the caecal lumen (Pumberger et al, 2000). Koumanidou et al in 2001 argued that the sonograhic appearance of multiple concecntric hypoechoic and hyperechoic rings is not characteristic of appendiceal intussusception but intussusception in general. She also claimed that visualization of the appendix within the head of the intussusception may be considered characteristic only when a small cyst or a "target-like" mass is demonstrated, having an outer diameter which should not exceed 6mm (Koumanidou et al, 2001). Tseng et al in 2006 reported a case of preoperative appendiceal intussusception diagnosis with endoscopic sonography, which revealed a multiconcentric ring structure in the region of the caecal base (Tseng et al, 2006).
Appendicidal intussusception has been described as having a target, layered, sausage-shaped, or reniform appearance on CT; when present, this appearance is virtually pathognomonic (Luzier et al, 2006). Moreover, CT scans may reveal a mass lesion within the caecum, a thickened "sausage shaped" caecum and the pathognomonic bowel-within-bowel configuration (Fernandez-Rey et al, 2010). The limitations of CT primarily relate to its use of ionizing radiation and the risk of allergy to contrast material. However, CT can provide excellent anatomic detail in addition to assessing the presence of complications of intussusception. Last but not least, with modern CT scanners, isotropic voxel reconstructions in nonaxial planes provide additional diagnostic certainty by allowing direct visualization and differentiation of the distal ileum and ileocecal valve from the caecal tip and appendix (Luzier et al, 2006).
Sonographic and CT scanning images from a case of an intussuscepted appendiceal mucocele encountered by our clinic are shown in **Figure 4** below.

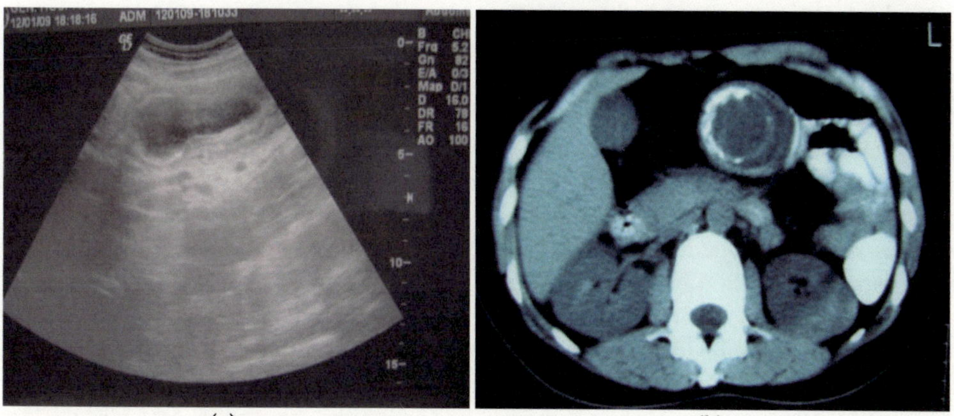

(a) (b)

Fig. 4. **(a)** Abdominal ultrasound image, showing the intussuscepted appendiceal mucocele mentioned in previous figures, in a longitudinal cross section. **(b)** Abdominal CT scanning image, showing the calcified base of the same appendiceal mucocele intussuscepted into the lumen of the transverse colon. Pathognomonic "bowel-within-bowel" configuration. (From our clinic's photo archive).

Finally, colonoscopy can play a very important role in the correct preoperative diagnosis of appendiceal intussusception. Most characteristic colonoscopical findings include a "mushroom-like", polypoid lesion within the caecal lumen, which appears erythematous and surrounds a central dimple corresponding to the appendiceal orifice. When air is insufflated, the dimple and mass may change appearance, becoming smaller or larger with peristalsis, or may even occur a total reduction of the appendiceal intussusception. If the intussusception has reduced on its own at the time of endoscopy, a central depression at the base of the caecum corresponding to the appendiceal lumen surrounded by an area of a halo type erythema can be seen (Ozuner et al, 2000). Therefore, careful endoscopical examination, with identification of the appendiceal orifice, should be required in all cases that recognition of a caecal polyp happens. Endoscopical removal of this lesion is associated with a high risk of subsequent peritonitis (Khawaja, 2002). Visualization of an appendiceal intussusception as a caecal polyp could also be achieved by means of CT colonogram scanning (Salehzadeh et al, 2010)

2.4.8 Differential diagnosis

Differential diagnosis of appendiceal intussusception includes the case of an appendiceal abscess, a duplication cyst or the presence of an asymptomatic inverted appendiceal stump. Of the appendiceal or other regional malignant tumors, lymphomas are the most common in the pediatric age group. Other primary malignancies most commonly found in adults include adenocarcinomas and carcinoid tumors. Benign tumors comprising lipomas, leiomyomas, fibromas and hemangiomas are scarcely encountered. Mucoceles of the appendix are more frequent in female patients and occur in adults (Atkinson et al, 1976, Christianakis et al, 2008; Wang et al, 2010).

In a case of caecocolic intussusception involving a calcified mucocele participating in the intussusception that was encountered by our surgical clinic, differential diagnosis included an inflammed Meckel's diverticulum and a mesenteric cyst. Final diagnosis was achieved intraoperatively after the reduction of the intussuscepted mucocele (Varsamis et al, 2010).

2.4.9 Methods of treatment

The treatment of the intussuscepted appendix can be conservative, minimally invasive or surgical. The choice must be done according to the patient's age, co morbidities, recurrence and risk of a neoplasm.

The intussuscepted appendix may be reduced with a barium enema if the diagnosis is certain, especially in children. However, there is a high recurrence rate (Kleiman, 1980). No more than 90 cm of hydrostatic pressure should be applied to avoid complications. Alternatively, air may be introduced via a rectal tube to produce caecal distention. If the attempt is successful and the appendix is completely filled, a close follow-up is indicated to early diagnose recurrence. Unlike children, reduction by barium enema or air is not suggested for adults, especially for patients over 60 years old. The reason is that adults have leading points which are frequently neoplastic (Patton & Ferrera, 2000).

Minimally invasive treatment includes colonoscopy, which should be done when the diagnosis of appendiceal intussusception is suspected. During colonoscopy, the intussusception may be reduced by performing several insufflations of air. This would result in a halo-like erythematous region surrounding the appendiceal lumen (Tavakkoli et al, 2007). It is crucial to avoid endoscopic removal because perforation and subsequent peritonitis are common and serious complications (Fazio et al, 1982). Resection with looping and snare retrieval should be performed by experienced gastroenterologists and when the

diagnosis is certain. If partial intussusception exists, colonoscopical appendectomy should be avoided (de Hoyos et al, 2006; Tavakkoli et al, 2007).
The treatment of choice for the appendiceal intussusception is surgical removal of the appendix either with laparotomy or laparoscopically. Appendectomy is the most common treatment in adults. If it is possible, an attempt to reduce the appendix should be made. The surgeon should try to milk out the intussuscepted appendix in a distal to proximal direction (Wolff & Boller, 2008). If the intussusception is not reducible, caecotomy (along a taenia band) should be performed to reduce it manually. Simple appendectomy should follow in every case (Nycum et al, 1999).
In pediatric patients the treatment of choice is the laparoscopic approach. In these cases, laparoscopic reduction is successful in 50% to 65% (Poddoubnyi et al, 1998; Schier, 1997). Inversion appendectomy is an option due to its aseptic benefit (Arora et al, 2008). However, the complication of intussusception after inversion appendectomy has been reported in 0,08% to 8% in children (Kidd et al, 2000).
Exploratory laparotomy is the management of choice if there is any suspicion of appendiceal mass, caecal neoplasm or compound ileocaecal-appendiceal intussusception. Right hemicolectomy with lymph node resection is the treatment of choice when the tumor is larger than 2 cm in diameter or when malignancy is suspected. Otherwise, simple appendectomy may be sufficient (Chen & Chiang, 2000). Special care must be taken in cases of mucoceles. Benign mucinous tumors are cured with appendectomy (simple excision); malignant lesions require right hemicolectomy if they are resectable (Connor et al, 1998; Rutledge & Alexander, 1992). The surgeon must avoid tumor rupture because mucinous cystadenocarcinoma can cause pseudomyxoma peritonei (Holder et al, 1989). In case of pseudomyxoma peritonei, treatment should include appendectomy, omentectomy and in females bilateral oophorectomy. Intraperitoneal chemotherapy may be useful (Hinson & Ambrose, 1998).
Other procedures include ileocaecal resection and partial caecectomy. In the latter case, a caecal cuff or a bigger part of the caecum should be resected. These procedures have the advantage of eliminating the appendiceal stump and resecting any appendiceal lesion in a safe margin (Chaar et al, 2009). In cases of mobile caecum or ascending colon, these structures could be attached to the lateral abdominal wall by sutures (Bridger, 1956).
Finally, some authors suggest that surgical intervention may be unnecessary in patients with long-standing asymptomatic appendiceal intussusception. A close follow up is indicated in these cases (Salehzaden et al, 2010).

2.4.10 Complications

The majority of patients suffering from appendiceal intussusception that received a surgical procedure had an uneventful postoperative course according to the literature. Only few cases had vague abdominal pain or discomfort. The symptoms subsided with conservative treatment.
Serious complications emerged after colonoscopical intervention in some cases of appendiceal intussusception. These included symptoms of pain and tenderness in the right lower abdominal quadrant or even bowel perforation and peritonitis after endoscopic removal of the intussuscepted appendix. Treatment of these patients varied from simple antibiotic medication to emergent surgical exploration (Fazio et al, 1982; Wirtschafter & Kaufman, 1976). In addition, systemic bacterial infection with fever and shivering has also been described in the literature, after simple endoscopic biopsies taken from an

intussuscepted appendix. Symptoms retreated with broad spectrum antibiotherapy (Seddik & Rabhi, 2011).
Special care should be taken in cases of simple appendectomy after reduction of the appendiceal intussusception, when the appendiceal stump is inverted with a purse-string suture into the caecal wall. It could act as the leading point for a new intussusception, as mentioned in a previous chapter of this essay.
Otherwise, potential complications are the same as those encountered after performing appendectomy or right hemicolectomy. Complications after appendectomy include injury to the bowel or to other adjacent structures, intra-abdominal abscess, surgical site infection and colonic fistula.
Complications after right hemicolectomy could be divided in three categories: intraoperative and technical, early and late postoperative complications. Intraoperative and technical complications include injury to the right ureter, to the duodenum, to the other bowel (such as deserosalizations), inadequate blood supply to the anastomosis, anastomosis under tension, stool and tumor cell spillage. Early postoperative complications include surgical site infection, anastomotic leak, intra-abdominal abscess and colocutaneous fistula. Late postoperative complications include anastomotic stricture, incisional and internal hernia, ureteral stricture and adhesions (Minter & Doherty, 2010).

3. Conclusions

Early recognition of appendiceal intussusception is important in avoiding misdiagnosis and misguided attempts at endoscopical removal or inappropriate surgery. An appendiceal intussusception may be mistaken for a polyp or carcinoma, and failure to accurately diagnose this condition has resulted in patients undergoing colonoscopical polypectomy with resultant perforation and peritonitis. Alternatively, patients have also undergone unnecessary hemicolectomy when the intussuscepted appendix is regarded as a malignancy.
Although reduction of the intussuscepted appendix may occur via increased caecal luminal pressure from barium enema or colonoscopy, the definitive treatment requires surgical resection. Finally, in those cases involved by a concurrent malignant tumor, reduction at laparotomy or laparoscopy with subsequent appendectomy and right hemicolectomy is the surgical treatment of choice (Duncan et al, 2005).
Complete invagination of the appendix is a condition with rare occurrence. If the appendix on laparotomy or laparoscopy cannot be found, this diagnosis should be considered and actively ruled out. Negative laparoscopy for acute appendicitis can only be negative if a normal appendix is seen (Vogelaar et al, 2004).
Finally, many surgeons continue to perform inversion appendectomy due to its aseptic benefit. This benefit, though potentially important, has never been strongly proven in the literature. With the advent of new stapling devices and the increased experience with laparoscopic appendectomies, the need for inversion appendectomy should be readdressed, since the inverted appendiceal stump has been described in literature as the leading point for ileo-colic intussusception (Arora et al, 2008).

4. References

Anson B.J, Mc Vay C.B (1971). *Surgical anatomy*, (5th ed.) W. B. Saunder Company, pp. 745-834, ISBN 0721612954, Philadelphia-USA.

Arora A, Caniano AD, Hammond S, Besner GE (2008). Inversion appendectomy acting as a lead point for intussusceptions. *Pediatric Surgery International,* Vol. 24, No. 11, (November 2008), pp. 1261-1264, ISSN 1437-9813.

Atkinson GO, Gay BB, Naffis D (1976). Intussusception of the appendix in children. *American Journal of Roentgenology,* Vol. 126, No. 6 , (June 1976), pp. 1164-1168, ISSN 0361–803X.

Bachman AL., Clemett AR (1971). Roentgen aspects of primary appendiceal intussusception. *Radiology,* Vol. 101, No. 3 , (December 1971), pp. 531–538, ISSN 1527-1315.

Bridger JE (1956). Ileo-colic intussusception after appendicectomy. *British Medical Journal,* Vol. 2, No. 4995, (September 1956), pp. 755, ISSN 0959-8138.

Chaar CI, Waxelman B, Zuckerman K, Longo W (2009). Intussueception of the appendix: a comprehensive review of the literature. *The American Journal of Surgery,* Vol. 198, No.1 , (July 2009), pp. 122-128, ISSN 0002-9610.

Chen YC, Chiang JM (2000). Appendiceal intussusception with adenocarcinoma mimicking a cecal polyp. *Gastrointestinal Endoscopy,* Vol. 52, No. 1, (July 2000), pp. 130-131, ISSN 1097-6779.

Christianakis E, Sakelaropoulos A, Papantzimas C, Pitiakoudis M, Filippou G, Filippou D, Rizos S, Pascalidis N (2008). Pelvic plastron secondary to acute appendicitis in a child presented as appendiceal intussusceptions. A case report. *Cases Journal,* Vol. 1, No. 1 , (September 2008), pp. 135-138 , ISSN 1757-1626.

Collins DC (1963). 71.000 human appendix specimens. A final report, summarizing forty years' study. *American journal of Proctology,* Vol. 14, (December 1963), pp. 265-281, ISSN 0002-9521.

Connor SJ, Hanna GB, Frizelle FA (1998). Appendiceal tumors: retrospective clinicopathologic analysis of appendiceal tumors from 7,970 appendectomies. *Diseases of the Colon and Rectum,* Vol. 41, No. 1, (January 1998), pp. 75-80, ISSN 1530-0358.

de Hoyos A, Monroy MA, Gallegos C, Checa G (2006) . Intussusception of the appendix resected at colonoscopy. *Endoscopy,* Vol. 38, No. 7, (March 2006), pp. 763, ISSN 0013726X.

Dunavant D, Wilson H (1952). Intussusception of the appendix, with complete inversion of the appendix and protrusion from the anus. *Annals of Surgery,* Vol. 135, No. 2, (February 1952), pp.287–288, ISSN 1528-1140.

Duncan JE, DeNobile JW, Sweeney WB (2005). Colonoscopic Diagnosis of Appendiceal Intussusception: Case Report and Review of the Literature. *Journal of the Society of Laparoendoscopic Surgeons,* Vol. 9, No. 4, (October-December 2005), pp. 488-490, ISSN 1086-8089.

Fazio RA, Wickremesinghe PC, Arsura EL, Rando J (1982). Endoscopic removal of an intussuscepted appendix mimicking a polyp-an endoscopic hazard. *American Journal of Gastroenterology,* Vol. 77, No. 8, (August 1982), pp. 556-558, ISSN 1572-0241.

Fernandez-Rey CL, Garcia C, Alvarez Blanco AM (2010). Appendicular mucocele as cause of intestinal intussusception: diagnostic by computer tomography. *Revista Espanola De Enfermedades Digestivas,* Vol. 102, No. 10, (October 2010), pp. 604-605, ISSN 1130-0108.

Fink VH, Al S, Goldberg SL (1964). Intussusception of the appendix. Case reports and reviews of the literature. *American Journal of Gastroenterology,* Vol. 42, (October 1964), pp. 431–4 41, ISSN 0002-9270.

Gilpin D (1989). Intussusception of the appendix. *The Ulster Medical Journal,* Vol. 58, No. 52, (October 1989), pp 193-195, ISSN 0041-6193.

Hanson EL, Goodkin L, Pfeffer RB (1967). Ileocolic intussusception in an adult caused by a granuloma of the appendiceal stump: report of a case. *Annals of Surgery,* Vol. 66, No. 1, (July 1967), pp. 150-152, ISSN 1528-1140.

Hinson FL, Ambrose NS (1998). Pseudomyxoma peritonei. *The British Journal of Surgery,* Vol. 85, No. 10, (October 1998), pp. 1332-1339, ISSN 1365-2168.

Holder PD, Fehir KM, Schwartz MR, Smigocki G, Madewell JE (1989). Primaty mucinous cystadenocarcinoma of the appendix with pseudomyxoma peritonei manifested as a splenic mass. *Southern Medical Journal,* Vol.82, No. 8, (August 1989), pp. 1029-1031, ISSN 1541-8243.

Holt S, Samuel E (1978). Multiple concentric ring sign in the ultrasonographic diagnosis of intussusceptions. *Gastrointestinal Radiology,* Vol. 3, No. 3, (August 1978), pp. 307–309, ISSN 0364-2356.

Jacobs R (1963). Intussusception of the appendix. *Canadian Medical Association Journal,* Vol. 89, (September 1963), pp. 620 -621, ISSN 1488-2329.

Jevon GP, Daya D, Qizilbash AH (1992). Intussusception of the appendix: a report of four cases and review of the literature. *Archives of Pathology & Laboratory Medicine,* Vol. 116, No. 9, (September 1992), pp. 960–964, ISSN 1543-2165.

Khawaja FI (2002). Diseases of the appendix recognized during colonoscopy. *Saudi Journal of Gastroenterology,* Vol. 8, No. 2, (May 2002), pp. 43–52, ISSN 1319-3767.

Kidd J, Jackson R, Wagner CW, Smith SD (2000) Intussusception following the Ladd procedure. *Archives of Surgery,* Vol. 135, No. 6, (June 2000), pp. 713-715, ISSN 0096-6908.

Kim YH, Blake MA, Harisinghani MG et al (2006). Adult intestinal intussusceptions: CT appearances and identification of a causative lead point. *Radiographics,* Vol. 26, No. 3 , (June 2006), pp. 733-744, ISSN 1527-1323.

Kleinman PK (1980). Intussusception of the appendix: hydrostatic reduction. *American Journal of Roentgenology,* Vol. 134, No. 6, (June 1980), pp. 1268-1270, ISSN 1546-3141.

Komine N, Yasunaga C, Nakamoto M, Shima I, Iso Y, Takeda Y, Nakamata T (2004). Intussusception of the appendix that reduced spontaneously during follow-up in a patient on hemodialysis therapy. *Internal Medicine,* Vol. 43, No. 6, (June 2004), pp. 479-483, ISSN 1349-7235.

Koumanidou C, Vakaki M, Theofanopoulou M, Nikas J, Pitsoulakis G, Kakavakis K (2001). Appendiceal and appendiceal-ileocolic intussusception: sonographic and radiographic evaluation. *Pediatric Radiology,* Vol. 31, No. 3, (March 2001), pp. 180-183, ISSN 1432-1998.

Levine MS, Trenkner SW, Herlinger H, et al (1985). Coiled-spring sign of appendiceal intussusception. *Radiology,* Vol. 155, No. 1, (April 1985), pp. 41–44, ISSN 1527-1315.

Lipskar A, Telemb D, Masseauxc J, Midullab P, Dolgina S (2008). Failure of appendectomy to resolve appendiceal intussusception. *Journal of Pediatric Surgery,* Vol. 43, No. 8, (August 2008), pp. 1554-1556, ISSN 1531-5037.

Lu IT, Ko CW, Chang CS, Hou TC (2009). Asymptomatic intussusceptions secondary to a giant appendiceal mucocele treated via a laparoscopic approach. *Gastrointestinal Endoscopy,* Vol. 70, No. 5 (Novenber 2009), pp. 1026-1027, ISSN 1097-6779.

Luzier J, Verhey P, Dobos N (2006). Preoperative CT diagnosis of appendiceal intussusception. *American Journal of Roentgenology,* Vol. 187, No. 3, (September 2006), pp. 325-326, ISSN 1546-3141.

Marinis A, Yiallourou A, Samanides L, Dafnios N, Anastasopoulos G, Vassiliou I, Theodosopoulos T (2009). Intussusception of the bowel in adults: A review. *World Journal of Gastroenterology,* Vol.15, No.4, (January 2009), pp. 407-411, ISSN 1007-9327.

McKidd J (1858). Case of invagination of caecum and appendix. *Edinburgh Medical Journal,* Vol. 4, pp.793–797, ISSN 0367-1038.

Minter R, Doherty G (2010). Appendectomy, Colectomy. In: *Current procedures: Surgery,* (1st ed), Mc Graw Hill, pp. 156-160 & 180-191, ISBN 978-0-07-145316-5, USA.

Nycum LR, Moss H, Adams JQ, Macri CI (1999). Asymptomatic intussusceptions of the appendix due to endometriosis. *Southern Medical Journal,* Vol. 92, No. 5, (May 1999), pp. 524-525, ISSN 1541-8243.

Okuda I, Matsuda M, Noguchi H, Kokubo T, (2008). Massive mucinous cystadenoma of the appendix with intussusception in an adult: usefulness of reconstructed computed tomography images. *Radiation Medicine,* Vol. 26, No. 2, (February 2008), pp. 88-91, ISSN 0288-2043.

Ozuner C, Davidson P, Church J (2000). Intussusception of the vermiform appendix: preoperative colonoscopic diagnosis of two cases and review of the literature. *International Journal of Colorectal Disease,* Vol. 15, No. 3 , (June 2000), pp. 185-187, ISSN 1432-1262.

Patton KR, Ferrera PC (2000). Intussusception of a normal appendix. *American Journal of Emergency Medicine,* Vol. 18, No. 1, (January 2000), pp. 115-117, ISSN 0735-6757.

Poddoubnyi IV, Dronov AF, Blinnikov OI, Smirnov AN, Darenkov IA, Dedov KA(1998). Laparoscopy in the treatment of intussusceptions in children. *Journal of Pediatric Surgery,* Vol. 33, No. 8, (August 1998), pp. 1194-1197, ISSN 1531-5037.

Pumberger W, Hormann M, Pomberger G, Hallwirth U (2000). Sonographic diagnosis of intussusception of the appendix vermiformis. *Journal of Clinical Ultrasound,* Vol. 28, No. 9, (November-December 2000), pp. 492- , ISSN 1097-0096.

Rutledge RH, Alexander JW (1992). Primary appendiceal malignancies: rare but important. *Surgery,* Vol. 111, No. 3, (March 1992), pp. 244-250, ISSN 1816-3211.

Ryu BY, Kim TH, Jeon JY, Kim HK, Choi YH, Baik GH (2005). Colonoscopic Diagnosis of Appendiceal Intussusception: A Case Report. *Journal of Korean Medical Science,* Vol. 20, No.4, (August 2005),pp.680-682, ISSN 1011-8934.

Salehzadeh A, Scala A, Simson JNL (2010).Appendiceal intussusceptions mistaken for a polyp at colonoscopy: case report and review of the literature. *Annals of Royal College of Surgeons England,* Vol.92, No.6 , (September 2010), pp. 46-48, ISSN 1478-7083.

Sbarounis C (1991). Diseases of the vermiform appendix. In: *General Surgery,* (1st ed.), University studio press, pp. 874-885, ISBN: 960-12-0303-6, Thessaloniki-Greece.

Schier F (1997). Experience with laparoscopy in the treatment of intussusceptions. *Journal of Pediatric Surgery,* Vol. 32, No. 12, (December 1997), pp. 1713-1714 , ISSN 1531-5037.

Schumpelick V, Dreuw B, Ophoff K, Prescher A (2000). Appendix and cecum. Embryology, anatomy and surgical applications. *The Surgical Clinics of North America*, Vol. 80, No. 1, (February 2000), pp. 295-318, ISSN 0039-6109.

Seddik H, Rabhi M (2011). Two cases of appendiceal intussusception : a rare diagnostic pitfall in colonoscopy. *Diagnostic and Theraupetic Endoscopy*; 2011:198984. Epub 2011 Apr 12, ISSN 1070-3608.

Snell S.R (2008). The Abdomen: Part II-The Abdominal Cavity In: *Clinical anatomy by regions*, (8th ed.), Lippincott Williams & Wilkins, pp. 230-232, ISBN-13: 978-0-7817-6404-9, ISBN-10: 0-7817-6404-1, Philadelphia/Baltimore-USA.

Taban S, Dema A, Lazar D, Sporea I, Lazar E, Cornianu M (2006). An unusual "tumor" of the cecum: the inverted appendiceal stump. *Romanian Journal of Morphology and Embryology*, Vol. 47, No. 2, (September 2006), pp. 193-196, ISSN 1220-0522.

Tavakkoli H, Sadrkabir SM, Mahzouni P (2007). Colonoscopic diagnosis of appendiceal intussusceptions in a patient with intermittent abdominal pain: a case report. *World Journal of Gastroenterology*, Vol. 13, No. 31, (August 2007), pp. 4274-4277, ISSN 1007-9327.

Tseng PH, Lee YC, Chiu HM, Wu MS, Lin JT, Wang HP (2006). Appendiceal intussusception diagnosed with endoscopic sonography. *Journal of Clinical Ultrasound*, Vol. 34, No. 7, (September 2006), pp. 348-351, ISSN 1097-0096.

Varsamis N, Theodosiou A, Voulalas G, Papadopoulou H, Pakataridis A, Manafis K, Christodoulidis K(2010). Caecocolic Intussusception Involving Calcified Mucocele of the Appendix. *Hellenic Journal of Surgery*, Vol. 82, No. 2, (July - August 2010), pp. 252-256, ISSN 0018 - 0092.

Vogelaar FJ, Molenaar IQ, Adhin S, Steenvoorde P (2004).Invagination of the appendix: Diagnostic laparoscopy? *Digestive Diseases and Sciences*, Vol. 49, No. 2, (February 2004), pp. 351-352, ISSN 1573-2568.

Wang SM, Huang FC, Wu CH, Ko SF, Lee SY, Hsiao CC (2010). Ileocecal Burkit's Lymphoma presenting as ileocolic intussusceptions with appendiceal invagination and acute appendicitis. *Journal of the Formosan Medical Association*, Vol. 109, No. 6, (June 2010), pp. 476-479, ISSN 0929-6646.

Wirtschafter SK, Kaufman H (1976). Endoscopic appendectomy. *Gastrointestinal Endoscopy*, Vol. 22, No. 3, (February 1976), pp. 173–174, ISSN 1097-6779.

Wolff BC, Boller AM (2008). Large bowel obstruction. In:. *Current surgical therapy*, (9th ed.), Cameron JL , Mosby Elsevier, pp. 189-192, ISBN 978-1-4160-3497-1, Philadelphia-USA.

Yeager GH (1947). The appendiceal stump. *Annals of Surgery*, Vol.126, No. 5, (November 1947), pp. 814-819, ISSN 1528-1140.

Part 2

Diarrhoea

4

Management of Secretory Diarrhea

Claudia Velázquez[1], Fernando Calzada[2],
Mirandeli Bautista[1] and Juan A. Gayosso[1]
[1]*Universidad Autónoma del Estado de Hidalgo*
[2]*Edificio CORCE 2° piso, CMN S XXI, IMSS*
México

1. Introduction

"Diarrhea is the passage of 3 or more loose or liquid stool per day, or more frequently than is normal for the individual. It is usually a symptom of gastrointestinal infection, which can be caused by a variety of bacterial, viral and parasitic organisms, infection is spread through contaminated food or drinking-water, or from person to person as a result of poor hygiene" (WHO). Diarrheal diseases affect all races, sexes, ages and geographic areas, has high impact on mortality and morbidity worldwide, an estimated 2-4 billion episodes of infectious diarrhea occurred each year and are especially prevalent in infants (Hodges and Gill 2010; Farthing 2002). In 2005, 1.8 million people died worldwide from diarrheal diseases (WHO, 2007). In México, in the past 6 years, the gastrointestinal infection has been a serious health problem and was the second cause of morbidity among all age groups (SS, 2008).

2. Pathophysiology classification of diarrhea

- Osmotic; is caused by poorly absorbable solutes (eg. sorbitol, magnesium salts) remaining in the gastrointestinal lumen retain water and electrolytes resulting in reduced water reabsorption
- Altered Motility; caused slowing of the motor function of the small intestine as with narcotic use, scleroderma, diabetic autonomic neuropathy and amyloidosis
- Exudative; the intestinal epithelium's barrier function is compromised by loss of epithelial cells or disruption of tight junctions (eg. *E. coli, Salmonella, Shigella, Yersinia, Campilobacter, Mycobacteryum tuberculosis, Clostridium difficile y Entamoeba histolytica*), inflammatory disease process as in ulcerative colitis and Crohn's disease
- Secretory; is caused by an increase in water and electrolytes (Chloride or bicarbonate) movements to the intestinal lumen, the final effect is the increase of secretion and decrease of absorption of net sodium and water (Navaneethan and Giannella, 2010).

2.1 Secretory diarrhea

Secretory diarrhea occurs when the balance between absorption and secretion in the small intestine is disturbed by excessive secretion caused by bacterial enterotoxins, is a net movement from mucous intestinal to lumen, the volume exceed 10 mL/Kg/day, and the osmolarity is similar with plasma. It is the leading cause of death in infants in developing countries and currently accounts for an estimated of three million deaths each year among under 5 years old children (Casburne-Jones and Farthing, 2004; Filbin 2004). Most causes of secretory diarrhea alter the second messenger system through alteration in cAMP, cGMP or intracellular calcium regulated ion transport pathways, alterations in these mediators cause CFTR-mediated Cl^- secretion an inhibition of small intestinal-coupled Na^+-Cl^- transport (Navaneethan and Giannella, 2010)

2.1.1 Secretory diarrhea noninfectious

Some of these include

- Tumors (pancreatic islet, which secrete vasoactive intestinal peptide (VIP), carcinoid which elaborate serotonin, bradykinin, substance P and prostaglandins, medullary carcinoma of thyroid-secreting calcitonin)
- Neurotransmitters are also potent secretory stimuli, such as histamine in systemic mastocytosis and inflammatory cytokines
- Malabsorbed bile salts and fatty acids (hydroxyl fatty acids also stimulate colonic secretion)
- The congenital absence or alterations in the numerous transporters that maintain the constant flux of the ions and water
- Rare congenital syndromes: congenital chloridorrhea, there is a defect in brush border Cl^-/HCO_3^- exchange in the ileum and the colon and hence impaired absorption of chloride, congenital sodium diarrhea results from a congenital defect in Na^+-bile acid absorption in the colon (Navaneethan and Giannella, 2010; Filbin 2004)

2.1.2 Secretory diarrhea caused by pathogens

Microbial causes include rotavirus, norovirus, *Cryptosporidium*, its affects the absorptive villi inhibiting sodium absorption. Enterotoxigenic *E. coli* (ETEC), *V. cholera* elaborate enterotoxins that stimulate intestinal chloride secretion along with impaired sodium absorption, *Giardia lambia* adhere to the mucosa disrupting the absorptive/secretary process of enterocyte producing active secretion (Navaneethan and Giannella, 2010)

2.1.2.1 Enterotoxigenic bacteria

- *Vibrio cholerae*
- *Enterotoxigenic Escherichia coli*
- *Clostridium perfringes*
- *C. botulinum*
- *Campylobacter jejuni*
- *Klepsiella pneumoniae*
- *Aeromonas hydrophila*
- *Yersinia enterocolitic*

2.1.2.2 Enteroinvasive bacteria

- *Enteroinvasive Escherichia coli*
- *Salmonella typhi*
- *S. enteritidis*
- *Shigella spp*

- *Campylobacter jejuni*
- *Plesiomonas shigeloids*
- *Yersinia enterocolitic*
- *Vibrio parahaemolyticus*

2.1.2.3 Viruses

- *Group A rotaviruses, G1 and G serotypes*
- *Norovirus (old term of Nolwalk virus)*
- *Parvoviruses (Hawai, Colorado, Ditchilling*
- *Enteric adenoviruses 40 and 41*
- *Coronaviruses*
- *Calciviruses*
- *Astroviruses*

2.1.2.4 Parasites

- *Gardia lamblia*
- *Entamoeba histolityca*
- *Cryptosporidium parvum*
- *Isospore belli*
- *Sarcosystis sp*
- *Cyclospore cayetanensis*
- *Blastocystis hominis*
- *Microsporidie*

2.2 Diarrhea caused by enterotoxins

A number of several bacteria cause diarrhea by the production of potent enterotoxins, such as enterotoxigenic Escherichia coli, Salmonella typhi, S. typhimurium, clostridium difficile, C. freundii, Aeromonas hydrophila, Yersinia enterocolic, Camphylobacter jejuni and Vibrio cholera. Enterotoxins have their effect on the enterocyte functions by stimulating the secretion of transepitelial electrolytes, increasing the osmotic flux of water and ions to the intestinal lumen, specifically, heat-labile (LT) and heat stable (ST) enterotoxins from E. coli, V. cholera and C. jejuni increase net fluid secretion by affecting the enzymes adenylate cyclase or guanilate cyclase by activation of the cAMP (cyclic 3',5'-adenosine monophosphate) in the mucosal epithelium which induces an increase of intestinal secretion and causes diarrhea.(Casburn-Jones and Farthing 2004, Amstrong and Cohen, 1999).

2.2.1 *Vibrio cholerae* enterotoxin

Vibrio cholerae enterotoxin is an oligomeric protein which is composed by two subunits, A subunit of 27.2 KDa composed as A1 and A2 subunits, and B subunit composed by five subunits B of 11.6 KDa each one, AB_5 complex Fig 1. (Sixma, 1991)

2.2.2 *Vibrio cholerae* enterotoxin mechanism

Mechanisms proposed to secretory diarrhea caused by *V. cholera* enterotoxin involves the union of subunits B to the oligosaccharide portion of the receptor GM1, present in the apical surface of enterocytes, this union lend the entrance of A subunit of toxin to the enterocyte for acidic endosomes, which pick up the golgi apparatus and endoplasmic reticulum,

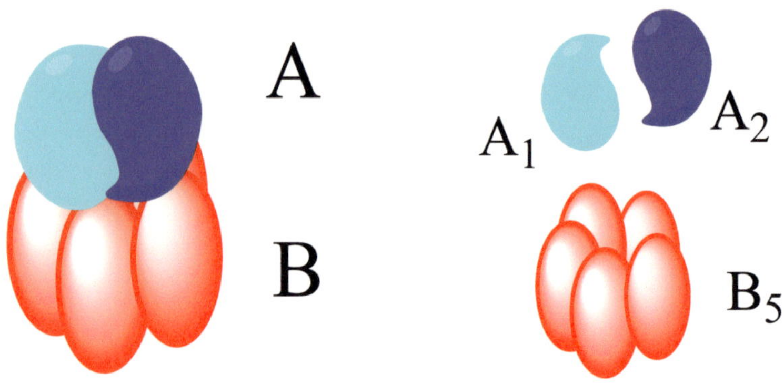

Fig. 1. *Vibrio cholerae* enterotoxin AB_5 complex

inside of enterocyte disulphure bond between A1-A2 is dissolved by protein disulfide isomerase, it causes release of A1 which is capable of binding NAD and catalyzing the NADP-ribosylation of $G_{s\alpha}$, a GTP-binding regulatory protein associated with adenylate cyclase. A1 subunit stimulates increasing of 1000 times production of cAMP second messenger, cAMP active protein cinase A, which phosphorile and activate transmembranal chloride channels of the enterocytes located on intestinal crypts, it causes massive secretion of water and electrolytes to intestinal lumen, in villus cell there is a decrease of absorption of Na^+ and Cl^- ions (Kopic 2010). Fig 2. shows the proposed mechanism to the action of *Vibrio Cholerae* enterotoxin. At 5 to 10 minutes to the exposure of V. cholera toxin cause intestinal hypersecretion of water and electrolytes for several hours (Thiagarajah, 2005; Spangler, 1992). The symptoms are manifested as severe cramp and the copious "rice water" diarrhea characteristic of the disease.

2.3 Dehydration

During diarrhea there is an increased loss of water and electrolytes (sodium, chloride, potassium and bicarbonate) in the liquid stool; dehydration occurs when these losses are not replaced adequately and a deficit of water and electrolytes develops. The degree of dehydration is graded according to signs and symptoms that reflect the amount of fluid lost:

- In the early stages of dehydration, there are no signs or symptoms
- As dehydration increases, signs and symptoms develop. Initially these include: thirst, restless or irritable behavior, decreased skin turgor, sunken eyes, and sunken fontanel (in infants).
- In severe dehydration, these effects become more pronounced and the patient may develop evidence of hypovolemic shock, including: diminished consciousness, lack of urine output, cool moist extremities, a rapid feeble pulse, low or undetectable blood pressure, and peripheral cyanosis.
- Death follows soon if rehydration is not started quickly (WHO, 2005).

2.4 Secretory diarrhea treatment

2.4.1 Oral rehydration

To control diarrhea disease, a sufficient hydration of the patient should be procure and provide the necessary ions to maintain electrolyte balance, the treatment of choice is oral

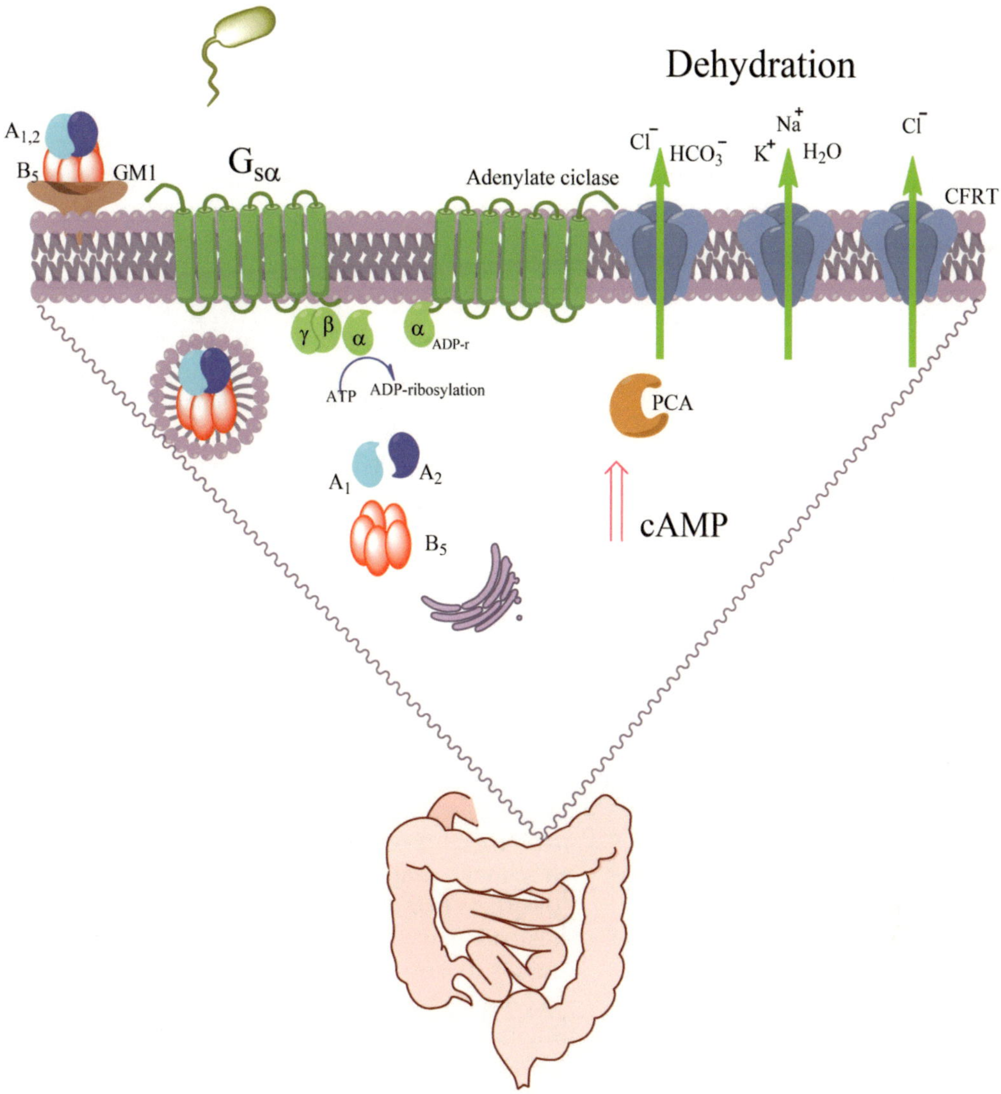

Fig. 2. Cholera toxin mechanism proposed by Velázquez et al., $A_{1,2}$ B_5 (subunits), GM1 (ganglioside receptor) , Gsα (G protein), cAMP (cyclic AMP), CFTR (cystic fibrosis transmembrane conductance regulator).

rehydration solution (ORS), it has reduced the levels of mortality in children and elderly by dehydration, but not morbidity (Turvill et al., 2000), the treatment is based by active absorption of glucose by smooth intestine, during the intestinal infection lend to the co-transport of Na^+ ions and water absorption. WHO and UNICEF guidelines recommend their use, is important to notice that ORS, is useful to treat dehydration caused by diarrhea, but it not decrease the amount and duration at the same. Depends of severity of diarrhea, in some cases ORS is not enough and antibiotic, spasmolytic, and antiprotozoal drugs should be used. WHO recommended use of secure and effective drugs to the pediatrics (Marion et al., 2010).

2.4.2 Drugs used to treat secretory diarrhea

To treat the secretory diarrhea there are some drugs which reduce the intestinal movement such as codeine (**1**), loperamide (**2**), diphenoxylate (**3**), lidamidine (**4**), bismuth subsalicylate (**5**), racecadotril (**6**) and clonidine (**7**) Table 1.; which are capable to stimulate absorption direct and reduce secretion of water and electrolytes in gastrointestinal tract, to decrease propulsion, contact time of intestinal content with mucosal surface increase, it favors the absorption. They act not premised release of prostaglandins too (Marion et al., 2010; Martindale 2009).

Structure	Effect
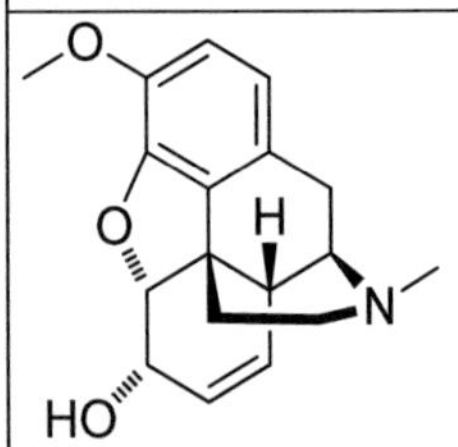 Codeine (**1**)	Has a high antidiarrheal action but, produces secondary effects such as nauseas, dizziness and acts against central nervous system, it can be used carefully in children, continuous use can induce physical dependence and addiction
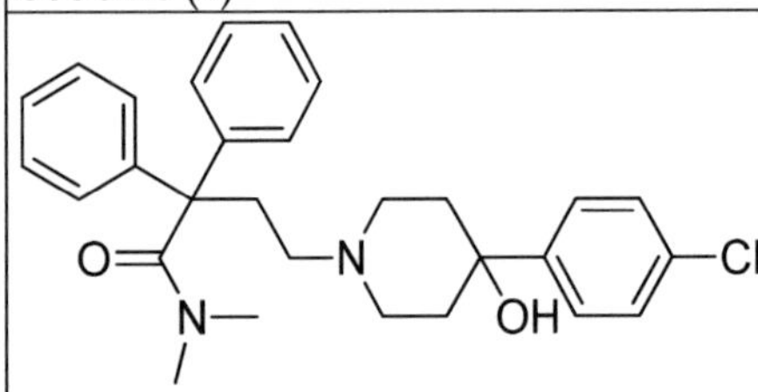 Loperamide (**2**)	Decrease intestinal motility and present antisecretory effect by activation of calmodulin, increase the water and electrolytes absorption to the intestinal lumen. It should not be administrated to children under six years old, patients with constipation, atony or intestinal obstruction, should avoid its use on bacterial infective severe and in acute dysentery. Frequent adverse reactions induced are hypersensibility reactions (cutaneous eruption), gastrointestinal disorders (constipation, colic, abdominal distention, nauseas and vomit), fiver and dry mouth, is a non-prescription drug for children because can cause CNS depression
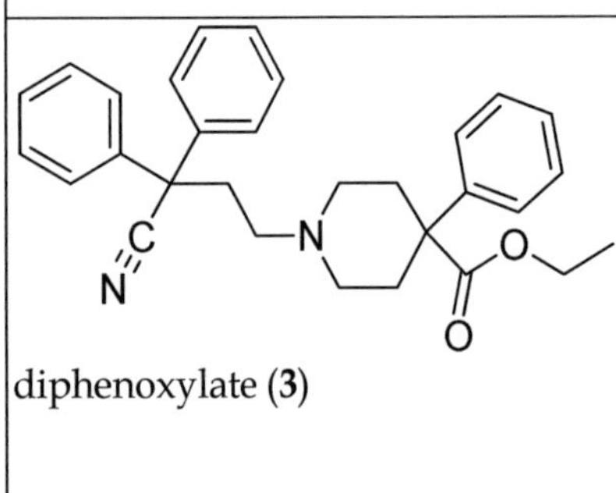 diphenoxylate (**3**)	Inhibits intestinal propulsion and fecal excretion velocity, cause decrease of intestinal transit, to therapeutic doses it induces adverse reactions in central nervous system (confusion, sedation, depletion, cephalea), allergic reactions (anaphylaxis, prurite) on gastrointestinal apparatus (toxic megacolon, paralytic ileum, vomit, nauseas and abdominal pain) It can cause euphoria and has analgesic effect. Difenoxilate is contraindicated in children younger than 2 years old.
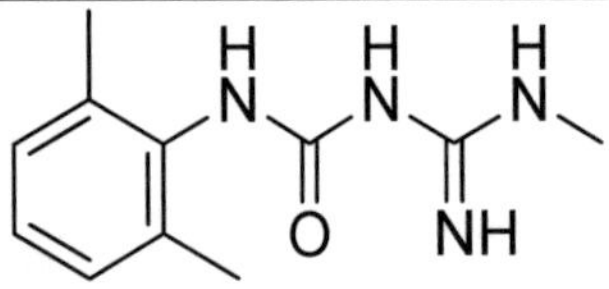 Lidamidine (**4**)	Improve the absorption of water and electrolytes in intestinal velocities and reverse their secretion to level on intestinal crypts.

Structure	Effect
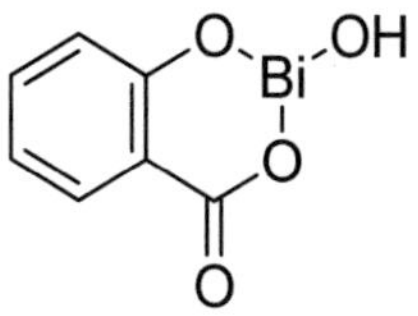 Bismuth subsalicylate (**5**)	Showed antisecretor effect for the inhibition of prostaglandins, reduce depositions number and reduce abdominal pain, causes adverse reactions (dizziness, cephalea, constipation, dark stools, ataxia, tremor, encephalopathy, confusion, delirium and convulsions).
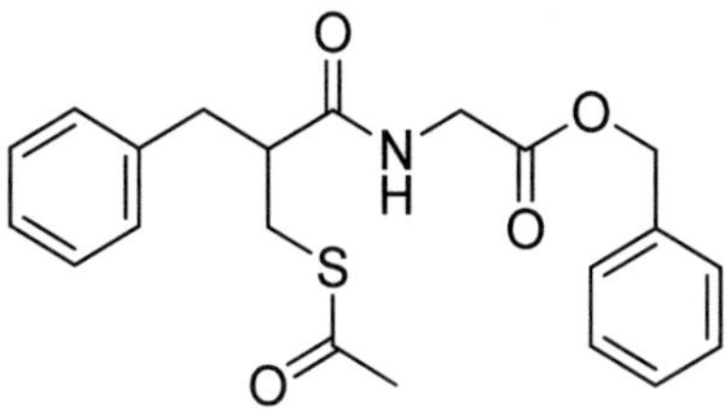 Racecadotril (**6**)	Decrease intestinal hipersecretion of water and electrolytes to intestinal lumen, inhibits release of encephalinse endogenus witch act on opiaceus receptors γ decreasing cAMP level (decrease water and electrolytes secretion), cause some adverse reactions such as hypokalemia, bronchospasm, fever, vomit and otitis.
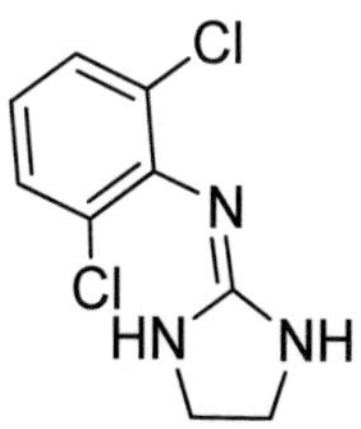 Clonidine (**7**)	Stimulates sodium and chloride absorption and inhibits chloride secretion by interaction with its receptor on enterocyte, causes an alteration of gut motility with effect on intestinal transport, it causes hypotension

Table 1. Drugs used to treat secretory diarrhea

On the other hand, there are some compounds that showed inhibitory properties on the intestinal secretion Fig 3. such as berberine (**8**), chlorpromazine (**9**), nicotinic acid (**10**), indomethacin (**11**), somatostatin (**12**) and ethacrinic acid (**13**) but they were not developed as antidiarrhoeal drugs (Fedorack and Field, 1987). Thus, the research for new antisecretory agents that should be effective and safe to treat diarrhea is still a necessary goal.

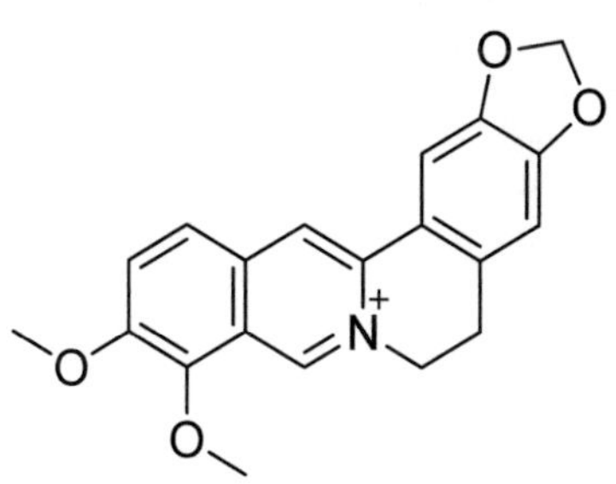

berberine 8

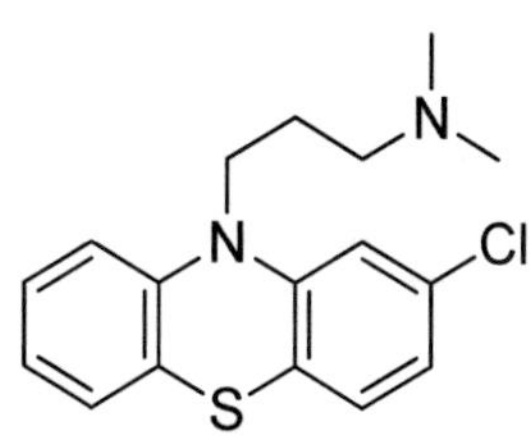

chlorpromazine 9

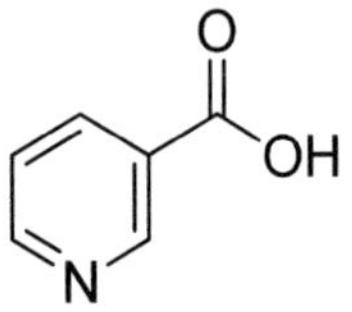

nicotinic acid **10**

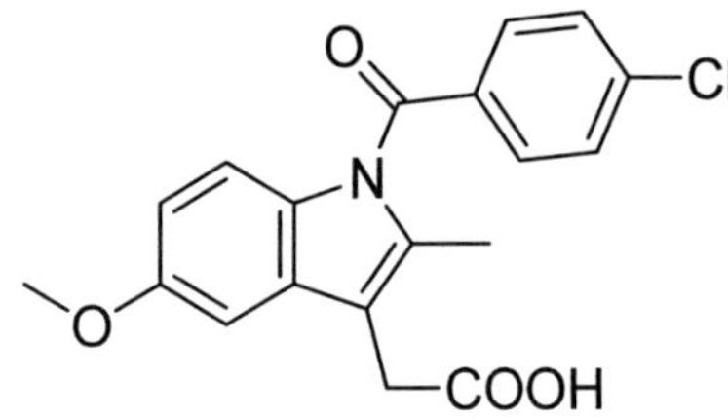

Indomethacin **11**

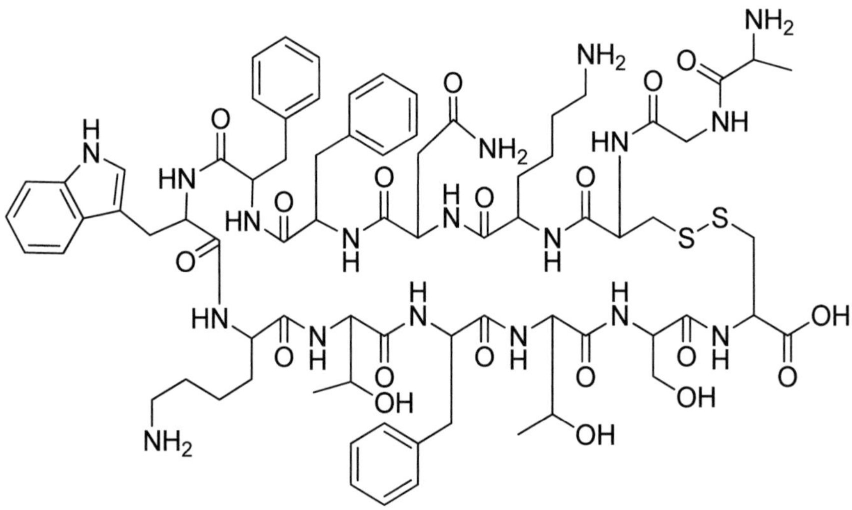

somatostatin 12

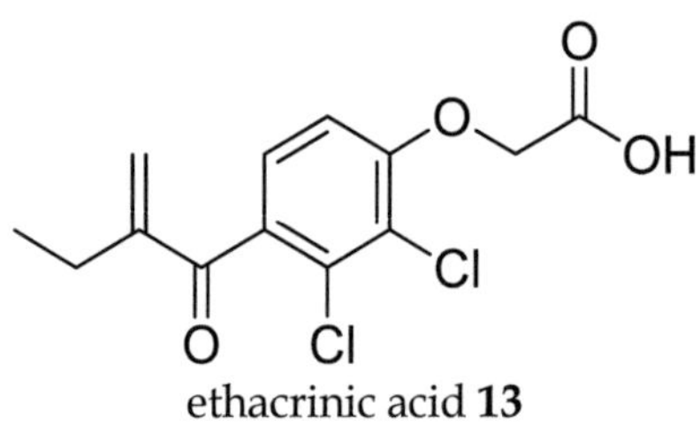

ethacrinic acid **13**

Fig. 3. Compounds with inhibitory properties on the intestinal secretion

2.4.3 Potential target areas to design therapeutic agents on *Vibrio cholerae* toxin

During the last two decades there has been a continuous research of drugs that inhibit the secretory process in the enterocyte to help to the control of diarrhea, but only a few candidates have emerged, and none has found a place in the routine management of secretory diarrhea. Particularly to cholera toxin its mechanism of action revel several potential target areas to design therapeutic agents such as:

a. The inhibition of adenylate cyclase
b. The blockage of the active site of the enzyme located in the A subunit
c. The disruption of the assembly of the holotoxin by interrupting the A_2-B interaction
d. The interception of the receptor binding to the bottom of the B pentamer (Guangtao Z., 2009).

e. Inhibitors of enkephalinase and of the cystic fibrosis transmembrane conductance regulator (Thiagarajah, 2005).
f. Inhibition of transport proteins involved in cAMP activated chloride secretion

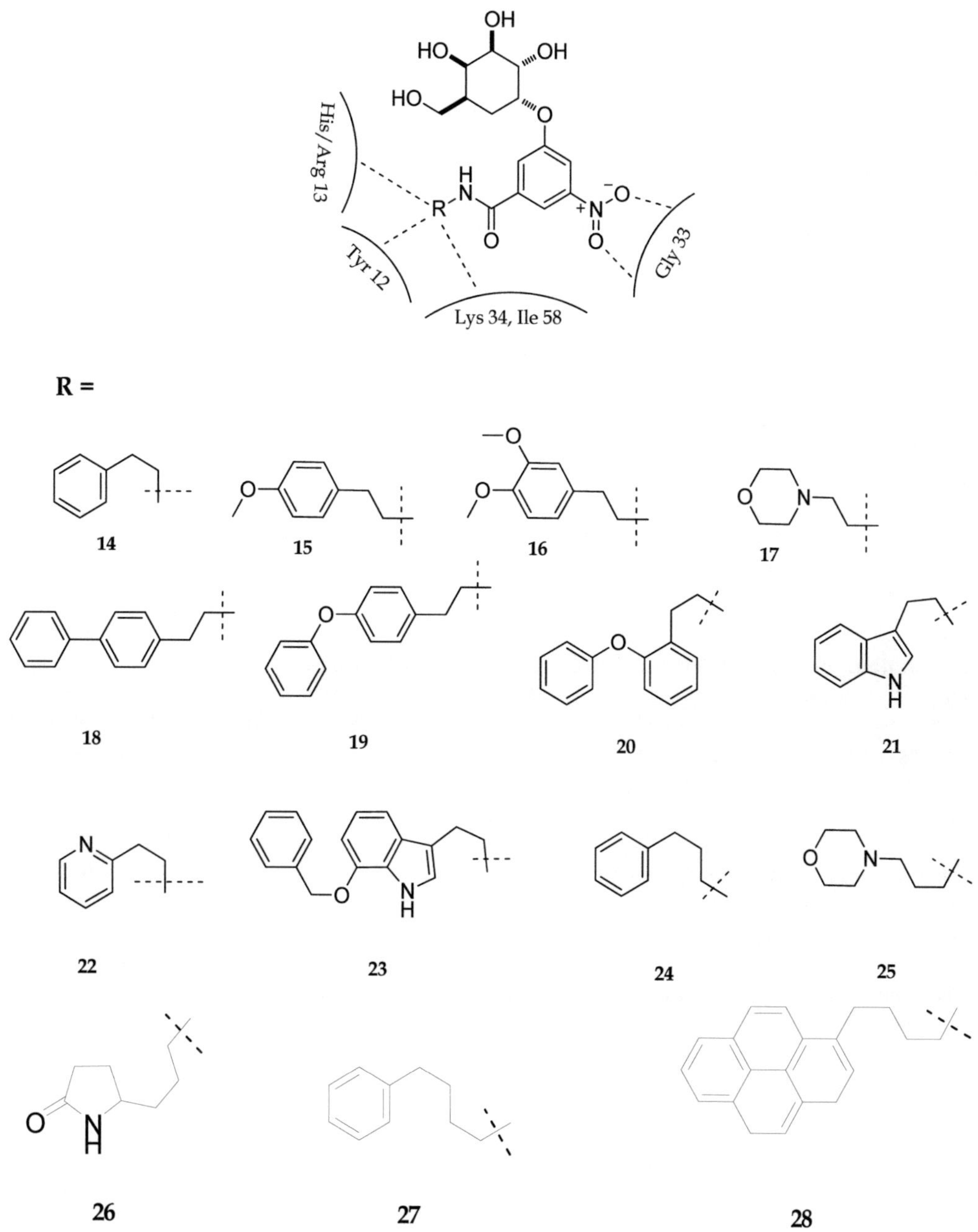

Fig. 4. Synergism of structure-based drug design with combinatorial chemistry for the design of receptor antagonist of cholera toxin
http://www.bmsc.washington.edu/WimHol/figures/figs2/WimFigs2.html

2.5 Medicinal plants as a source of antidiarrheal compounds

Diarrheal diseases are a health problem because affect a large number of the population mainly children and elderly. In México the use of medicinal plants to treat gastrointestinal disorders including diarrhea occupied the first place, there are few pharmacological and chemical studies which support their use. Approximately 80% of the world's population uses medicinal plants to treat immediately health problems, is clear the importance of multidisciplinary research of our natural sources. The study of medicinal plants with the propose to provide pharmacological evidence that may explain its therapeutic use

There are some *in vitro* models such as isolated ileum of guinea pig, isolated jejune of rabbit, ileum and duodenum isolated of rat or rabbit and *in vivo* reduction of intestinal motility using charcoal meal, Castor oil, PGE_2, $MgSO_4$ induced diarrhea, and Enteropooling models. Antispasmodic activity has been demonstrate for some flavonoids such as quercetin, quercitrin, genistein, sakuranetin, rutin and bisabolol; terpenoids such as himachalol, coleonol, β-damascenone, ε-fitol, capsidiol, β-eudemol, hinesol, huatriwaico acid, camaldulin and tymol; essential oils such as, 1,8-cineol, eugeol, timol, carvacrol, estragolanetol, α y β pinenes, nonanal, and linalool; alkaloids such as himbacine, protopine, coptisine, cantleyine, mitraginine, vertine, retuline, cavidine and metuenine (Astudillo et al., 2009).

There are a great number of natural remedies for diarrhea control, historically *Papaver somniferum* preparations are efficient and powerful against diarrhea, as the derivative codeine, alkaloids are ones of major substances explored form natural products and they give to pharmaceutical industry a big number of patents, another class of compound explored therapeutically are flavonoids and has been used as complement in treatment of cancer, heart diseases, venous insufficiency, venous ulcers, hemorrhoids and diarrhea. (Martindale 2009)

2.5.1 Antisecretory compounds isolated from medicinal plants

Some studies have been performed in order to find antisecretory compounds from several plants used in traditional medicine to treat several kinds of diarrheas. In this sense the extracts from *Croton urucurana, C. lechleri, Berberis aristata* and *Guazuma ulmifolia* were studied against intestinal secretion caused by *V. cholera* toxin, in the cases of *C. lechleri, B. aristata* and *G. ulmifolia* the isolated compounds were oligomeric proantocyanidins and berberine, respectively. From *C. urucurana* saponins, steroids, alkaloids, antocianidins and catechins have been isolated. Prontocianidins and catechins probably can be associated with their antisecretory activity.

Steviol (**29**) and dihydroisosteviol (**30**) can inhibit cAMP-activated chloride secretion in human's intestine cells by targeting CFTR (Pariwat 2008). Penta-*m*-digalloyl-glucose (PDG) (**31**) isolated of Chinese gallnuts showed efficacy in reducing enterotoxin-induced intestinal fluid secretion in mice (Wongsamitkul et al., 2010)

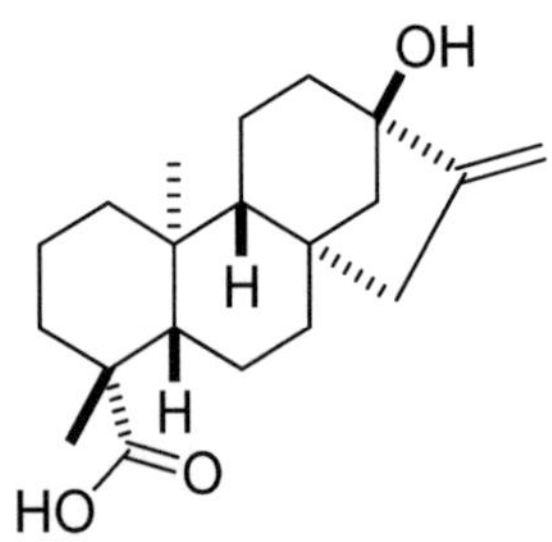

Steviol **29**

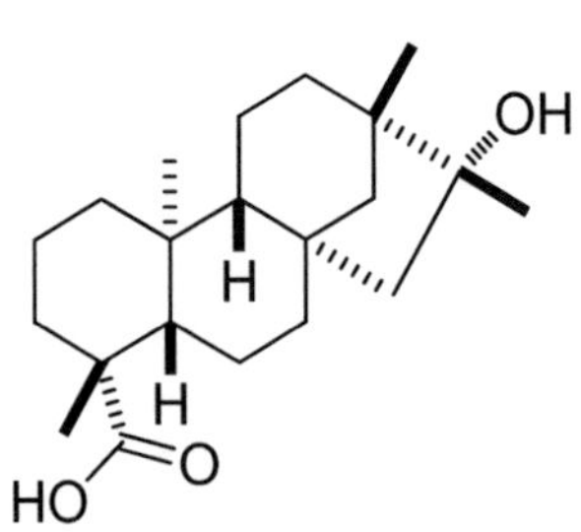

dihydroisosteviol **30**

Crofelemer (**32**) is a proanthocyanidin oligomer obtained from *Croton lechleri* (dragon's blood), the sap has been used to treat diarrheas including dysentery and cholera, pharmacological studies have shown that it reduces fluid secretion in cell culture and mouse models (Gabriel et al., 1999), it has been reported that the antisecretory mechanism of action of crofelemer involves dual inhibition of The cystic fibrosis transmembrane regulator conductance (CFTR), a cAMP stimulated Cl- channel, and calcium-activated Cl- channels (CaCC) at the luminal membrane of enterocytes (preliminary studies showed that crofelemer (**32**) may reduce watery stool output in patients with infectious diarrhea such as cholera. But it needs further Phase 3 clinical trials are still necessaries (Crutchley et al., 2010).

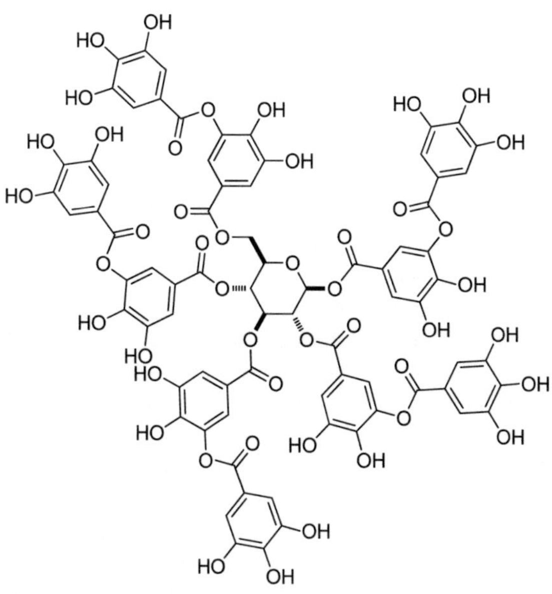

Penta-*m*-digalloyl-glucose (PDG) (**31**)

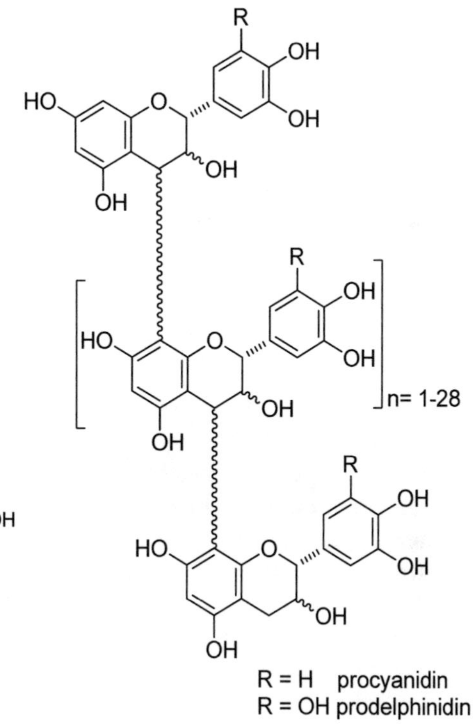

Crofelemer (**32**)

We continue with the research of compounds with antisecretory activity useful to treat diarrhea. Medicinal plants used in Mexican traditional medicine to treat gastrointestinal disorders could be a source of compounds with therapeutic utility. In México, the use of medicinal plants to treat gastrointestinal disorders such as diarrhea and dysentery is widespread (Aguilar et al., 1994). However most of these plants have not been investigated from a pharmacological point of view to demonstrate their antisecretory properties, which could lead to support their use as antidiarrheal and anti-dysenteric drug in traditional medicine. We screened aqueous and methanol extracts from 26 Mexican medicinal plants to assess their antisecretory activity using the cholera toxin-induced intestinal secretion in rat jejunal loops model. None of this species or their isolated compounds has been previously evaluated as antisecretory agents (Velázquez et al., 2006).

2.5.2 Material and methods

2.5.2.1 Plant materials

The plants used in that study were collected from different regions in Mexico: Mexico City, States of Hidalgo, Mexico, Sinaloa, Guanajuato and Yucatan, all of them were selected according to their use in Mexican traditional medicine to treat gastrointestinal disorders. Voucher herbarium specimens were deposited in Herbarium IMSSM of Instituto Mexicano del Seguro Social and were authenticated by MS Abigail Aguilar.

2.5.2.2 Preparation of crude extracts

The air-dried plant material (20g) was extracted by maceration with 300 mL of MeOH for 1 week. Then the macerate was filtered and concentrated under reduced pressure at 40°C. For aqueous extracts, 20 g of air-dried plant material were extracted by decoction with 100 mL of distilled water for 30 min, the solution was filtered and lyophilized.

2.5.2.3 Cholera toxin

Lyophilized powder (1mg) of Cholera toxin (SIGMA) containing approximately 220,000 units/mg of protein was suspended in 1 mL of sterile water. Aliquots of the toxin solution were dissolved in a 1x PBS (NaCl 8g, KCl 0.2 g, Na2HPO4.7H2O o.115 g, KH2PO4 0.2 g/L) solution with 1% bovine serum albumin (SIGMA) to obtain a concentration of 3 μg/mL.

2.5.2.4 Antisecretory assay

The antisecretory activity of the extracts was tested using a method described by Torres et al., in 1993. Briefly, male Sprague-Dawley rats (200-250 g) were obtained from the animal house of the IMSS. The experimental protocols were in accordance with the official Mexican norm NOM 0062-ZOO-1999 entitled technical specifications for the production, care and use of laboratory animals (SAGARPA 2001). The antisecretory effect of the extract was studied on intestinal secretion indirectly by measuring the fluid accumulation in the intestine following cholera toxin administration to rats. Two jejuna loops were prepared in the rats and inoculated with 3 μg/mL of cholera toxin dissolved in 1x PBS with 1 % bovine albumin. Rats (*n*=4 per group by duplicated) were treated orally with each extract (300 mg/Kg in 1 mL of a 2 % DMSO solution in water). Loperamide (10 mg/Kg) was used as antidiarrhoeal drug. After 4 h, the animals were sacrificed using ethyl ether. The antisecretory activity of the extracts was measured as the fluid accumulation in the loops and expressed in percentage of inhibition. Values are expressed as mean ± SEM. Statistical significance was determinate using Mann-Whitney U-test. Values with $p<0.05$ were considered significant.

2.5.2.5 Results

We tested 56 aqueous and methanol crude extracts obtained from 26 medicinal plants used in Mexican traditional medicine for the treatment of gastrointestinal disorders. The antisecretory activity was tested using the cholera toxin-induced intestinal secretion in rat jejunal loops model. Only the principal antisecretory activity of the extracts tested is shown in Table 2, the full list is showed in Velázquez et al., 2006.

In traditional medicine since infusions or decoctions are usually taken three times per day when diarrhea occurs, our results can be related with their traditional use because the used dose is approximately one cup of plant tea which is recommended by Mexican people to treat gastrointestinal disorders (Aguilar et al., 1994).We found that both extracts from *Chiranthodendron pentadactylon, Hippocratea excelsa* and *Ocimum basilicum* were the most active with inhibition values ranging from 68.0 to 87.6% at 300 mg/kg. Methanol extract of *Geranium mexicanum* (aerial parts) and the aqueous extract of *Bocconia frutescens* were active too with inhibition values of 93.4 and 86.0%, respectively. On the other hand, the methanol extract of *Chenopodium ambrosioides* green variety (aerial parts), *Lygodium venustum, Punica granatum* and *Ruta chalepensis,* the aqueous extracts of *Aloysia triphylla, Chenopodium ambrosioides* green variety (aerial parts), *Dorstenia contrajerva* and *Schinus molle* shown inhibitory activity with values ranging from 43.4 to 79.5%. The 87% of the extracts tested showed inhibitory activity of the intestinal secretion; only seven extracts did not show any antisecretory activity. In general, among the researched extracts, the methanol extracts exhibited the highest antisecretory activity.

Family	Plant specie	Part used	Voucher number	Extract	% Inhibition
Verbenaceae	*Aloysia triphylla* (L'Hér) Britton	AP	126110	Methanol Aqueous	7.8± 4.7 80.4±22.8
Papaveraceae	*Bocconia frutescens*L.	AP	12618	Methanol Aqueous	24.1±15.4 86.0± 9.8
Chenopodiaceae	*Chenopodium ambrosioides* L., green variety	AP	14402	Methanol Aqueous	43.4 ±6.5 48.7 ±11.6
Sterculiaceae	*Chiranthodendron pentadactylon* Larreat	F	14104	Methanol Aqueous	87.6± 15.3 84.8 ±17.4
Moraceae	*Dorstenia contrajerva* L.	AP	14406	Methanol Aqueous	24.4±16.4 44.8± 5.9
Geraniaceae	*Geranium mexicanum* H. B. & K.	AP	14405	Methanol Aqueous	93.4 ±6.7 42.1±15.2
Hippocrateaceae	*Hippocratea excels* H. B. & K.	R	14394	Methanol Aqueous	80.3 ±21.3 75.0 ±24.9
Schizaeaceae	*Lygodium venustum* Sw.	AP	1270	Methanol Aqueous	51.6±15.6 0
Labiatae	*Ocimum basilicum* L.	AP	14393	Methanol Aqueous	68.7 ±9.7 68.0±20.8
Punicaceae	*Punica granatum* L.	EF	14403	Methanol Aqueous	55.9 ±3.6 19.1 ±6.9
Rutaceae	*Ruta chalepensis* L.	AP	14400	Methanol Aqueous	73.7 ±.01 23.6 ±9.27
Anacardiaceae	*Schinus molle* L.	AP	14408	Methanol Aqueous	0 79.5±17.7

Table 2. Antisecretory activity of methanol and aqueous extracts of Mexican medicinal plants on intestinal secretion response to cholera toxin, AP: aerial parts, EF: fruit exocarpus, F: flowers, R: roots.

2.6 Antisecretory study of Chiranthodendron penthadactylon

We selected *Chiranthodendron pentadactylon* Larreat (Sterculiaceae) to perform bio-guided assay fractionation. *C. pentadactylon* know in Mexico as "flor de manita"has been used in Mexican traditional medicine since Aztecs ancient times to treat heart illness, epilepsy, diarrhea and dysentery (Linares et al., 1988, Argueta et al., 1994). This study lend to the isolation of some compounds with *in vivo* antisecretory activity (Velázquez et al., 2009).

2.6.1 Isolation of active compounds

The flowers of *C. pentadactylon* were ground and extracted by maceration at room temperature with methanol, the extract was suspended in 10 % MeOH-water and successively partitioned with CH_2Cl_2 and EtOAc, the aqueous residual layer was lyophilized. The fractions were tested for antisecretory activity at doses of 50 mg/Kg. The most active fraction was AcOEt with 88.2 % of Inhibition. In order to isolate the active compounds, it was subjected to column chromatogaphy on Sephadex (Pharmacie) using $CHCl_3$ in EtOH, MeOH and Water to give eight secondary fractions, further chromatography lend to the isolation of tiliroside (**33**), astragalin (**34**), isoquercitrin (**35**), (+) catechin (**36**), and (-) epicatechin (**37**). All the isolated compounds were identified by comparison of spectroscopic data (^1H and ^{13}C NMR, UV, IR, [α], and TLC and HPLC with authentic samples available in our laboratory (Kuroyanagui et al., 1978; Lee et al., 1992; Lui et al., 1999; Calzada et al., 2007).

2.6.2 Antisecretory activity of isolated compounds

Antisecretory activity of the isolated compounds from the AcOEt fraction was tested on cholera toxin-induced intestinal secretion in rat jejunal loops model (table 3). Among the isolated compounds (-) epicatechin (**37**) showed the best antisecretory activity on the intestinal secretion with an ID_{50} of 8.3 μM /mL, its antisecretory activity was like of loperamide (**2**) (ID_{50} 6.1 μM/mL), isoquercitrin (**35**) and (+)-catechin (**36**) showed moderate and weak antisecretory activity, respectively. Tiliroside (**33**) and astragalin (**34**) were inactive at doses tested table 3. Flavonoids such as flavan-3-ols and flavonol glycosides have been considered as the active principles of many antidiarrheal plants. Isoquercitrin isolated from *Psidium guajava* showed spasmolytic effect on guinea pig ileum (Morales et al., 1994). Tiliroside (**33**) and (-)-epicatechin (**37**) obtained from *Helianthemum glomeratum* and *Rubus coriifolius*, respectively, showed antiprotozoal activity against *Entamoeba histolytica* and *Giardia lamblia* (Alanis et al., 2003; Barbosa et al., 2007). Data obtained in this investigation suggest that (-)-epicatechine (**37**), isoquercitrin (**35**) and tiliroside (**33**) may play an important role in antidiarrheal of *C. penthadactylon* in Mexican traditional medicine. Also, our results are in agreement and could explain the result previously obtained by Hör et al., 1995, with antisecretory oligomeric proantocianidins from *Guazuma ulmifolia* which monomeric unit are (+)-catechin (**36**) and (-)-epicatechin (**37**). The antiprotozoal activity together with the antisecretory activity is evidences that support the use of these plants to treat diarrhea in Mexican traditional medicine.

Further studies are carried on in order to determinate the action mechanism of active compounds against intestinal secretion caused by *Vibrio cholerae* toxin (non publicated results), Additionally we are studying some medicinal plants used to treat gastrointestinal disorders in Mexican traditional medicine from Hidalgo, using intestinal propulsion (charcoal meal), castor oil induced diarrhea and castor oil induced intestinal fluid accumulation models in vivo.

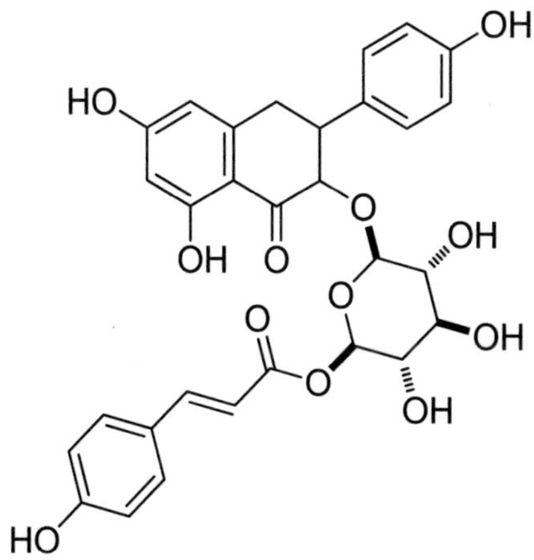

tiliroside 33

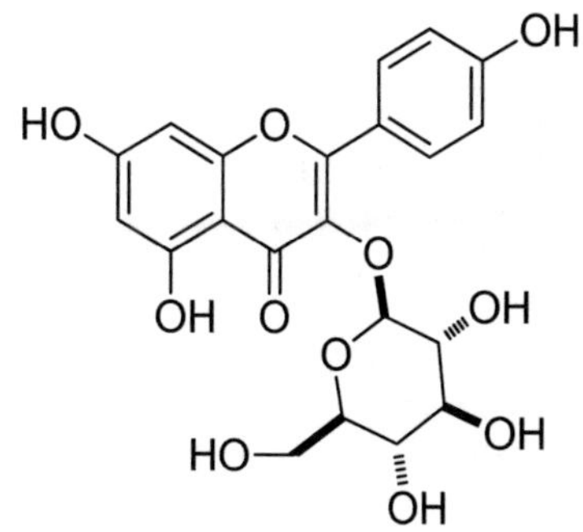

astragalin 34

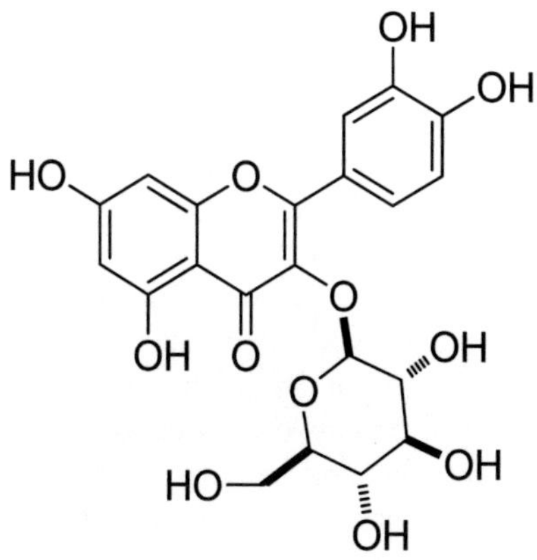

Isoquercitrin (35)

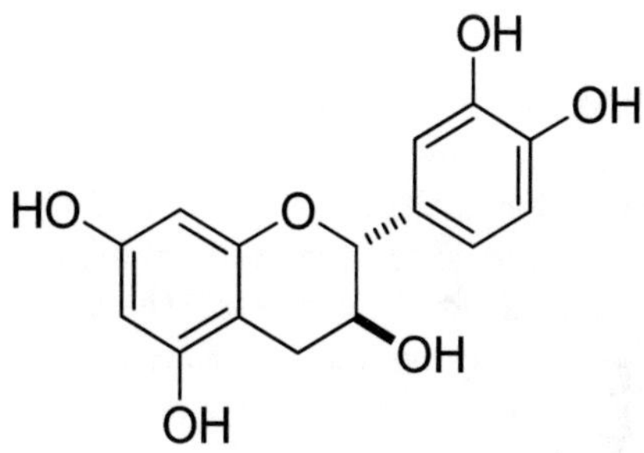

(+)-catechin (**36**)

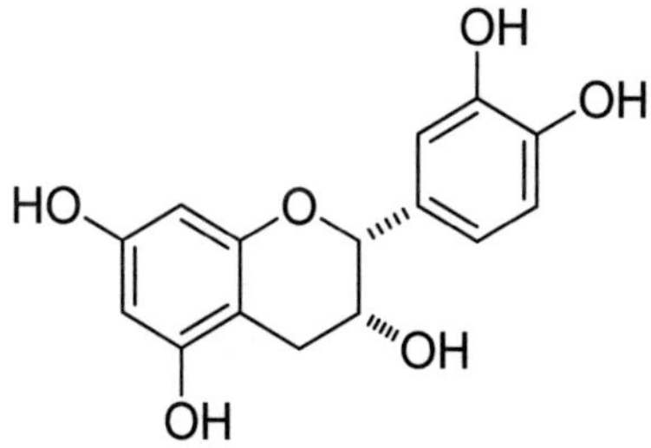

(-) epicatechin **(37)**

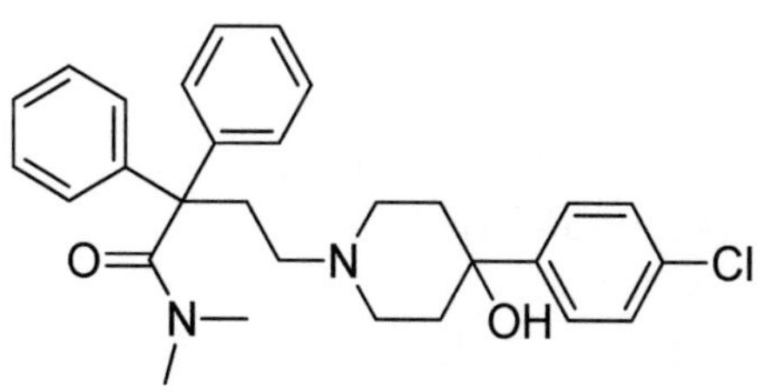

loperamide **(2)**

Compound	Doses (mg/Kg)	% of Inhibition	ID_{50} (μM/Kg)
MeOH extract	300	*87.1 ±14.5*	-
EtOAc fraction	50	*88.2±9.5*	-
Tiliroside (**33**)	10	-	Inactive
Astragalin (**34**)	10	-	Inactive
Isoquercitrin (**35**)	10	-	19.2
(+)-catechin (**36**)	10	-	51.7
(-)-epicatechin (**37**)	10	-	8.3
Loperamide (**2**)	10	-	6.1

Table 3. Antisecretory activity of MeOH extract, EtOAc fraction and isolated compounds from *Chiranthodendron pentadactylon*

3. Conclusion

Some of the medicinal plants tested showed antidiarrheal activity in the model used. Both extracts of *Annona cherimola, Chiranthodendron pentadactylon, Hippocratea excelsa, Ocimum basilicum, Geranium mexicanum* (aerial parts), methanol extract of *Ruta chalepensis, Lygodium venustum, Punica granatum,* and the aqueous extract of *Bocconia frutescens, Aloysia triphylla, Dorstenia contrajerva* and *Schinus molle* showed better antisecretory activity than loperamide. The active extracts found in this study will be an option to develop novel phytodrugs useful to treat fluid loss in diarrhea. These results allows to propose these species as a potential sources of antisecretory compounds and should be therefore subjected to further bioassay-guided phytochemical studies to obtain their active principles, the antisecretory compounds isolated from medicinal plants combined with ORS might be useful in decreasing the mortality caused by dehydration. The properties previously described of (-)-epicatechin suggest that it may be a leading compounds in the development of novel antidiarrheal agents. The results obtained give some scientific support to the use of some medicinal plants tested for the treatment of gastrointestinal disorders such as diarrhea.

4. Acknowledgment

MS Abigail Aguilar, IMSS herbarium, for authentication of plant material and MS Carlos Carrillo. This study was supported by CONACyT (grant: 3800-M); IMSS-FOFOI (FP-2001-05) and PROMEP (PROMEP/103.5/10/7313).

5. References

Aguilar A., Camacho, R., Chino S., Jáquez P., Lopez E. (1994). Herbario medicinal del Instituto Mexicano del Seguro Social. IMSS. P 43

Alanis A., Calzada F., Cedillo-Rivera R., Meckes M.(2003). Antiprotozoal activity of the constituents of Rubuscoriifolius.*Phytotherapy Research,* 17, 681-682

Amstrong D., Cohen J. (1999). Infectious diseases, vol 2. Mosby, Spain, pp35: 35.1-35.70

Argueta A., Cano L., Rodarte M (1994). Atlas de las plantas de la medicina tradicional mexicana. Vols I-III. Instituto Nacional Indigenista. Mexico. Pp 644-645

Astudillo A., Mata R., Navarrete A. (2009). El reino vegetal, fuente de agentes antiespasmodicos gastrointestinales y antidiarreicos. *Rev Latinoamer. Quím.*, 37, 1, 7-44

Barbosa E., Calzada F., Campos R. (2007). In vivo antigiardial activity of three flavonoids isolated of some medicinal plants used in Mexican traditional medicine for the treatment of diarrhea. *J of ethnoph* 109. 552-554

Calzada F., Alanis AD. (2007). Additional antiprotozoal flavonol glycosides of the aerial parts of Helianthemum glomeratum.*Phytotherapy research*, 21, 78-80

Capasso F., Grandolini G., Izzo A., (2006) FitoterapiaImpiegoRazionaledlleDrogheVegetali (TirthEdition) Springer , ISBN 10: 88-470-0302-4, Printed in Italia.

Casburn-Jones C., Farthing, M. (2004). Management of infectious diarrhoea.*Gut*, 5.296-305.

Crutchley R., Miller J., Garey K. (2010).New drug developments: Crofelemer, a Novel Agent for treatment of secretory diarrhea. *Ann Pharmacother*. 44, 878-884

Farthing M. (2002). Novel targets for the control of secretory diarrhea Gut 50. Iii15-iii18

Fedorack R., Field M.(1987). Anthidiarrheal therapy prospects for new agents. *Digestive disease and sciences* 32. 195-205.

Filbin, M., Lee, L., Shaffer B., Caughey A. (2004).*Blueprints Pathophysiology: Pulmonary, gastrointestinal and rheumatology*. Blakwell publishing, ISBN: 1-4051-0351-5, p 66

Guangtao, Z. (2009). Desing and in silico screening of inhibitors of the cholera toxin. Expert Opinion on Drug Discovery.*InformaHealthcarpublisher* ,Vol 4, No. 9, pp 923-938

Kopic S., Geibel J. (2010). *Toxin mediated diarrhea nin the 21st century: The pathophysiology of intestinal ion transport in the course of ETEC, V. cholerae and Rotavirus infection.* Toxins 2, 2132-2157 ISSN 2072-6651 (www.mdpi.com/journal/toxins)

Kuroyanagui, M., Fukuoka, M., Yoshihira, K. (1978). Confirmation of the structure of tiliroside, an acylatedkaemperol glycoside by 13C,-nuclear magnetic resonance. *Chemical & Pharmaceutical Bull*, 26, 3593-3596

Lee, W., Maremoto, S., Nonaka G., Noshioka, I. (1992).Flavan-3-ol gallates and proanthocyanidins from Pithecellebiumlobatum.*Phytochemistry*, 31, 2117-2120

Liu, H., Orjalata, J., Sticher, O. (1999). Acylatedflavonol glycosides from the leaves of Stenochlaenapalustris, *Journal of Natural Products* 62, 70-75

Linares E., Flores B., Bye R. (1988). Selección de plantas medicinales de México. Limusa. México, p 44

Marion K., Scarlett H., Webber K. (2010) Clinical Drug Therapy for Canadian Practice. 2nd edition, Lippincott Williams & Wilkins Editor. ISBN 1605475173, chapter 16, section 9, p 991

Martindale (2009)*The Complete Drug Reference* (Thirty-sixth edition) ,Pharmaceutical Press, ISBN 978 0 85369 840 1, Printed in China by Everbest Printing Co. Ltd

Morales MA., Tortoriello J., Meckes M. (1994). Calcium antagonist effect of quercetin and its relation with the spasmolytic properties of Psidium guajava. Archives Medical Research 25, 17-21.

Sixma T. K., Pronk S. E., Kalk K. H., Wartna E. S., Zanten B A., Witholt B., Hoi W. G. (1991) *Nature*. 351, 371-377.

Navaneethan U., Giannella R. (2010). *Diarrhea Diagnostic and therapeutic advances.* Chapter 1 in Guandalini S. and Vaziri H. editors, e-ISBN 978-1-60761-183-7. Springer science+Busines media p 1-16

SAGARPA (Secretaria de agriculturaganaderíadesarrollorural pesca y alimentación) 2001. Norma oficialmexicana (NOM-062-ZOO-1999).Especificacionestécnicaspara la producción, cuidado y uso de los animales de laboratorio. Diariooficial, México, pp 16-20, 5, 6, 8-45.

Spangler, B. (1992).Structure and function of Cholera toxin and the related *Escherichia coli* Heat-labile enterotoxin.*Microbiological rewiews,* vol. 56, No. 4, p 622-647.

SS (Secretaría de Salud) 2008. SistemaNacional de VigilanciaEpidemiológica.Epidemiologia 34, semana 4, ISNN: 1405-2636.

Thiagarajah, J. R.,Verkman, A. S. (2005). New Drug Targets for Cholera Toxin.*PharmacolSci,* Vol. 26, No.4, pp. 172-5

Velázquez C., Calzada F., Torres J., González F., Ceballos G. (2006). Antisecretory activity of plants used to trat gastrointestinal disorders in Mexico. *Journal of Ethnopharmacology,* 10, 66-70

Velázquez, C., Calzada, F., Esquivel, B., Barbosa, E., Calzada, S. (2009).Antisecretory activity from the flowers of *Chiranthodendronpentadactylon* and its flavonoids on intestinal fluid accumulation induced by Vibrio cholerae toxin in rats.*Journal of Ethnopharmacology,* 126, 455-458

5

Clostridia Difficile Diarrhea

Enoch Lule
Medical Center Of Central Georgia
USA

1. Introduction

The term antibiotic associated diarrhea is usually reserved for diarrhea caused by infection with the organism Clostridia Difficile. Infection is thought to take place after the normal intestinal flora is altered by antibiotic use allowing for proliferation of Clostridia Difficile. Worryingly, the incidence and severity of illness caused by Clostridia Difficile is on the increase.

2. Pathophysiology

Clostridia difficile is a gram positive, spore forming anaerobic bacilli[1] Infection occurs when the organism is ingested. Though initially thought of as a nosocomial infection, community acquired clostridia difficile infection is increasingly recognized.[2]

Clostridia Difficile produces a variety of toxins, toxin A (enterotoxin) and B (cytotoxin) are the toxins most frequently linked to disease. They cause inflammation and disrupt cell cytoskeleton synthesis leading to colonic cell disruption.[3,4,5] A new strain, termed NAP1 or BI or 027 (depending on the technique used to identify it) was identified in the early 2000s the cause of selected outbreaks. This strain of clostridia difficile is associated with clinically more severe disease, innate resistance to quinolones and higher amounts of toxin production.[6]

3. Epidemiology

Clostridia difficile infection was linked to the development of pseudomembranous colitis in the 70's.[7] Initial cases were mostly linked to clindamycin but since then the range antibiotics linked with development of Clostridia Difficile has widened and cephalosporins and floroquinolones are thought to be the major causes.[8]

Though less often thought of as a cause of diarrhea in developing countries, pathogenic C. Difficile has been noted in South Africa[9] and India.[10]

The incidence rate of C. Difficile infection in the US was about 30 to 40 cases per hundred thousand.[11]

One research group noted an increasing rate of colectomies following C. Difficile infection.[12]

Canadian authors noted a four fold increase in background prevalence of C. Difficile between when the period before 2002 was compared to 2003.[13]

4. Clinical presentation

Presentation may range from asymptomatic carrier state[14] to fulminant colitis.[15]
Symptomatic patients typically present with watery diarrhea and lower abdominal pain.[16] Severe diarrhea with leucocytosis, fever, abdominal pain and distention occurs in the severely ill[16,17]. Surgical management with colectomy may be required in severe cases[18]. C. Difficile colitis was increasingly listed as the cause of death in an English population.[19]
Rises in white cell count to above 30,000 or a doubling of serum creatinine have been suggested as harbingers complicated disease.[20]

5. Diagnosis

C. Difficile diagnosis is usually done with laboratory testing in a patient suspected to be having the infection.
One of the most sensitive and specific tests available is the cell cytotoxycity assay, which had a sensitivity of 98% and specificity of 99% when compared to clinical and laboratory criteria.[21] This test is unfortunately technically demanding and may not be the first choice of many laboratories.
Many laboratories will use EIAs for detection of toxin A and B. These tests are insensitive when compared to cell culture or cytotoxicity assay but they are cheaper and produce results in hours rather than days.[22] Due to the lower positive predictive value of these tests a 2 step approach with a sensitive screening test followed by confirmation by culture or cell cytotoxicity may be appropriate.[23]
Testing for glutamate dehydrogenase, an enzyme produced by C. Difficile is sensitive (96 to 100%) [24], cheap, and rapid but it only detects presence of organism rather than toxin production.
Though its usually unnecessary, direct visualization of colitis by endoscopy is virtually diagnostic as they are few other infections that would cause pseudomembrane formation.[25] Endoscopy carries the risk of perforation in fulminant colitis.

6. Treatment

First line therapy for C. Difficile infection has long been considered to be a choice between metronidazole or vancomycin. Resolution of disease was seen in over 90% of patients taking a 10 day course of either therapy.[26]
More recently, metronidazole has been associated with therapeutic failure rates as high as 50 percent if persistence of disease and recurrence are conbined.[27] That said, oral metronidazole at a dose of 500mg, three times daily for ten to fourteen days remains the initial recommended therapy for mild disease.[28] Oral or rectal vancomycin (500mg four times a day) is recommended for more severe disease.[28] Patients who cannot tolerate oral therapy may be treated with intravenous metronidazole.[29]
Up to 25% of patients may have recurrent infection[16] believed to occur because of germination of spores or ingestion of new spores.
Many approaches have been taken to recurrent symptomatic C Difficile infection. A tapered or pulsed course of oral vancomycin may reduce recurrence rates[30].

Other approaches include fecal transplants[31], immunization against C difficile toxins[32], cholestyramine[33], rifampin[34] or probiotics[35]. There isn't sufficient data to recommend any of these approaches.
Recently fidaxomicin (200 mg oral, twice daily for ten days), a macrolide antibiotic, was shown to be non inferior to vancomycin.[36] During the trial referenced, patients were noted to have a lower recurrence rate when they were treated using fidaxomicin rather than vancomycin (13.3% vs. 24.0%)

7. Prevention

Judicious use of antibiotics has been shown to reduce the rates of C. difficile infection.[37, 38] Washing hands with soap and water, using gloves when touching patients and use of disposable thermometers have been recommended as control measures with good quality evidence of efficacy.[39] Alcohol hand washing gels are not effective in preventing disease spread.[40]

8. References

[1] Ryan KJ, Ray CG (editors) (2004). *Sherris Medical Microbiology* (4th ed.). McGraw Hill. pp. 322–4. ISBN 0-8385-8529-9.

[2] Epidemiology of community-acquired Clostridium difficile-associated diarrhea. Hirschhorn LR, Trnka Y, Onderdonk A, Lee ML, Platt R. J Infect Dis. 1994 Jan;169(1):127-33.

[3] Just I, Selzer J, Wilm M, von Eichel-Streiber C, Mann M, Aktories K. Glucosylation of Rho proteins by Clostridium difficile toxin B. Nature. 1995;375(6531):500.

[4] Clostridium difficile toxin A. Interactions with mucus and early sequential histopathologic effects in rabbit small intestine. Lima AA, Innes DJ Jr, Chadee K, Lyerly DM, Wilkins TD, Guerrant RL. Lab Invest. 1989;61(4):419.

[5] Clostridium difficile toxin-induced inflammation and intestinal injury are mediated by the inflammasome. Ng J, Hirota SA, Gross O, Li Y, Ulke-Lemee A, Potentier MS, Schenck LP, Vilaysane A, Seamone ME, Feng H, Armstrong GD, Tschopp J, Macdonald JA, Muruve DA, Beck PL. Gastroenterology. 2010 Aug;139(2):542-52, 552.e1-3. Epub 2010 Apr 13.

[6] Toxin production by an emerging strain of Clostridium difficile associated with outbreaks of severe disease in North America and Europe. Warny M, Pepin J, Fang A, Killgore G, Thompson A, Brazier J, Frost E, McDonald LC. Lancet. 2005;366(9491):1079

[7] Role of Clostridium difficile in antibiotic-associated pseudomembranous colitis. Bartlett JG, Moon N, Chang TW, Taylor N, Onderdonk AB. Gastroenterology. 1978;75(5):778.

[8] Narrative review: the new epidemic of Clostridium difficile-associated enteric disease. Bartlett JG Ann Intern Med. 2006;145(10):758.

[9] PCR detection of Clostridium difficile triose phosphate isomerase (tpi), toxin A (tcdA), toxin B (tcdB), binary toxin (cdtA, cdtB), and tcdC genes in Vhembe District, South

Africa. Samie A, Obi CL, Franasiak J, Archbald-Pannone L, Bessong PO, Alcantara-Warren C, Guerrant RL. Am J Trop Med Hyg. 2008 Apr;78(4):577-85.
[10] Dhawan B, Chaudhry R, Sharma N. Incidence of Clostridium difficile infection: a prospective study in an Indian hospital. J Hosp Infect. 1999;43:275-280. Abstract
[11] McDonald LC, Owings M, Jernigan JB. Clostridium difficile infection in patients discharged from US short-stay hospitals, 1996 to 2003. Emerg Infect Dis 2006;12:409-415 Ricciardi R, Rothenberger DA, Madoff RD, Baxter NN.
[12] Increasing prevalence and severity of Clostridium difficile colitis in hospitalized patients in the United States. Arch Surg. 2007;142:624-631; discussion 631.
[13] Pepin J, Valiquette L, Alary ME, et al. Clostridium difficile-associated diarrhea in a region of Quebec from 1991 to 2003: a changing pattern of disease severity. CMAJ 2004;171:466-472
[14] Nosocomial acquisition of Clostridium difficile infection. McFarland LV, Mulligan ME, Kwok RY, Stamm WE. N Engl J Med. 1989;320(4):204.
[15] Severe Clostridium difficile colitis. Rubin MS, Bodenstein LE, Kent KC. Dis Colon Rectum. 1995;38(4):350.
[16] Clostridium difficile Colitis. Ciaran P. Kelly, Charalabos Pothoulakis, and J. Thomas LaMont. N Engl J Med 1994; 330:257-26
[17] Leukocytosis as a harbinger and surrogate marker of Clostridium difficile infection in hospitalized patients with diarrhea. Bulusu M, Narayan S, Shetler K, Triadafilopoulos G. Am J Gastroenterol. 2000;95(11):3137.
[18] Fulminant Clostridium difficile: An Underappreciated and Increasing Cause of Death and Complications. Ramsey M. Dallal, Brian G. Harbrecht, Arthur J. Boujoukas, Carl A. Sirio, Linda M. Farkas Kenneth K. Lee,Richard L. Simmons, Ann Surg. 2002 March; 235(3): 363–372.
[19] United Kingdom national statistics. Newport, United Kingdom: Office for National Statistics, UK Statistics Authority. (Accessed October 6, 2008, at http://www.statistics.gov.uk.)
[20] Predictors of Serious Complications Due to Clostridium difficile Infection. D. Gujja; F. K. Friedenberg. Alimentary Pharmacology & Therapeutics. 2009;29(6):635-642.
[21] Connor D, Hynes P, Cormican M, Collins E, Corbett-Feeney G, Cassidy M. Evaluation of methods for detection of toxins in specimens of feces submitted for diagnosis of Clostridium difficile–associated diarrhea. J Clin Microbiol 2001;39:2846-9.
[22] Clinical Recognition and Diagnosis of *Clostridium difficile* Infection. John G. Bartlett and Dale N. Gerding. Clin Infect Dis. (2008) 46 (Supplement 1): S12-S18. doi: 10.1086/521863
[23] Planche T, Aghaizu A, Holiman R, et al. Diagnosis of Clostridium difficile infection by toxin detection kits: a systematic review. Lancet Infect Dis 2008;8:777-784
[24] Ticehurst JR, Aird DZ, Dam LM, Borek AP, Hargrove JT, Carroll KC. Effective detection of toxigenic Clostridium difficile by a two-step algorithm including tests for antigen and cytotoxin. J Clin Microbiol 2006;44:1145-9.

[25] Kawamoto S, Horton KM, Fishman EK. Pseudomembranous colitis: spectrum of imaging findings with clinical and pathologic correlation. Radiographics 1999;19:887-97.

[26] Wenisch C, Parschalk B, Hasenhundl M, Hirschl AM, Graninger W. Comparison of vancomycin, teicoplanin, metronidazole, and fusidic acid for the treatment of *Clostridium difficile*-associated diarrhea [published correction appears in Clin Infect Dis 1996;23:423]. *Clin Infect Dis*. 1996;22:813–8.

[27] Musher DM, Aslam S, Logan N, et al. Relatively poor outcome after treatment of Clostridium difficile colitis with metronidazole. Clin Infect Dis 2005;40:1586-1590

[28] Shea-idsa guideline. Clinical Practice Guidelines for Clostridium difficile Infection in Adults: 2010 Update by the Society for Healthcare Epidemiology of America (SHEA) and the Infectious Diseases Society of America (IDSA). Stuart H. Cohen, Dale N. Gerding, Stuart Johnson, Ciaran P. Kelly, Vivian G. Loo, L. Clifford McDonald, Jacques Pepin, Mark H. Wilcox. Infect Control Hosp Epidemiol 2010; 31(5):000-000

[29] Bolton RP, Culshaw MA. Faecal metronidazole concentrations during oral and intravenous therapy for antibiotic associated colitis due to Clostridium difficile. Gut 1986;27:1169-1172

[30] McFarland LV, Elmer GW, Surawicz CM. Breaking the cycle: treatment strategies for 163 cases of recurrent Clostridium difficile disease. Am J Gastroenterol 2002;97:1769-1775

[31] Aas J, Gessert CE, Bakken JS. Recurrent Clostridium difficile colitis: case series involving 18 patients treated with donor stool administered via a nasogastric tube. Clin Infect Dis 2003;36:580-585Tedesco FJ. Treatment of recurrent antibiotic-associated pseudomembranous colitis. Am J Gastroenterol 1982;77:220-221

[32] Leung DY, Kelly CP, Boguniewicz M, Pothoulakis C, LaMont JT, Flores A. Treatment with intravenously administered gamma globulin of chronic relapsing colitis induced by Clostridium difficile toxin. J Pediatr 1991;118:633-637

[33] Zimmerman MJ, Bak A, Sutherland LR. Treatment of Clostridium difficile infection. Aliment Pharmacol Ther 1997;11:1003-1012

[34] Buggy BP, Fekety R, Silva J Jr. Therapy of relapsing Clostridium difficile-associated diarrhea and colitis with the combination of vancomycin and rifampin. J Clin Gastroenterol 1987;9:155-159

[35] Probiotics for treatment of Clostridium difficile-associated colitis in adults. Anjana Pillai, Richard L Nelson. Intervention review, The Cochrane Library. DOI: 10.1002/14651858.CD004611.pub2

[36] Fidaxomicin versus Vancomycin for *Clostridium difficile* Infection. Thomas J. Louie, Mark A. Miller, Kathleen M. Mullane, D.O., Karl Weiss, Arnold Lentnek, Yoav Golan, Sherwood Gorbach, M.D., Pamela Sears, Youe-Kong Shue. N Engl J Med 2011; 364:422-431

[37] Carling P, Fung T, Killion A, Terrin N, Barza M. Favorable impact of a multidisciplinary antibiotic management program conducted during 7 years. *Infect Control Hosp Epidemiol*. 2003;24:699–706.

[38] Climo MW, Israel DS, Wong ES, Williams D, Coudron P, Markowitz SM. Hospital-wide restriction of clindamycin: effect on the incidence of *Clostridium difficile*-associated diarrhea and cost. *Ann Intern Med.* 1998;128(12 pt 1):989–95.

[39] Prevention of Endemic Healthcare-Associated *Clostridium difficile* Infection: Reviewing the Evidence. J Hsu, C Abad, M Dinh, N Safdar. *Am J Gastroenterol* 6 July 2010; doi: 10.1038/ajg.2010.254

[40] Leischner J, Johnson S, Sambol S, Parada J, Gerding DN. Effect of alcohol hand gels and chlorhexidine hand wash in removing spores of Clostridium difficile from hands [abstr]. In: Program and abstracts of the 45th interscience conference on antimicrobial agents and chemotherapy. Washington, DC: American Society for Microbiology, 2005:LB-29.

6

Introduction and Classification of Childhood Diarrhoea

Angela Ine Frank-Briggs
University of Port Harcourt Teaching Hospital, Port Harcourt, Rivers State, Nigeria

1. Introduction

1.1 Diarrhoea is a global problem

Diarrhoea is one of the most common causes of morbidity and mortality in children worldwide. The word diarrhoea is derived from the Greek "diarrhoia", meaning to flow through. In clinical terms, diarrhoea refers to either an increased stool frequency or a decreased stool consistency, typically a watery quality. The World Health Organization (WHO) defines a case as the passage of three or more loose or watery stools per day. Nevertheless, absolute limits of normalcy are difficult to define; any deviation from the child's usual pattern should arouse some concern (particularly when the passage of blood or mucus, or dehydration occurs) regardless of the actual number of stools or their water content.

Diarrhoeal illness is the second leading cause of child mortality; among children younger than 5 years, it causes 1.5 to 2 million deaths annually. In 1982, on the basis of a review of active surveillance data from studies conducted in the 1950s, 1960s and 1970s, it was estimated that 4.6 million children died annually from diarrhoea. In 1992, a review of studies conducted in the 1980s suggested that diarrhoeal mortality had declined to approximately 3.3 million annually. It was noted that children in the developing world experienced a median of between two and three episodes of diarrhoea every year. Where episodes are frequent, young children may spend more than 15% of their days with diarrhoea. About 80% of deaths due o diarrhoea occur in the first two years of life. The main cause of morbidity from acute diarrhoea is dehydration, which results from loss of fluid and electrolytes in the diarrhoeal stools. In severe cases this could lead to vascular collapse, shock and eventually death. Other causes of death include malnutrition from loss of nutrients from the stool, effects of infection on metabolism and the withholding or modification of food during diarrhoea which is a common practice.

Diarrhoeal illnesses may have a significant impact on psychomotor and cognitive development in young children. Early and repeated episodes of childhood diarrhoea during periods of critical development, especially when associated with malnutrition, co-infections, and anemia may have long-term effects on linear growth, as well as on physical and cognitive functions.

Worldwide childhood death secondary to diarrhoea declined from an estimated five million per year in 1980 to less than two million in 1999. The decline is generally attributed to global improvements in sanitation and the use of oral rehydration therapy, as well as zinc and vitamin A therapy.

In developing countries, infants experience a median of six episodes annually; children experience a median of three episodes annually. Diarrhoeal illness may consist of acute watery diarrhoea, invasive (bloody) diarrhoea, or chronic diarrhoea (persistent ≥14 days). The major causes and the prevalence of chronic diarrhoea differ between developed and developing countries. In the developing world, chronic diarrhoea is typically associated with serial enteric infections and malnutrition; it is manifested by a chronic enteropathy, with impaired mucosal healing and diminished digestive and absorptive capacity.

In developed countries, children are less likely to be exposed to serial enteric infections and malnutrition. In these populations, chronic diarrhoea is more likely to be induced by underlying disease causing malabsorption or maldigestion. However, enteric infections (particularly in immunocompromised patients), malnutrition, and dietary factors (eg, excessive consumption of juice), play a role in some cases. Figure 1 below shows the relationship between malnutrition and diarrhoea.

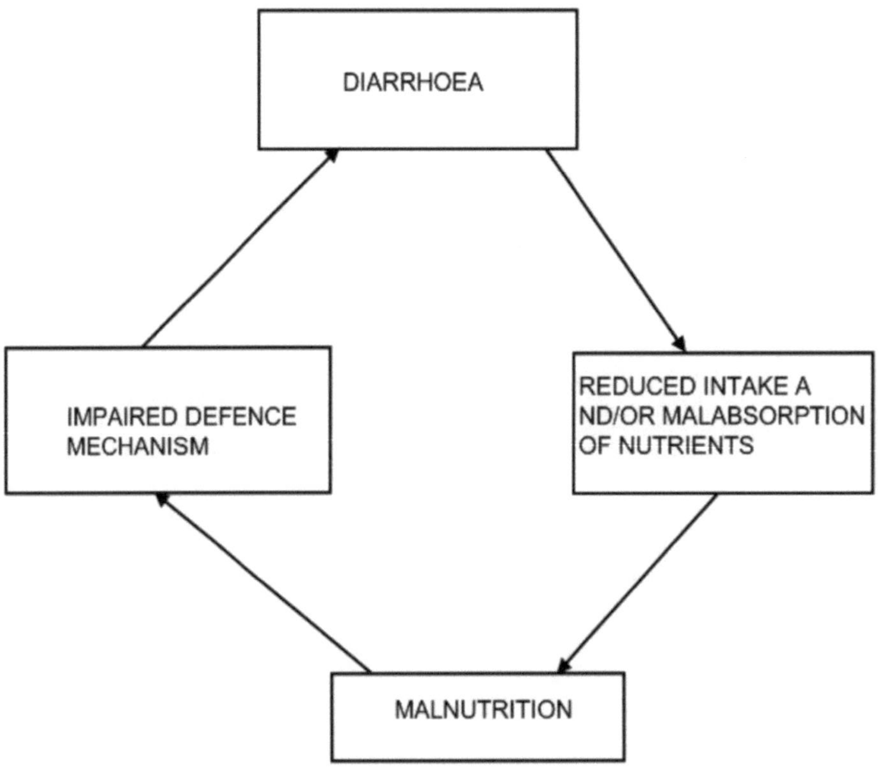

Fig. 1. The vicious cycle of diarrhoea and malnutrition.

2. Classification of diarrhoea

Classification facilitates the approach to management of childhood diarrhoea.

Issues related to the etiology, clinical assessment, treatment, and prevention of different types of diarrhoea are better analyzed when classified.

Diarrhoea is defined in epidemiological studies as the passage of three or more loose or watery stools in a 24- hour period; a loose stool being one that would take the shape of the container. Exclusively breastfed infants normally pass several soft, semi-liquid stools; for them, it is practical to refer to diarrhoea as an increase in stool frequency or liquidity that is considered abnormal by the mother.
Diarrhoea can be classified based on duration of each diarrhoeal episode, aetiological factor, pathophisiological mechanism and systemic diseases contributing to diarrhoea.
The distinction, supported by the World Health Organization (WHO), has implications not only for classification and epidemiological studies but also from a practical standpoint because protracted diarrhea often has a different set of causes, poses different problems of management, and has a different prognosis.

3. Classification based on duration

3.1 Acute watery diarrhoea

This term refers to diarrhoea that begins acutely, lasts less than 14 days (most episodes last less than seven days), and involves the passage of frequent loose or watery stools without visible blood. Vomiting may occur and fever may be present. Acute watery diarrhoea causes dehydration; when food intake is reduced it also contributes to malnutrition. When death occurs, it is usually due to acute dehydration. The most important causes of acute watery diarrhoea in young children in developing countries are rotavirus, enterotoxigenic Escherichia coli, Shigella, Campylobacter jejuni, and Cryptosporodium. In some areas vibrio cholerae 01, Salmonella and enteropathogenic E. Coli are also important.

3.2 Persistent diarrhoea

This is diarrhoea that begins acutely but is of unusually long duration (at least 14 days). The episode may begin either as watery diarrhoea or as dysentery. Marked weight loss is frequent. Diarrhoeal stool volume may also be great, with a risk of dehydration. There is no single microbial cause for persistent diarrhoea; enteroadherent E. coli, Shigella and Cryptosporidium may play a greater role than other agents. Persistent diarrhoea should not be confused with chronic diarrhoea, which is recurrent or long lasting diarrhoea due to non infectious causes, such as sensitivity to gluten or inherited metabolic disorders.

3.3 Intractable (protracted) or chronic diarrhoea

Is a term applied to diarrhoea episodes which are of long duration, (more than 4 weeks), for which no known cause can be found and which does not respond to specific or non specific form of treatment. Chronic diarrhoea is defined as stool volume of more than 10 grams/kg/day in infants and toddlers, or more than 200 grams/day in older children for more than 14 days. This typically translates to persistent loose or watery stools occurring at least three times a day, where the change in stool consistency is more important than stool frequency. Some authors make a distinction between chronic diarrhoea, which they define as having a gradual onset, from persistent diarrhoea, which they define as having a sudden onset. However, it is frequently difficult to identify the time of onset of the diarrhoea and delineation of the two entities can be problematic. Chronic diarrhoea is a common condition. Diarrhoea lasting more than two to four weeks occurs in up to 3 to 5 percent of the population worldwide. It is generally more frequent in males, with a male-to-female ratio of 1.2 to 2.6:1 in the age range of 6 to 24 months.

In the developed world, the prevalence of chronic diarrhoea is substantially lower. In the United States, there is approximately one case of persistent diarrhoea per five person-years in infants and young children. Most of these cases are self-limited, with fewer than 28 percent presenting for medical care. Fewer than 100 per 10,000 children are hospitalized in the United States for diarrhoeal disease, and this figure includes many cases of acute diarrhoea.

4. Classification based on pathophysiology

4.1 Secretory diarrhoea

Secretory diarrhoea occurs when there is active secretion of water into the gut lumen.
This type of diarrhoea is often caused by a secretagogue, such as cholera toxin, binding to a receptor on the surface epithelium of the bowel and thereby stimulating intracellular accumulation of cyclic adenosine monophosphate or cyclic guanosine monophosphate. Also there are many other infectious and non-infectious causes. Examples of the latter include those mediated by gastrointestinal peptides (such as vasoactive intestinal peptide and gastrin). Certain substances, such as bile acids, fatty acids, and laxatives, also can produce a secretory diarrhoea, as can congenital problems (eg, congenital chloride diarrhea). Diarrhoea not associated with an exogenous secretagogue may also have a secretory component (congenital microvillus inclusion disease). Secretory diarrhoea tends to be watery and of large volume; the osmolality of the stool can be accounted for by the presence of electrolytes. Secretory diarrhoea generally persists even when no feedings are given by mouth.

4.2 Osmotic diarrhoea

This occurs after ingestion of a poorly absorbed solute. The solute may be one that is normally not well absorbed such as magnesium, phosphate, lactulose, and sorbitol or one that is not well absorbed because of a disorder of the small bowel (lactose with lactase deficiency or glucose with rotavirus diarrhoea). This results in a higher than normal concentration of the solute in the gut lumen, altering the gradient of water absorption toward fluid retention in the intestinal lumen. Enteric infections that cause damage to intestinal epithelial cells leading to malabsorption may cause diarrhoea with an osmotic component. Rotavirus and shigella are examples. Rotavirus selectively invades mature enterocytes causing a disruption of absorptive capacity. Shigella produces a "shiga" toxin which can cause villous cell destruction leading to malabsorption.
Malabsorbed carbohydrate is fermented in the colon, and short-chain fatty acids (SCFAs) are produced. Although SCFAs can be absorbed in the colon and used as an energy source, the net effect is to increase the osmotic solute load. This form of diarrhoea is usually of lesser volume (quantity) than secretory diarrhoea and stops with fasting. The osmolality of the stool will not be explained by the electrolyte content, because another osmotic component is present. Motility disorders can be associated with rapid or delayed transit and are not generally associated with large-volume diarrhoea. Slowed motility can be associated with bacterial overgrowth as a cause of diarrhoea.

4.3 Inflammatory

Diarrhoea can be caused by intestinal inflammation. Exudation of mucus, protein, and blood into the gut lumen leads to water and electrolyte loss and subsequent diarrhoea.

The most common cause of inflammatory diarrhoea is infection. The initial event in the pathogenesis of acute infection is the ingestion of the offending organism. After ingestion, the organism colonizes the intestinal epithelium and adheres to the enterocyte. One of two pathways are generally followed depending upon the offending organism, either mucosal invasion or production of an enterotoxin.

Intestinal inflammation can also be caused by chronic diseases, such as inflammatory bowel disease and celiac disease. It can also be caused by tuberculosis, colon cancer, and enteritis. Diarrhoea in these disorders is multifactorial but is due in part to the mucosal inflammation, which leads to malabsorption. Malabsorbed substances produce an osmotic load in the gut lumen resulting in diarrhoea. Several bacterial infections of the gastrointestinal tract produce diarrhoea secondary to preformed toxins. Examples include the enterotoxins produced by Clostridia perfringens and Clostridia difficile, and the shiga-like toxins of Escherichia coli, Staphylococcus aureus, and Shigella species. Viral enterotoxins also have been described. As an example, rotavirus produces a viral enterotoxin, the non-structural glycoprotein (NSP4). NSP4 causes calcium-dependent transepithelial chloride secretion from the crypt cells, with resultant secretory diarrhoea.

4.4 Impaired motility

Motility disorders are relatively uncommon causes of acute diarrhoea. Changes in gastrointestinal motility can influence absorption. This could be hypermotility or hypomotility. Hypermotility is caused by the rapid movement of food through the intestines. If the food moves too quickly through the gastrointestinal tract, there is no enough time for sufficient nutrients and water to be absorbed. Hypermotility can be observed in people who have had portions of their bowel removed, allowing less total time for absorption of nutrients. Motility related diarrhoea can also be due to a vagotomy or diabetic neuropathy, or a complication of menstruation. Hyperthyroidism can produce hypermotility and lead to pseudodiarrhoea and occasionally real diarrhoea. This type of diarrhoea can be treated with antimotility agents (such as loperamide).

Hypomotility, or the severe impairment of intestinal peristalsis, results in stasis, with subsequent inflammation, bacterial overgrowth, and secondary bile acid deconjugation and malabsorption.

5. Classification based on systemic diseases

5.1 Infectious causes

5.1.1 Postenteritis syndrome

Most enteric infections in otherwise healthy children resolve within 14 days and do not develop into a chronic diarrhoeal illness. However, in a minority of patients, an acute gastroenteritis can trigger persistent diarrhoea by causing mucosal damage to the small intestine, termed a "postenteritis syndrome". The mechanisms underlying this syndrome are not fully understood. Contrary to previous hypotheses, sensitization to food antigens and secondary disaccharidase deficiency, including lactase deficiency (causing lactose intolerance), are uncommon. Therefore, international guidelines discourage the use of hypoallergenic or diluted milk formulas during acute gastroenteritis. Recurrent or sequential enteric infections may be responsible for some of these cases. In some cases, treatment with probiotic bacteria may facilitate recovery from postenteritis syndrome.

5.1.2 Bacterial infection

In immunocompromised patients, common infectious causes of acute diarrhoea, such as Campylobacter or Salmonella, can cause persistent diarrhoea. Chronic infections with these pathogens are uncommon in immunocompetent hosts. Bacterial cultures should be part of the initial diagnostic evaluation for all patients if the stool contains blood, or for immunocompromised patients regardless of fecal blood.

In children recently treated with antibiotics, Clostridium difficile may cause a colitis characterized by "pseudomembrane" formation. The enzyme immunoassay available in most laboratories detects C. difficile toxins A and B with high specificity but only moderate sensitivity. Polymerase chain reaction (PCR) based diagnostic methods can enhance the detection rate.

Enterotoxigenic strains of Staphylococcus aureus typically cause acute gastrointestinal symptoms in children or adults, due to the effects of ingested pre-formed toxin produced in contaminated food.

5.1.3 Parasitic infections

Intestinal parasites sometimes cause diarrhoea especially among children in developing countries. However, they are an uncommon cause of chronic diarrhoea in developed countries, except among individuals with an immunodeficiency. Specific antigen assays for Giardia and examination from the stool for parasites is imperative for children with known immunodeficiencies or with a history of travel to endemic areas. An step in the evaluation of immunocompetent children if initial testing fails to determine a cause of the chronic diarrhoea.

When a specific parasite is identified, treatment with specific medications is generally indicated, although the organism may not always be the cause of the diarrhoea. Empiric therapy for enteric pathogens is generally not advisable, except in cases with special characteristics in developing countries.

5.2 Syndromic persistent diarrhoea

Occasionally children in developed countries will develop a pattern in which enteric infection triggers a cycle of undernutrition, immune compromise and re-infection, resembling the syndromic persistent diarrhoea that is more commonly seen in developing countries. This pattern is uncommon in developed countries except in children with an underlying immunodeficiency.

5.2.1 Immune deficiency

Chronic diarrhoea may present as a complication of a known immune deficiency such as HIV disease. In this case, the evaluation should focus on potential infectious causes of the diarrhoea, particularly parasites and opportunistic infections such as Cryptosporidium, Isospora, and Cyclospora. These children also are at risk for persistent infectious pathogens that typically cause acute diarrheas, such as rotavirus.

Chronic diarrhoea also may be a presenting symptom of immune deficiency in a child. When a patient is infected with an unusual pathogen, or has multiple or recurrent infections of the gastrointestinal tract or elsewhere, further evaluation for immune deficiency is required. In rare instances, live vaccines may call attention to the potential diagnosis of immunodeficiency by inducing chronic infection. As an example, vaccine-acquired chronic rotavirus diarrhoea has been observed in infants with severe combined immunodeficiency

5.3 Abnormal immune response

5.3.1 Celiac disease

Celiac disease (also known as gluten-sensitive enteropathy or nontropical sprue) is an immune-mediated inflammation of the small intestine caused by sensitivity to dietary gluten and related proteins in genetically sensitive individuals. The disorder is common, occurring in 0.5 to 1 percent of the general population in most countries. Celiac disease often presents as chronic diarrhoea, with or without malnutrition, during late infancy or early childhood.

5.3.2 Inflammatory bowel disease

Ulcerative colitis and Crohn's disease

These are idiopathic chronic inflammatory diseases of the bowel. These disorders typically present with gradual onset of chronic diarrhoea, with or without blood, from mid-childhood through adulthood.

Allergic enteropathy

An abnormal immune response to food proteins can cause a proctitis/colitis or an enteropathy. The former tends to present as bloody diarrhoea and is frequently triggered by cow's milk protein in infants. The latter presents as non bloody diarrhoea and/or failure to thrive.

Eosinophilic gastroenteritis

This is an incompletely understood disorder that is sometimes but not always associated with an identifiable dietary antigen. Approximately one-half of patients have allergic disease, such as asthma, defined food sensitivities, eczema, or rhinitis; some patients have elevated serum IgE levels; rare patients have IgE antibodies directed against specific foods.

Microscopic and collagenous colitis

Microscopic colitis typically presents with chronic watery non bloody diarrhoea. It typically occurs in middle-aged adults, but occasionally presents in children. The endoscopy is grossly normal, but histopathology reveals abnormal inflammatory findings, characterized by a collagenous colitis or lymphocytic colitis, sometimes with an eosinophilic infiltrate. In some cases, this disorder may represent an overlap with the eosinophilic gastroenteropathies.

Collagenous colitis is a related form of colitis that has been reported in a few children. The colon appears grossly normal, but biopsies show a thickened subepithelial collagenous band in the colonic mucosa.

Autoimmune enteropathies

Autoimmune enteropathies are rare disorders that may present as severe diarrhoea during infancy or toddler hood. The diarrhoea may be isolated, or may occur in association with diabetes mellitus as part of the IPEX syndrome (Immune dysregulation, Polyendocrinopathy and Enteropathy, X-linked), which is associated with mutations in the

FOXP3 gene. IPEX is characterized by chronic diarrhoea, which usually begins in infancy, dermatitis, autoimmune endocrinopathy (diabetes mellitus, thyroiditis).
Autoimmune polyendocrine syndrome 1 (APS-1), also known as autoimmune polyendocrinopathy-candidiasis ectodermal dystrophy (APECED), is one of several autoimmune disorders caused by mutations in the autoimmune regulator gene (AIRE). Features include hypoparathyroidism and adrenal insufficiency, and about 25 percent of patients develop autoimmune enteritis.

5.3.3 Maldigestion of fat

Cystic fibrosis

Cystic fibrosis is the most common cause of pancreatic exocrine insufficiency in children. The disease may present at birth with meconium ileus, or may be suggested later by gastrointestinal symptoms of fat malabsorption, failure to thrive, rectal prolapse (particularly in the setting of diarrhoea) or pulmonary symptoms.

Other causes of pancreatic insufficiency

Other causes of pancreatic exocrine insufficiency include Shwachman-Diamond syndrome (associated with bone marrow failure and skeletal abnormalities), and two rare disorders, Pearson syndrome and Johanson-Blizzard syndrome.

Cholerheic diarrhoea

Patients who have undergone resection of the terminal ileum have impaired absorption of bile acids. If sufficient bile acids enter the colon, they may cause a secretory diarrhoea.
Similarly, patients who have had a cholecystectomy can develop cholerheic diarrhoea because the continuous drainage of bile into the small bowel may overcome the terminal ileum's reabsorptive capacity.

Gastrointestinal protein loss

Signs and symptoms of gastrointestinal protein loss include hypoalbuminemia and reduced concentrations of serum immune globulins. When severe, clinically evident edema is present.

Mucosal disease

Many diseases affecting the intestinal mucosa may cause excessive loss of protein through the gastrointestinal tract. Protein losses may be caused by inflammatory exudation through mucosal erosions (eg, inflammatory bowel disease), or to increased mucosal permeability without erosions (eg, celiac disease). In most cases the protein loss will be accompanied by other signs and symptoms pointing to the cause of the diarrhoea.

Lymphatic obstruction

Obstruction of the intestinal lymphatic impairs lymph flow and increases pressure in the intestinal lymphatics. This leads to leakage of lymph into the intestinal lumen, reduced recirculation of intestinal lymphocytes into the peripheral circulation, and decreased absorption of fat-soluble vitamins.
Primary intestinal lymphangiectasia is characterized by diffuse or localized ectasia of enteric lymphatics.

Secondary intestinal lymphangiectasia may be caused by cardiac diseases, and chemotherapeutic, infectious, or toxic substances that are associated with inflammatory processes that cause retroperitoneal lymph node enlargement, portal hypertension or hepatic venous outflow obstruction.

Bowel obstruction or dysmotility

Partial bowel obstruction or dysmotility may present with diarrhoea.
Hirschsprung's disease – This disorder may present with dysmotility and diarrhoea, and may progress to life-threatening toxic megacolon.
Intestinal pseudo obstruction – This disorder of intestinal motility typically presents with constipation, but patients also may have periods of diarrhoea, particularly if bacterial overgrowth supervenes.

6. Classification based on congenital disorders

6.1 Congenital secretory and osmotic diarrhoeas

Congenital diarrhoea can be caused by a variety of inherited disorders that disrupt nutrient digestion, absorption, or transport, enterocyte development and function, or entero endocrine function. Specific genes have been identified for some of these disorders.

Secretory diarrhoea

Congenital secretory diarrhoea is rare and is characterized by profuse watery diarrhoea beginning at birth. The diarrhoea is so watery that it may be mistaken for urine in the diaper.

Congenital chloride diarrhoea

Congenital chloride diarrhoea is caused by a variety of mutations in the SLC26A3 (solute-linked carrier family 26 member A3) gene, which encodes for an epithelial anion exchanger. Most reported cases are in Finland, Poland, or Arab populations. Because of excessive fecal losses of fluid and electrolytes, affected individuals present in the neonatal period with hyponatremia, hypochloremia, and metabolic alkalosis; there may be a history of polyhydramnios. The diagnosis of CCD is based on the finding of excessive fecal secretion of chloride, in which the chloride concentration exceeds the concentration of cations. However, this finding is only reliable when the patient is in fluid and electrolyte balance. In the untreated patient, the volume and chloride content of the diarrhoea may be artificially reduced.
Congenital sodium diarrhoea – Congenital sodium diarrhoea (CSD) has a syndromic form which includes choanal or anal atresia and is associated with mutations in the SPINT2 gene, which are not seen in patients with isolated CSD. The stool is alkaline and fecal sodium concentrations are high; metabolic acidosis and hyponatremia are typically present; there may be a history of polyhydramnios.
Microvillus inclusion disease – Microvillus inclusion disease (MID) also called microvillus atrophy) was associated with mutations in type Vb myosin motor protein (MYO5B) in several kindreds. The disorder typically presents with intractable secretory diarrhoea shortly after birth, rapidly progressing to hypotonic dehydration and metabolic acidosis. A milder form of MID presents a few months later.
Tufting enteropathy – Tufting enteropathy (also known as intestinal epithelial cell dysplasia) appears to be caused by mutations in the EpCAM (epithelial cell adhesion

molecule) gene. The disorder presents with secretory diarrhoea shortly after birth; the diarrhoea volume is often less than in MID, and may partially respond to fasting.

Epithelial tufts also may be observed in congenital diarrhoea associated with other gene defects, such as in the case of SPINT2-related disease. In such cases, genetic testing can be particularly helpful to define the diagnosis, prognosis, and potential therapy.

Enteric anendocrinosis — Enteric anendocrinosis (also known as congenital malabsorptive diarrhoea 4) is caused by mutations in neurogenin-3 (NEUROG3) and is associated with a paucity of enteroendocrine cells in the pancreas and intestine. It is characterized by an osmotic diarrhoea and later development of insulin-deficient diabetes, without anti-islet cell antibodies. Enteroendocrine and/or enterochromaffin cell paucity can be caused by a variety of other mechanisms.

Osmotic diarrhoea — In contrast with the secretory diarrhoea described above, congenital osmotic diarrhoea ceases during fasting or upon exclusion of certain dietary components that are maldigested by the patient.

Glucose-galactose malabsorption — Glucose-galactose malabsorption presents with severe life-threatening diarrhoea and dehydration during the neonatal period, caused by deficiency in the intestinal sodium/glucose transporter. Patients are symptomatic as long as their diet includes lactose or it's hydrolysis products, glucose and galactose. The diagnosis is suspected if the diarrhoea resolves promptly when these sugars are eliminated, and confirmed by a positive glucose breath hydrogen test and normal intestinal biopsy.

Congenital sucrase-isomaltase deficiency — Congenital sucrase-isomaltase deficiency is rare in most populations, except among individuals of Eskimo or Canadian Native descent. Infants are asymptomatic if their diet contains only lactose (eg, exclusively breast-fed infants), but typically develop chronic diarrhoea after sucrose-containing formulas or foods are introduced. A number of mutations in the gene encoding sucrase-isomaltase have been described in affected individuals.

Steatorrhoea

Defects in pancreatic enzyme activity and lipid trafficking tend to present with chronic low-volume diarrhoea and failure to thrive during infancy, caused by fat malabsorption. These include abetalipoproteinemia and defects of bile acid absorption (eg, primary bile acid malabsorption, or of pancreatic enzyme production (eg, pancreatic lipase deficiency). Neurologic symptoms may ensue, particularly in abetalipoproteinemia.

Chylomicron retention disease (also known as Anderson disease) is characterized by failure to secrete chylomicrons across the basolateral membrane of the enterocyte. Patients generally present with fat malabsorption, steatorrhoea, and failure to thrive during infancy. The lipid distension of the enterocytes causes secondary malabsorption of carbohydrates and amino acids, which may improve with a low-fat diet.

7. Classification based on tumors

7.1 Neuroendocrine tumors

Neuroendocrine tumors affecting the gastrointestinal tract are rare in children; they tend to cause secretory diarrhoea.

Gastrinoma — In this syndrome, also known as Zollinger-Ellison syndrome, unregulated secretion of gastrin causes hypersecretion of gastric acid, with consequent peptic ulcer disease and chronic diarrhoea. Fewer than 5 percent of patients present during adolescence. The disorder may be suspected in a patient presenting with unexplained peptic ulcer disease and/or with a secretory diarrhoea and fat malabsorption. Fasting serum gastrin levels are elevated 5 to 10 fold.

VIPoma – Unregulated hypersecretion of vasoactive intestinal polypeptide (VIP) causes watery diarrhoea, hypokalemia, and achlorhydria. VIPomas are very rare in children, but may occur as ganglioneuromas and ganglioneuroblastomas in the sympathetic ganglia and in the adrenal glands (rather than in the pancreas where they are often found in adults).

Mastocytosis – In children, this disorder usually takes the form of cutaneous mastocytosis, consisting only of the skin lesions of urticaria pigmentosa, and is often self-limited. A few children, particularly those presenting after 2 years of age, have systemic mastocytosis, which may include histamine-induced gastric hypersecretion and chronic diarrhoea.

8. Non specific

Factitious diarrhoea

Factitious diarrhoea may be characterized by a true increase in stool volume, which is self-induced (eg, laxative abuse), or the creation of an apparent increase in stool volume by the addition of various substances to the stool (eg, water or urine). Diagnosing factitious diarrhoea is often difficult and requires alertness to this possibility, exclusion of other diseases, and may be aided by specific testing.

Functional diarrhoea

Functional diarrhoea is defined as the painless passage of three or more large, unformed stools during waking hours for four or more weeks, with onset in infancy or the preschool years, and without failure to thrive or a specific definable cause. This common, benign disorder has also been termed chronic nonspecific diarrhoea of childhood or toddler's diarrhoea.

Children with functional diarrhoea usually pass stools only during waking hours. Early morning stools typically are large and semi-formed, then stools become progressively looser as the day progresses. Virtually all children develop normal bowel patterns by four years of age. In some cases, the diarrhoea is associated with excessive intake of fruit juice, sorbitol, or other osmotically active carbohydrates, and will improve when the intake of these foods is moderated. Other than this precaution, restrictions to the diet or other interventions are not necessary or helpful. In particular, restriction of dietary fat may be counter-productive.

Dysentery

This is diarrhoea with visible blood in the faeces of any duration. Important effects of dysentery include anorexia, rapid weight loss and damage to the intestinal mucosa by the invasive bacteria. A number of other complications may occur. The most important cause of acute dysentery is Shigella; other causes are Campylobacter jejuni and, infrequently, enteroinvasive E. coli or Salmonella. Entamoeba hystolitica can cause serious dysentery in young adults but is rarely a cause of dysentery in young children.

Irritable bowel syndrome

Another possible type of diarrhoea is irritable bowel syndrome (IBS) which usually presents with abdominal discomfort relieved by defecation and unusual stool (diarrhoea or constipation) for at least 3 days a week over 3 months. About 30% of patients with diarrhoea-predominant IBS have bile acid malabsorption. Symptoms of diarrhoea-predominant IBS can be managed through a combination of dietary changes, soluble fiber supplements, and/or medications such as loperamide or codeine.

9. References

[1] Black, RE, Morris SS, Bryce J: Where and why are 10 million children dying every year? Lancet 2003; 361: 2226–2234.

[2] Mortality and Burden of Disease Estimates for WHO Member States in 2004". World Health Organization. http://www.who.int/entity/healthinfo/global_burden_disease/gbddeathdalycountryestimates 2004.

[3] Navaneethan U, Giannella RA. "Mechanisms of infectious diarrhea". Nature Clinical Practice. Gastroenterology & Hepatology 2008; 5 (11): 637–47.

[4] WHO | Diarrhoeal Diseases (Updated February 2009)". World Health Organization. http://www.who.int/vaccine_research/diseases/diarrhoea.

[5] A.I. Frank-Briggs, A.R. Nte. Diarrhoeal Disease: The Trend In A Southern Nigerian City West African Journal of Medicine 2009; 28(4): 211-215.

[6] Patel MM, Hall AJ, Vinjé J, Parashar UD (January 2009). "Noroviruses: a comprehensive review". Journal of Clinical Virology 44 (1): 1–8.

[7] Greenberg HB, Estes MK. "Rotaviruses: from pathogenesis to vaccination". Gastroenterology 2009; 136 (6): 1939–1951.

[8] Mitchell DK. "Astrovirus gastroenteritis". The Pediatric Infectious Disease 2002; 21 (11): 1067–1069.

[9] Frank- Briggs A.I, George I.O. Knowledge of use of zinc in the treatment of Diarrhoeal Diseases among practicing Doctors: The Port Harcourt Experience. The Nigeria Health Journal, 2005; (5): 314-317.

[10] Viswanathan VK, Hodges K, Hecht G. "Enteric infection meets intestinal function: how bacterial pathogens cause diarrhoea". Nature Reviews. Microbiology2009; 7 (2): 110–119.

[11] Rupnik M, Wilcox MH, Gerding DN. "Clostridium difficile infection: new developments in epidemiology and pathogenesis". Nature Reviews. Microbiology 2009;7 (7): 526–536.

[12] Kiser JD, Paulson CP, Brown C. "Clinical inquiries. What's the most effective treatment for giardiasis?". The Journal of Family Practice 2008; 57 (4): 270–272.

[13] Dans L, Martínez E. "Amoebic dysentery". Clinical Evidence 2006; (15): 1007–1013.

[14] Alam NH, Ashraf H. "Treatment of infectious diarrhea in children". Paediatr Drugs 2003; 5 (3): 151–165.

[15] Longstreth GF, Thompson WG, Chey WD, Houghton LA, Mearin F, Spiller RC. "Functional bowel disorders". Gastroenterology 2006; 130 (5): 1480–1491.

[16] Wedlake, L; A'Hern, R, Russell, D, Thomas, K, Walters, JR, Andreyev, HJ. "Systematic review: the prevalence of idiopathic bile acid malabsorption as diagnosed by SeHCAT scanning in patients with diarrhoea-predominant

irritable bowel syndrome.". Alimentary pharmacology & therapeutics 2009; 30 (7): 707-17.

[17] Ejemot RI, Ehiri JE, Meremikwu MM, Critchley JA. Hand washing for preventing diarrhoea. Cochrane Database of Systematic Reviews 2008, Issue 1. Art. No.: CD004265.

[18] King CK, Glass R, Bresee JS, Duggan C. "Managing acute gastroenteritis among children: oral rehydration, maintenance, and nutritional therapy". MMWR Recomm Rep 2003; 52 (RR-16): 1-16.

[19] Schiller LR. "Management of diarrhea in clinical practice: strategies for primary care physicians". Rev Gastroenterol Disord.2007; 7 Suppl 3: S27-38.

[20] Dryden MS, Gabb RJ, Wright SK. "Empirical treatment of severe acute community-acquired gastroenteritis with ciprofloxacin". Clin. Infect. Dis. 1996; 22 (6): 1019-1025.

[21] de Bruyn G. "Diarrhoea in adults (acute)". Clin Evid (Online) 2008.

[22] DuPont HL, Ericsson CD, Farthing MJ, Gorbach S, Pickering LK. "Expert review of the evidence base for self-therapy of travelers' diarrhea". J Travel Med 2009; 16 (3): 161-171.

[23] Pawlowski SW, Warren CA, Guerrant R. "Diagnosis and treatment of acute or persistent diarrhea". Gastroenterology 2009; 136 (6): 1874-1886.

[24] Lazzerini M, Ronfani L. Oral zinc for treating diarrhoea in children. Cochrane Database of Systematic Reviews 2008, Issue 3. Art. No.: CD005436.

[25] Kale-Pradhan PB, Jassal HK, Wilhelm SM. "Role of Lactobacillus in the prevention of antibiotic-associated diarrhea: a meta-analysis". Pharmacotherapy 2010; 30 (2): 119-126.

[26] Guarino A, Albano F, Guandalini S, Working Group on Acute Gastroenteritis. Oral rehydration: toward a real solution. J Pediatr Gastroenterol Nutr 2001; 33 Suppl 2:S2.

[27] Boschi-Pinto C, Velebit L, Shibuya K. Estimating child mortality due to diarrhoea in developing countries. Bull World Health Organ 2008; 86:710.

[28] Kosek M, Bern C, Guerrant RL. The global burden of diarrhoeal disease, as estimated from studies published between 1992 and 2000. Bull World Health Organ 2003; 81:197.

[29] Bryce J, Boschi-Pinto C, Shibuya K, Black RE and the WHO Child Health Epidemiology Reference Group. WHO estimates of the causes of death in children. Lancet 2005; 365:1147.

[30] Ryan ET, Dhar U, Khan WA, Salam WA, Faruque ASG, Fuchs GJ. Mortality, morbidity, and microbiology of endemic cholera among hospitalized patients in Dhaka, Bangladesh. Am J Trop Med Hyg 2000; 63:12.

[31] Karim AS, Akhter S, Rahman MA, Nazir MF. Risk factors of persistent diarrhea in children below five years of age. Indian J Gastroenterol 2001; 20:59.

[32] Binder HJ. Causes of chronic diarrhea. N Engl J Med 2006; 355:236.

[33] Ochoa TJ, Salazar-Lindo E, Cleary TG. Management of children with infection-associated persistent diarrhea. Semin Pediatr Infect Dis 2004; 15:229.

[34] Wedlake L, A'Hern R, Russell D, Thomas K, Walters JR, Andreyev HJ. "Systematic review: the prevalence of idiopathic bile acid malabsorption as diagnosed by SeHCAT scanning in patients with diarrhoea-predominant irritable bowel syndrome". Alimentary pharmacology & therapeutics 2009; 30 (7): 707–17.

7

Traveller's Diarrhoea and Intestinal Protozoal Diarrhoeal Disease

Constantine M. Vassalos and Evdokia Vassalou
National School of Public Health, Athens
Greece

1. Introduction

Traveller's diarrhoea is usually a mild gastrointestinal disorder. It is generally acute and short-term, but in 10 percent of all cases symptoms last for more than a week. Bacterial and viral agents are responsible for more than 80 percent of cases of acute traveller's diarrhoea. Though incriminated in only one to three percent of cases of acute traveller's diarrhoea, parasites –mainly protozoa– account for about 30 percent of cases of persistent diarrhoea in travellers (Leder, 2009; Okhuysen, 2001). Recent acceleration and expansion of international travel for business, leisure, philanthropic or other purposes has contributed to an increase in cases of intestinal protozoal disease in the developed world (Topazian & Bia, 1994; Vassalou & Vassalos et al., 2010).

2. Traveller's diarrhoea

Since the 1950s, a decade which saw an increase in trips to exotic locales, the prospect of developing diarrhoea has been a major concern for foreign travellers. It is believed that traveller's diarrhoea is the most common health problem of people journeying abroad for education, research, business, or pleasure. Traveller's diarrhoea is classically defined as the passage of three or more unformed stools in a 24-hour period with or without mild gastrointestinal symptoms including cramps, nausea and mild fever (Steffen, 2005). More serious gastrointestinal symptoms, such as vomiting and dysentery with blood and/or mucus in the stool, are rare. Owing to the brief incubation period that ranges from hours to a few days, it is most likely that traveller's diarrhoea will develop on the third or fourth day of the travel. A second peak is observed around the 10th day, although some digestive problems may occur at any time (Cailhol & Bouchaud, 2007).

3. Aetiological agents

Many non-infectious phenomena, such as a change in lifestyle, climate or eating habits, consumption of spicy foods, and psychosomatic conditions, have been incriminated as causes of diarrhoea in the traveller. However, traveller's diarrhoea is generally of an infectious origin. Bacteria account for approximately 60 to 80 percent of all cases, whereas viral agents and parasites, mainly protozoa, are responsible for about 10 to 20 percent and 5 to 10 percent of the cases, respectively (Ericsson et al., 2008). There are differences in causality among travel destinations, depending on the geographical distribution of pathogenic organisms. Enterotoxigenic *Escherichia coli*, or ETEC, is a major bacterial cause of traveller's diarrhoea worldwide. Several other bacteria, for instance *Shigella, Campylobacter, Salmonella, Aeromonas, Plesiomonas,* and non-cholera vibrio species, have also been involved (Shah, 2009). Rarely is *Vibrio cholerae* transmitted to western travellers. The risk of contracting cholera is estimated at one per 500,000 travellers to endemic areas (Synder & Blake, 1982). Enterotoxigenic *Bacteroides fragilis*, or ETBF, and *Arcobacter* strains including diarrhoeagenic *A. butzleri* as well as *A. cryaerophilus*, formerly considered non-pathogenic, have recently been shown to cause diarrhoea in those travelling to different parts of the Indian subcontinent and Latin America (Houf & Stephan, 2007; Jiang et al., 2010). In cruise ships and tourist resorts, there is high risk of acquiring viruses such as noroviruses (Domènech-Sánchez et al., 2009; Koo et al., 1996). Rotavirus, a common paediatric pathogen, has also been found in adults with traveller's diarrhoea (Anderson & Weber, 2004). *Giardia* is the most commonly encountered parasite among travellers with diarrhoea. *Cryptosporidium, Cyclospora, Isospora,* and microsporidia are emerging causes (Goodgame et al., 2005). Aetiological agents and their order of occurrence by different geographical regions are shown in Table 1.

Aetiological agents	Africa	Latin America	South Asia	Southeast Asia
Enterotoxigenic *Escherichia coli*	1	1	1	5
Enteroaggregative *E. coli*		2	2	
Enteropathogenic *E coli*	4	4		2
Campylobacter			4	1
Salmonella			5	3
Shigella	3		3	
Non-cholera vibrios				4
Norovirus	2	3		
Rotavirus	5	5		

Table 1. Traveller's diarrhoea: aetiological agents and their order of occurrence (from 1 to 5) among different geographical regions (adapted from Shah et al., 2009).

3.1 Pathogenicity

A variety of pathogens have been shown to contribute to traveller's diarrhoea. Based on the pathophysiological mechanism responsible for the diarrhoea, their pathogenicity can be divided into non-inflammatory, enteroinvasive, and inflammatory types. However, irrespective of the mechanism involved, the host defence system is evaded and modulated. Concerning traveller's diarrhoea of bacterial origin, the non-inflammatory diarrhoeas are due to enterotoxin-producing organisms, such as *Vibrio cholerae* and ETEC, which adhere to the mucosa and disrupt the absorptive and secretory functions of the enterocyte. In the case of viral traveller's diarrhoea, viruses such as rotaviruses disrupt the digestive and absorptive functions of the enterocyte: therefore the diarrhoea caused by the rotavirus is classified as osmotic. Enteroinvasive organisms such as *Salmonella, Shigella, Campylobacter*, or *Entamoeba histolytica* produce diarrhoea by invading intestinal mucosal barriers, followed by the initiation of acute inflammatory reaction through activation of cytokines and other

Localization	Enteropathogens	Virulence factors	Mechanisms
Small bowel	Enterotoxinogenic *E.coli* (ETEC)	Colonization factors (CFs) (adherence) Heat-labile toxin (LT), Heat-stable toxin (ST) (toxins)	Secretory (toxinogenic)
	Enteroaggregative *E.coli* (EAEC)	AAFs, dispersin (adherence) EAST1, Pet, Pic, ShET1 (toxins)	
	Vibrio cholerae	ACF, TCP (adherence) Ace, CT, RTX toxin, Zot (toxins)	
	Vibrio parahaemolyticus	Vp-TDH, Vp-TRH, Vp-TDH/1 (haemolysins)	
	Rotavirus	VP4 (adherence) NSP4 (toxin)	Osmotic Apoptosis of enterocytes Absorptive villus Architecture disruption
	Norovirus	VP1-P2 domain (adherence)	
	Giardia spp.	Variant-specific surface proteins (VSPs), arginine deiminase	
	Cryptosporidium spp.	Unknown	
	Cyclospora	Unknown	
Large bowel	*Entamoeba histolytica*	Gal-specific adhesin , cysteine proteinases, amoebapores Gal/GalNAc lectin, amoebapore and cystein proteases	Invasive
Small bowel and large bowel ileocolonic	*Campylobacter* spp.	CadF, JlpA, LOS, MOMP, PEB1 capsule (adherence) CiaB (invasion) CDT (toxin)	Inflammatory Invasive
	Shigella spp.	IcP, (SopA), Pic, SigA (protease) ShET1, ShET2, Shiga toxin (*S. dysenteriae*) (serotype 1 only) (toxin)	
	Salmonella spp.	AgF, LpF, MisL, Pef, RatB, ShdA, SinH, Type 1 fimbriae (adherence) Vi antigen (*S. enterica*) (serovar typhi) (immune evasion) CdtB (*S. enterica*) (serovar typhi), Spv (toxin)	
	Aeromonas hydrophila	Cytotonic Alt [heat-labile] and Ast [heat-stable], cytotoxic Act (enterotoxin) aerolysin (cytotoxin), hyl H (haemolysin).	
	Yersinia enterocolitica	Ail, Invasin (invasion) Yst (toxin)	

Table 2. Traveller's diarrhoea: localization, mechanisms and virulence factors of enteropathogens.

inflammatory mediators. In addition to enteroinvasive organisms, inflammatory diarrhoea can also be caused by cytotoxin-producing non-invasive bacteria, such as EAEC and *Clostridium difficile*, which adhere to the intestinal mucosa, activate cytokines and release inflammatory mediators (Navaneethan and Giannella, 2008).

3.1.1 Virulence factors

All the classical virulence factors including endotoxins, fimbriae and flagella, plasmids, apoptotic inducers, pathogenic islands and complete types I, II, and III secretion systems have been identified as being responsible for traveller's diarrhoea. Virulence factors in strains of *E. coli, Shigella, Salmonella, Vibrio, Campylobacter, Aeromonas, Yersinia, E. histolytica, Giardia*, and norovirus, as well as genes encoding virulence factors in these enteropathogens have been analysed. These factors are listed in Table 2. Research continues into candidate virulence factors of *Cryptosporidium* spp., while virulence factors of *Cyclospora* are yet to be defined.

4. Epidemiological data

Each year 100 million people from industrialized countries travel to areas of high risk for contracting traveller's diarrhoea, the majority of which are in the developing world. And up to 40 million cases of diarrhoea are reported among such travellers. Approximately 15 to 50 percent of travellers to tropical and subtropical areas in Africa, the Caribbean and Latin America, or in South Asia may develop diarrhoea (Steffen, 2005). Traveller's diarhoea can affect men and women equally. It is rare in travellers over the age of 55, while it is more frequent in children and in young adults under the age of 30 (Pitzinger et al, 1991). A Geosentinel study indicated that in more than 17,000 international travellers acute and chronic diarrhoea were the most common syndromes —at a rate of 335 diarrhoeal cases per 1,000 returned travellers (Freedman et al., 2006). Travellers to South Central Asia are at the greatest risk of contracting acute diarrhoea. On the other hand, the highest rates of chronic diarrhoea were reported after a journey to West Africa and East Asia (Sanders et al., 2008). ETEC is the main causal agent of traveller's diarrhoea in Africa, Latin America, and South Asia, followed by enteroaggregative *E. coli*, or EAEC, in Latin America and South Asia, whereas *Campylobacter* predominates in Southeast Asia (Hill & Beeching, 2010). Of the viral agents, noroviruses were found in mixed infections with bacteria such as ETEC in one-third of diarrhoea cases among those travelling to Latin America (Chapin et al., 2005). Rotaviruses are also frequent causes of traveller's diarrhoea in Mexico and Jamaica (Steffen et al., 1999; Vollet e al., 1979,). Considering parasites, *Giardia* has been mostly found after travel to central parts of South Asia (Freedman et al., 2006). *E. histolytica*, like other parasites, is frequently encountered among travellers returning from Asia, however seldom found after a short stay in Mexico (Frachtman et al., 1982; Freedman et al., 2006). Study groups in Nepal, Haiti and Peru have shown that *Cyclospora* is endemic in the regions of South Asia, the Caribbean and Latin America, respectively (Yates, 2005). In most cases, traveller's diarrhoea is quite mild, benign, and lasts for a short period of time (Hill, 2000). However, in 40 percent of the cases, digestive disturbances may lead to a change in travel plan with a potential for serious negative impact on the travel objective, for instance that of a business traveller. In 20 to 30 percent of cases, travellers may be confined to bed for a period of time, while in some (<1%) hospitalization is required.

5. Sources and modes of transmission

Traveller's diarrhoea is most commonly contracted by ingesting food and/or beverage contaminated with faecal material of human or animal origin. Despite the popular belief that drinking water posed the most significant risk for traveller's diarrhoea, unsafe/contaminated food was shown to be the major vehicle for infection. Raw or rare meat, poultry and seafood, and also the fruit and vegetables eaten raw are the more likely vehicles to spread the pathogens. Direct contact with contaminated, unwashed hands and indirect transmission by non-biting flies, such as the house fly, play only secondary roles in the transmission of diarrhoea to the traveller.

6. Risk factors

There are a variety of environmental and host-related factors that can predispose travellers to diarrhoeal illness. These risk factors include those that are associated with travel destination, planning, or seasonality and those in relation with the traveller's age, eating habits, or susceptibility.

Environment has been considered to have an impact on traveller's diarrhoea. The wider hygiene gap between the country of origin with a higher level and that of the destination may put a traveller at greater risk of contracting traveller's diarrhoea. Travel destinations are classified into three groups according to their hygiene level. Group I includes developed countries such as the United States, Canada, Australia, New Zealand, Japan, and the North and Western European countries with high level of hygiene and consequent low risk for acquiring diarrhoea by travellers to those countries (at a rate less than eight percent). Group II consists of areas of intermediate risk (at a rate of eight to 20 percent): such as Eastern European countries, South Africa, tourist places in Thailand, the Caribbean, and the Mediterranean. Areas of low hygiene level and high risk (at a rate more than 20 percent), such as the most part of Asia, the Middle East, Africa, and Central and South America, belong to group III. Furthermore, individuals travelling to temperate regions in winter are less at risk: for instance, the rate for *Campylobacter* infection was 58 percent in autumn, while it was only eight percent in the wintertime (Mattila et al., 1992). A recent study indicated that the rate for both enteroaggregative and enteropathogenic *Escherichia coli* infections among visitors to Mexico in winter was similar to that recorded in summer, whereas the rate of ETEC traveller's diarrhoea increased by seven percent for each degree centigrade increase in weekly ambient temperature (Paredes-Paredes et al., 2011). In travellers to the Tropics, however, the occurrence of diarrhoea does not seem to follow a clear seasonal pattern: EAEC, *Shigella*, and rotavirus are mostly found during the dry season. And those travelling during the rainy season or post-moonson are at a high risk for acquiring traveller's diarrhoea due to ETEC or *Giardia*, but not viral diarrhoea. (Taylor & Echeverria, 1986). The effect of the El Niño/Southern Oscillation, or ENSO, climate phenomenon should also be considered: the rise in average annual temperatures related with ENSO event has been positively associated with risk of diarrhoeal disease (Lauerman, 2001; Lama et al., 2004; Sari Kovats et al., 2003).

Travel plans and itineraries are also related to the possibility of exposure. Campers and backpackers, people who have more contact with the rural population, are at a higher risk than are business travellers (Piyaphanee et al., 2011). Being busy and often confined to their hotel rooms, business travellers dine in their hotels. Organized travelling and planned itineraries may be considered safer. However, unforeseen situations may arise (Vassalos & Vassalou et al., 2011). For instance, travellers may end up eating food that has been on display for several hours or may try food from street vendors and local popular restaurants (Tjoa et al.,1977; Adachi, 2002). In the latter case, inadequate water supplies can lead to incorrect dish washing. Improper storage of food may also result from limited access to electricity. Recently, it has been shown that food contamination is widespread in developing countries despite the fact that food is cooked and served hot (Koo et al., 2008). Also, the individual traveller may or may not practise sound eating habits regarding consumption of food and/or water. Travellers visiting areas with access to clean drinking water and food are at lower risk for diarrhoea. In addition to all the foregoing, overcrowded areas such as campgrounds, military camps and cruise ships are particularly prone to diarrhoeal disease.

Besides environmental factors, host-related factors, viz personal factors and host genetic background, may also contribute to traveller's diarrhoea risk. Traveller's diarrhoea usually develops at the beginning of the tour. A longer stay may, however, increase the possibility of the occurrence of a gastrointestinal disorder (Piyaphanee et al., 2011). Young people are the ones most likely to develop diarrhoeal disease because of their keenness to explore the local flavours. Elderly travellers are less liable to contract diarrhoea, since they are more cautious about what they eat and drink (Alon et al., 2010). But they are also more likely to suffer complications because of their immunocompromised status from having debilitating, underlying medical conditions, such as diabetes, renal failure or hypochlorhydria induced by taking antacids. Rehydration therapy is important for the very young, elderly and those in cardiac glycosides or diuretics (DuPont & Khan, 1994). In contrast, healthy travellers visiting areas of low hygienic level may only experience mild gastrointestinal symptoms. The development of natural immunity plays a role in the lower rates of diarrhoeal disease among the locals in destination countries with relatively lower levels of socio-economic development. Similarly, earlier travel to an area of low hygienic level would also reduce the possibility of acquiring traveller's diarrhoea due to the immunity acquired from previous exposure to pathogens prevalent in such areas (DuPont et al., 1986). That is particularly important for travellers with high socio-economic status, who are less likely to develop protective immunity in their countries of origin.

Persons with blood type O are susceptible to developing cholera, whereas individuals with blood type A are more likely to get giardiasis (Harris et al., 2005; El- Ganayni et al., 1994). Differences in ABO, Lewis, secretor phenotypes seem to be associated with differences in susceptibility to infection caused by norovirus strains (Huang et al., 2002; Hutson et al., 2002; Marionneau et al., 2005). Several single nucleotide polymorphisms, or SNPs, have been investigated for possible association with traveller's diarrhoea. It was found that travellers with the T/T genotype in position codon 632 of the lactoferrin gene were more likely to develop traveller's diarrhoea (Mohamed et al., 2007). Polymorphism in the interleukin (IL)-8 promoter appears to be associated with susceptibility to EAEC (Jiang et al., 2003), whereas polymorphism in IL-10 promoter is likely to be associated with traveller's diarrohea due to ETEC (Flores et al., 2008). Osteoprotegerin, or OPG, is an immunoregulatory member of the tumour necrosis factor receptor superfamily. Polymorphism in the OPG gene has been found to be associated with increased susceptibility to traveller's diarrhoea (Mohamed et al., 2009).

7. Diagnostic approach

In a returned traveller with diarrhoea, a history of events is required to be established post-travel; a questionnaire concerning travel destination and conditions, eating habits, antimalarial chemoprophylaxis, onset of symptoms and other matters is suggested. In post-travel febrile diarrhoea, the traveller should be tested for malaria, given that malarial gastrointestinal manifestations are quite common. Once malaria is excluded, further work up should include routine haematological and biochemical testing, transabdominal ultrasound scan, stool culture and microscopy for cells, ova and parasites. For the isolation of *Escherichia coli, Campylobacter, Salmonella, Shigella, Aeromonas, Plesiomonas, Vibrio* and *Yersinia*, standard microbiological procedures are used. ETBF culture is carried out under anaerobic conditions. In the past, an aetiological agent remained unidentified in about 40 percent of such cases. Improved modern techniques have proven helpful in increasing the rate of identification of the cause of diarrhoea (Shah et al., 2009). The possibility of detecting *Shigella, Salmonella* or *Campylobacter* has increased substantially by using polymerase-chain-reaction (PCR)-based methods. Molecular techniques are used to detect the heat-labile and the heat-stable toxins of ETEC, aggR gene of EAEC , ipaH and invE genes of EIEC, and the genes of *B. fragilis* toxin of ETBF. To detect noroviruses, immunochromatography and reverse transcriptase PCR are employed. Diagnostic approach of traveller's diarrhoea is demonstrated in Figure 1.

8. Prevention

8.1 Hygiene measures

Traveller's diarrhoea is associated with inadequate sanitation and hygiene in countries being toured. Occurrence of traveller's diarrhoea is also related to the hygienic standards practised at the food preparation level. The challenge is to avoid faecal contamination of food and water. Furthermore, there is a need to minimize the burden of pathogen in the food and/or water just before consumption (Bandres et al., 1988). It has been shown that consumption of cold foods stored at a temperature that allows microorganisms to grow and produce toxins is responsible for small clusters of sickness even in luxury hotels.

The old adage 'boil it, cook it, peel it, or forget it' remains valid at the individual level. A traveller often wants to taste a local cuisine or to try vendor food, or a traveller may be forced to consume water of suspect quality. Table 3 shows a list of some foods and beverages that could be consumed safely during travel, and some others that are best avoided. Practical methods for water disinfection are: boiling for 1 min (or for 3 min at altitudes above 2, 000 m/6, 562 ft), or filtering through a 0.10 to 0.30 μm membrane in order to remove bacteria and protozoan parasites followed by chlorination or iodination to kill viruses. Travellers should remember to wash their hands with soap and running water or to use alcohol-based gels or solutions for a thorough hand-rub after going to the bathroom and before eating. In the case of infants, the best prevention measure is breastfeeding. Alternatively, infant formula should be prepared by using boiling hot water. Traveller's diarrhoea is also related to leisure activities such as swimming and diving in lakes or rivers, which are contaminated with human sewage or animal faeces. Consequently, travellers should choose to swim or dive in swimming-pools, which are kept properly sanitised and are regularly checked, even though protozoal cysts and viruses are resistant to usual levels of chlorination.

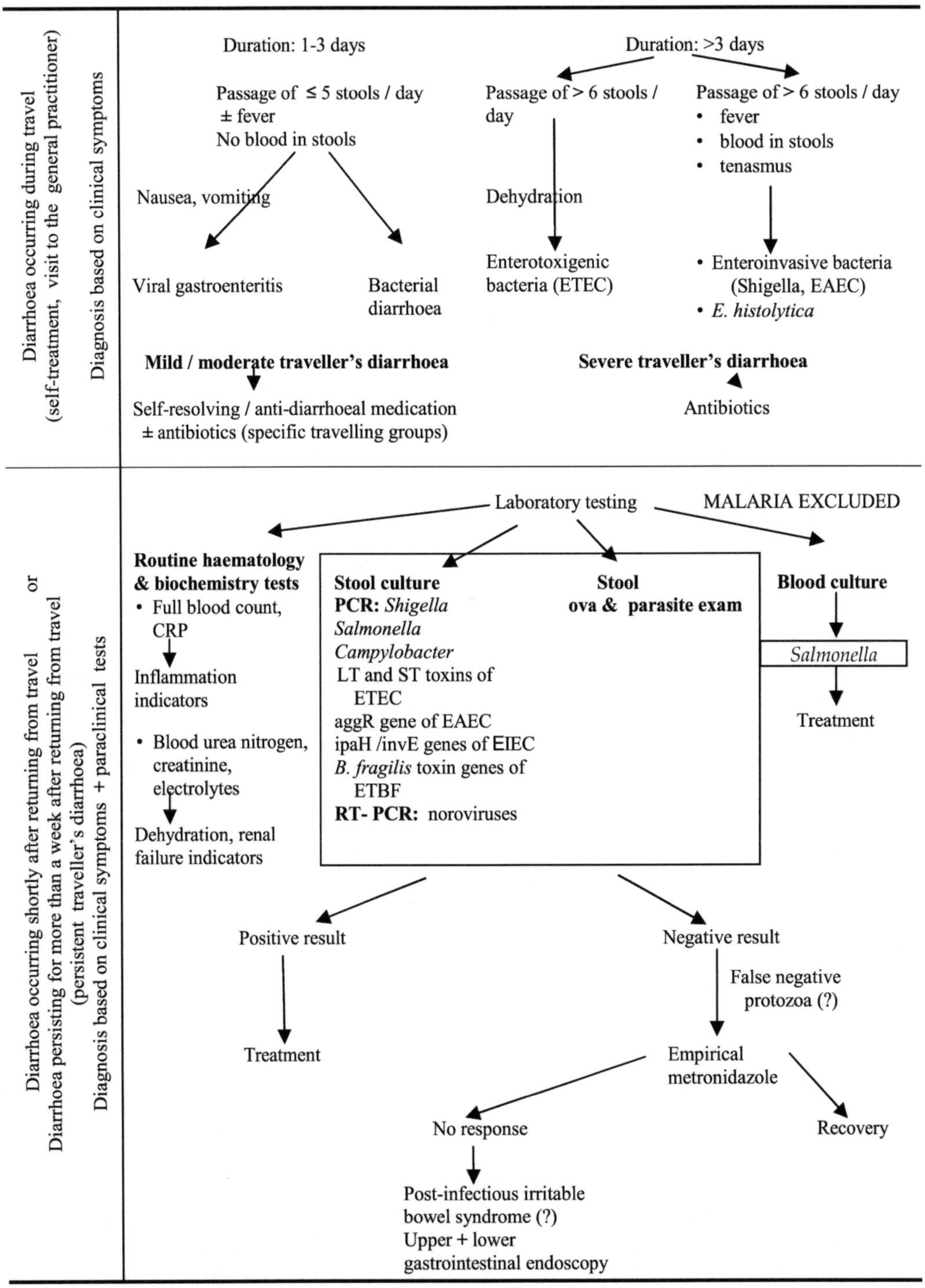

Fig. 1. Diagnostic approach and management of traveller's diarrhoea.

Foods and beverages that can be consumed	Foods and beverages that would be better avoided
Dry items such as bread, biscuits, or dry foods Syrups, jellies, jams, honey Any foods carefully prepared in one's own apartment or hotel Cooked foods consumed hot Beverages served steaming hot Decontaminated water (through filtration, chlorination or iodination) Bottled water with intact seal apparent on opening Bottled carbonated drinks including soft drinks and beer Fruits peeled by the traveller	Moist foods served at room temperature including vegetables and meats Underdone meat and fish Hot sauces on tabletop Seafood Ice-creams Salads Milk and dairy products Prepared foods eaten cold Any food served buffet-style maintained at room temperature Hamburgers not served hot or at fast food service restaurants with rapid turnover of prepared hamburgers (hamburger toppings are a major concern in these areas) Tap water even in hotels claiming filtration systems Large quantities of ice Non-bottled drinks Fruits and vegetables with intact skins: berries, tomatoes Pre-peeled fruit

Table 3. Examples of foods and beverages that can be consumed and the ones better avoided.

8.2 Chemoprophylaxis

8.2.1 Non-antimicrobial agents

Bismuth subsalicylate has been shown to provide a 65 percent protection rate in cases of traveller's diarrhoea, when the typical dosage of 525 mg is orally given four times daily. Bismuth subsalicylate cannot be used for a period more than three weeks. Bismuth subsalicylate should be avoided in travelling children and in travellers on anticoagulants owing to the activity of the salicylate ions (Diemert, 2006; Ericsson, 2005)

8.2.2 Probiotics

Probiotics, such as *Lactobacillus rhamnosum* strain GG, *L. acidophilus, L. bulgaricus,* and *Saccharomyces boulardii,* are live microorganisms capable of colonizing the intestine, and thus competing with enteric pathogenic microorganisms. These strains may secrete antimicrobial agents, induce the production of mucin or modulate immune response. Use of probiotics can be considered an alternative prophylaxis against traveller's diarrhoea, even though the protection provided by them is still quite low with a rate of only 47 percent (Hilton et al., 1997; McFarland, 2007). No side effects were observed; yet in elderly or immunocompromised travellers and in travellers with an underlying condition, probiotcs should be prescribed with caution (DuPont, 2008).

8.2.3 Antibiotics

Pre-travel medical consultation should make the decision regarding the need and modality of antibiotic prophylaxis. The doctor and traveller should first discuss the plan and duration of the journey. Antibiotic prophylactic is only recommended for a select group of travellers (DuPont & Ericsson, 1993). Such a group comprises those with immunodeficiency, including travellers with AIDS or neoplasia, travellers undergoing treatment with immunosuppressants, travellers with an underlying condition, i.e. diabetes, that could be worsened by the diarrhoeal illness, and those with achlorhydria or hypochlorhydria due to gastrectomy, administration of a H_2 receptor blocker or a proton pump inhibitor.

Antibiotic prophylaxis may also be recommended for certain important business travels of short duration. Situations where such a use can be justified are: travel for negotiating and signing important business deals, politicians gathering for summits, athletes participating in international meetings, speakers making presentations at international conferences, or students travelling for a short duration to appear in an examination or any other similar situation. Antibiotic prophylaxis can induce a false sense of security in a traveller who may consequently relax the adherence to hygiene and other precautions. This raises the possibility of infection by resistant organisms and worse outcomes. Hypersensitivity to the prescribed antibiotic can be a serious problem during travel. Vaginal candidiasis is not uncommon in such cases and pseudomembranous colitis due to *Clostridium difficile* can be a serious illness (DuPont et al., 2009). Antibiotic prophylaxis should be taken with caution and the administration should never exceed a period of two to three weeks. Although small, the risk of emerging resistant strains should also be taken into account, since the antibiotics used for traveller's diarrhoea prophylaxis and treatment are the same. Fluoroquinolones provide up to 90 percent protection. The oral administration of ciprofloxacin, 500 mg once a day, or norfloxacin, 400 mg once a day, starts upon arrival at travel destination and continues for 24 to 48 hours after departure from areas of elevated risk of traveller's diarrhoea. With fluoroquinolones taken as a short-term prophylaxis, the risk of side effects is small. Yet the emergence of resistance not just for Enterobacteriaceae strains such as *Campylobacter* spp. as found in Southeast Asia, but also for strains of *Salmonella* spp. and *Shigella* spp. is a major concern. Such an occurrence could reverse the progress made so far in the prevention and management of traveller's diarrhoea (Kuschner et al., 1998; Lindgren et al., 2009; Mensa et al., 2008). This has not been a concern when using rifaximin in a dose of 200 mg orally twice a day. Rifaximin given orally is poorly absorbed (Koo et al., 2010). It offers a 58 to 77 percent protection rate and does not affect intestinal flora even after continuous administration for a period of two weeks (DuPont et al., 2005). Also, it can be used to prevent traveller's diarrhoea in children who are at least 12 years old.

8.3 Immunoprophylaxis and vaccines

Although diarrhoea due to heat-labile toxin (LT) producing ETEC is more frequent in travellers, the development of vaccines that protect against more than one pathogenic strain is challenging. Today, oral, inactivated vaccine against cholera, which consists of killed whole cell, or WC, *Vibrio cholerae* and the non-toxic, recombinant cholera toxin B-subunit, or BS, is the only vaccine proven to fight a form of traveller's diarrhoea. But it is only administered to specific travelling groups such as people involved in humanitarian aid and military personnel deployed overseas, if travelling to an area where they are going to be at unavoidable risk of exposure to cholera. Nevertheless, the amino acid sequences of cholera toxin B subunit and LT toxin of ETEC share approximately 80 percent homology, thus implying that the WS/BS vaccine may also offer some protection against traveller's diarrhoea caused by enterotoxigenic *E. coli* (Hill et al., 2006). Unfortunately, since the temporary protection provided is moderate at a rate of only seven percent, the use of WC/BS vaccine against cholera is therefore not routinely recommended for the majority of travellers (Hill et al., 2006). Transcutaneous vaccine, comprising purified LT toxin of ETEC, does not appear to offer either statistically significant protection against ETEC or any in general protection against traveller's diarrhoea (Frech et al., 2008).

9. Treatment

Traveller's diarrhoea treatment includes rehydration, diet, antisecretory agents, antimotility drugs, and antibiotics.

9.1 Rehydration

Traveller's diarrhoea does not usually cause dehydration. If patients are otherwise healthy and are not dehydrated, they can drink water *ad libitum*. They can rehydrate by taking frequent, small sips of bottled/boiled water or a rehydration drink. Until diarrhoea subsides, patients should avoid consuming beverages with high osmolality or caffeine content. These drinks can aggravate diarrhoea (Ericsson et al., 2008). Fluid replacement with oral rehydration solution is necessary for the very young and the elderly travellers, since they are vulnerable to the effects of dehydration (Rose et al., 2010). Further, in potentially dehydrating diarrhoea cases, oral rehydration solution should be used by all age groups: excessive fluid loss is not a rare event among adult travellers to the developing countries, especially in South Asia, where enterotoxigenic *E. coli* is the predominant cause of traveller's diarrhoea (Table 1). In an attempt to maintain a good state of hydration, vigorous treatment of traveller's diarrhoea should start as soon as the diarrhoea begins (Ericsson et al., 2008; Rose et al., 2010).

9.2 Diet

Complete abstention from food is neither required nor recommended, since foods providing calories are necessary to facilitate renewal of mucosal cells lining the intestine (Lever & Soffer, 2009). Dietary restriction, on the whole, has been questioned lately except for food or drinks with high content of simple carbohydrates. Patients with traveller's diarrhoea have been advised to restrict lactose containing foods after correcting dehydration because of transient lactase deficiency (Ericsson et al., 2008). But no hard evidence has yet surfaced to support that dietary restriction benefits those travelling to developing countries (Gottlieb & Heather, 2011; Huang et al., 2004). Instead, frequent small meals, incorporating well cooked complex carbohydrates/starch such as mashed potatoes, rice or other cereals, are being generally encouraged. This may not be important for a well nourished adult traveller from a developed country but would be an important consideration in travellers, whose nutritional status is borderline and may be further affected by the loss of appetite (Ericsson et al., 2008).

9.3 Non-antimicrobial agents

Non-antimicrobial agents can be used in cases of travellers with mild to moderate diarrhoea. Bismuth subsalicylate is composed of a bismuth oxide core structure with salicylate ions attached to the surface. It exerts antisecretory, antimicrobial and adsorbent effects to control diarrhoea, even though its exact mechanism still remains unknown. It was shown that bismuth subsalicylate can alleviate non-specific symptoms such as nausea in patients with traveller's diarrhoea (Hill & Beeching, 2011). The dosage of 525 mg is orally given every half hour eight times daily. In travellers with acquired immunodeficiency syndrome or with chronic enteric disease, bismuth absorption may occur across the damaged mucosa (DuPont et al., 2009b). Serious neurotoxic and nephrotoxic adverse events may be attributable to the use of bismuth (Bao, 2006). The highest concentrations of absorbed bismuth are found in the kidneys and liver (Fowler & Sexton, 2007). Bismuth subsalicylate should not be used by travellers with renal or hepatic impairment. Antisecretory racecadotril, 100 mg after the first loose stool followed by 100 mg three times daily up to seven days, which acts as a peripherally acting enkephlalinase inhibitor, is prescribed in patients with traveller's diarrhoea. In pediatric patients, it is given as an adjunct to oral rehydration therapy. Antimotility agents may be good for relieving the symptoms of traveller's diarrhoea and used as adjuncts to antibiotic treatment. Loperamide, the most widely used antimotility drug, is an opioid-receptors agonist, which does not affect the central nervous system, acts on the opioid receptors of the myenteric plexus of the large intestine and decreases intestinal movements. Two capsules are recommended as the initial dose and subsequently one capsule is given after each unformed stool, with clinical improvement being seen within 48 hours. Although it may trap pathogens in the intestine, loperamide may help travellers who cannot afford to have diarrhoea during a short-term trip of critical importance. It should not be given in the presence of mucus or blood in the stool with or without fever, which represents diarrhoea due to enteroinvasive bacteria. Loperamide may cause narcotic intoxication and ileus in young children and be responsible for severe constipation in the elderly (Galleli et al., 2010; Li et al., 2007). The use of antimotility agents by the pediatric and geriatric population is not always without risk and should perhaps be avoided.

9.4 Antibiotics

Antibiotics are used in moderate and severe traveller's diarrhoea. Such antimicrobial agents are fluoroquinolones, azithromycin and rifaximin (Table 4).

Fluoroquinolones, which are synthetic broad spectrum antibiotics, are active against invasive bacteria including *Shigella*, even though, mainly in Southeast Asia, resistance of *Campylobacter* to fluoroquinolones has emerged. In the latter case, azithromycin, which is a subclass of macrolide antibiotics, is recommended; it has high intracellular concentrations and serum-based definition of resistance does not necessarily apply to controlling the disease in a clinical situation. If the traveller wishes for a prompt relief from afebrile, gastrointestinal symptoms, loperamide can be taken in combination with one of the antibiotics mentioned above. Among travellers visiting Mexico, loperamide combined with azithromycin was shown to reduce the time from the last unformed stool when compared to those who were administered only azithromycin (Ericsson et al., 2007). Rifaximin, a novel semi-synthetic derivative of rifamycin, is active against ETEC but not against invasive bacteria (Taylor et al., 2008).

9.5 Self evaluation and treatment

Traveller's diarrhoea usually develops shortly after arrival at the travel destination. Study indicates that 80 percent of patients with traveller's diarrhoea choose to treat themselves

Antibiotic per os[a]	Adults' dosage (normal renal function)	Children's dosage (normal renal function)[b]
Fluoroquinolones		
Norfloxacin	800 mg once or 400 mg b.i.d. for 1-5 days	-
Levofloxacin	500 mg once or 500 mg q.d. for 1-5 days	-
Ofloxacin	400 mg once or 200 mg b.i.d. for 1-5 days	-
Ciprofloxacin	750 mg once or 500 mg b.i.d for 1-5 days	10-15 mg kg^{-1} b.i.d. for 3 days
Macrolide		
Azithromycin	500-1000 mg [c] once or 500mg q.d. for 3 days	20 mg kg^{-1} q.d. for 3 days
Rifamycin derivate		
Rifaximin	200 mg t.i.d.[d]	-

[a] Antibiotics taking should be interrupted in case of improvement
[b] Children's dose should not exceed adult dose
[c] 1000 mg azithromycin dose can cause nausea
[d] Rifaximin should not be administered in bloody diarrhoea

Table 4. Antibiotics dosage for moderate or severe traveller's diarrhoea.

irrespective of the illness being mild or more severe (Hill, 2000). For that reason, during pre-travel consultation, travellers should be given information about the problem and importance of traveller's diarrhoea and instructed on how to proceed with self-evaluation. Local medical help should be sought if diarrhoea lasts for more than 48 hours or in case of fever, blood or mucus in the stool. Otherwise, travellers could replace lost fluids and electrolytes and take non-antimicrobial agents in their possession. In high risk areas with difficult access to medical services, travellers should promptly start taking antibiotics (immediately after the symptoms appear, and before they get worse). The choice of antibiotic should be determined by the locally prevalent predominant organisms and their sensitivity pattern. Fluoroquinolones are usually recommended for most travel destinations excepting South and Southeast Asia, where azithromycin can be a better choice because of prevalence of fluoroquinolones-resistant *Campylobacter* (Table 1). For self-treatment, a single dose of antibiotics can be given. If there is no improvement, administration can continue for three days (Tribble et al., 2007). An otherwise healthy adult can take the antibiotics in combination with loperamide to achieve a faster improvement of diarrhoea (Ericsson et al., 2007).

10. Clinical course

All patients suffering from traveller's diarrhoea develop similar symptoms, regardless of the causal agent. It usually occurs within the first week of travel and resolves upon returning to the country of origin. The onset of traveller's diarrhoea is usually sudden, although abdominal pain, anorexia, and malaise may sometimes occur before the diarrhoea begins. Other manifestations such as nausea and vomiting in 10 to 25 percent, mild fever in up to 30

percent, and blood in stool in one to 10 percent of the cases may accompany diarrhoea. Average duration is approximately four days. Fifty percent of patients begin to recover within 48 hours (Steffen et al., 1983).
Irrespective of the aetiology, mild traveller's diarrhoea is generally short-term: this is not the case with more severe attacks (Hill, 2000). It is estimated that up to 25 percent of the cases of traveller's diarrhoea have more than five bowel movements in a day, and 30 to 45 percent of the cases may have their trip interrupted or travel plan altered for at least 12 to 24 hours (Steffen et al., 1987). Some patients with traveller's diarrhoea need to seek medical help while travelling or upon returning to the country of origin.

10.1 Viral gastroenteritis

Viral gastroenteritis is an intestinal infection caused by a variety of viruses resulting in mild, short-term diarrhoea, with vomiting being a prominent feature. It is often clinically undistiguishable from bacterial acute diarrhoea. In popular travel destinations, however, viruses have been shown to be responsible for up to 10 percent of cases of traveller's diarrhoea (Apelt et al., 2010). Viruses, mostly incriminated in cases of gastroenteritis, include GI and GII norovirus strains (Ajami et al., 2010) and rotaviruses belonging to groups A and C (Peñaranda et al., 1989; Sheridan et al, 1981). Enteric adenoviruses type 40 and 41 as well as astroviruses, though being an important cause of acute infantile gastroenteritis, do not appear to be a major health problem in travellers. Viruses can be transmitted from person to person or through contaminated food and water. Outbreaks of norovirus gastroenteritis have occurred in case of travellers co-existing in relatively confined spaces, such as aboard cruise ships and in tourist resorts, thus being in close contact with other passengers and tourists, relatively (Widdowson et al., 2002; Kornylo et al., 2009) Noroviruses cause transient malabsorption of D-xylose and fat, while rotaviruses cause malabsorption of glucose through the mechanism of cAMP protein kinase (Karst et al., 2010; Lorrot & Vasseur, 2007). Antibiotics do not work on viral gastroenteritis. Notwithstanding this, non-antimicrobial agents have been found effective in the treatment of intestinal viral infection associated with traveller's diarrhoea. Studies have shown that mixed viral and bacterial infections are common in gastroenteritis (Marshall, 2002). Thus, combination therapy with loperamide plus antibiotic is given empirically for traveller's diarrhoea (Ostrosky-Zeichner & Ericsson, 2001).

10.2 Persistent traveller's diarrhoea

Traveller's diarrhoea generally resolves even without treatment. However, in 10 percent of cases, digestive disturbances tend to persist for more than two weeks after the onset of the diarrhoea. In persistent cases, the patient continues to complain of intermittent or continuous gastrointestinal symptoms, such as loose stools, abdominal pain, bloating or other non-specific symptoms. Continued intestinal infection, post-infectious mucosal damage, or chronic gastrointestinal functional disorder may be responsible for persistent traveller's diarrhoea. In most of these cases, tests for the presence of pathogens may fail if sampling is delayed for a period of time after the onset (Connor, 2011).

10.2.1 Functional disorders

Similar to any acute inflammatory process, traveller's diarrhoea may disrupt the brush border microvilli of intestinal epithelial cells where disaccharidases reside. Consequently, a transient lactose intolerance may occur. Likewise, transient malabsorption of xylose, folate and vitamin B12 may also occur (Lindenbaum, 1965). Another post-infectious sequela is the development of irritable bowel syndrome, or IBS. Among sufferers, five to 10 percent are likely to experience non-specific gastrointestinal symptoms that are compatible with those of irritable bowel syndrome. Also, it has been found that 10 percent of patients with irritable bowel syndrome have reported travelling abroad before the onset of their symptoms (DuPont et al., 2010). Travellers experiencing diarrhoea during their trip were five times more likely than travellers without to develop post-infectious irritable bowel syndrome, or PI-IBS (Stermer et al., 2006). In 15 percent of travellers, traveller's diarrhoea with serious symptoms can lead to post-infectious irritable bowel syndrome within a six month period (Okhyusen et al., 2004). Risk factors for developing post-infectious irritable bowel syndrome include female gender, young age, pre-existing anxiety or depression, fever or weight loss, and infection due to strains of *Campylobacter* with toxigenic properties (de la Cabada Bauche & DuPont, 2011). Following traveller's diarrhoea, transient changes in intestinal motility should may lead to stasis and small intestinal bacterial overgrowth. This can cause secondary diarrhoea, and other non-specific symptoms that resemble those of irritable bowel syndrome (Attar et al., 1999; Tureja et al., 2008).

10.2.2 Persistent intestinal infection

In acute traveller's diarrhoea, parasites account for only a small percentage of the cases. In persistent traveller's diarrhoea, by contrast, intestinal protozoa are the most frequently encountered aetiological agents. Where travellers develop persistent diarrhoea, the most commonly detected enteric protozoa are *Giardia, Cryptosporidium,* and *Entamoeba histolytica,* followed by a small percentage of cases caused by *Isospora belli* and microsporidia. In returning traveller patients, *Cyclospora cayetanensis* has also been suggested to cause diarrhoea that continues after travel. Risk factors that are associated with contracting intestinal protozoal infections while travelling abroad are quite well known: longer duration of stay, and the low level of hygiene and socio-economic development in the country travelled (Kansouzidou et al., 2004; Müller et al., 2001; Okhyunsen et al., 2001; Taylor et al., 1988).

11. Intestinal protozoal diarrhoeal disease

11.1 Giardiasis

Giardiasis is a disease of the small intestine caused by *Giardia;* it has recently been included in the World Health Organization 'Neglected Disease Initiative'. Clinical spectrum of *Giardia* infection may vary from asymptomatic carriage to acute and chronic diarrhoea with abdominal pain. *G. intestinalis* is a cosmopolitan flagellated protozoan of humans and other animals. Molecular analysis has demonstrated that *Giardia* isolates can be separated into at least eight genotypes or assemblages, namely A to H, that may show host preference (Lasek-Nesselquist et al., 2010). Humans are mostly infected by assemblages A and B. Genomic difference may underlie the often distinct difference in biology and clinical manifestations observed between the two assemblages. This implies that *Giardia* assemblage A and assemblage B may represent two distinct species (Franzén et al., 2009). *Giardia* infection is usually transmitted by ingesting cysts found in contaminated water or food, but human-to-human transmission has also been reported in situations of poor faecal–oral hygiene. Giardial encystation (when trophozoites pass through the small intestine to the colon) is successful only if *Giardia* cysts are able to excyst after ingestion and entry into the small intestine (Lauwaet et al., 2007).

11.2 Amoebiasis

Amoebic colitis is characterized by gradual onset and symptoms present over a period of one to two weeks. It can thus be distinguished from bacterial dysentery. The protozoan may be responsible for various symptoms such as bloody diarrhoea and non-specific symptoms i.e. weight loss, fatigue, and abdominal pain. Also, it may cause fulminating dysentery. *Entamoeba,* whose habitat is the large intestine, is one of the most commonly detected enteric protozoans worldwide. It has been demonstrated that it comprises two species, *E. histolytica* and *E. dispar* and these cannot be morphologically differentiated from each other under the light microscope (Clark, 2004). However, these two species can be differentiated by using zymodeme patterns, monoclonal antibodies, or DNA probes (Stanley, 2003). Most recently, *E. histolytica* genome sequence has been re-annotated and re-assembled and data have been compared to closely related organisms (Lorenzi et al., 2010). Infection with *E. histolytica* is considered more prevalent in developing countries. It is transmitted by contaminated water and/or food or by the faecal-oral route. Immunocompromised persons as well as persons with a mental illness housed in institutional settings are at high risk for acquisition of amoebiasis. *Entamoeba* has two stages in its life cycle: active and motile trophozoite and the dormant cystic form. Trophozoite or the trophic form can be detected in the fresh unformed stool from a host. By contrast, cysts can survive outside the host, in the environment i.e. in water, in soils, or in food. *E. histolytica* is considered to be pathogenic, as opposed to the non-pathogenic *E. dispar.* Since *E. dispar* is regarded as non-pathogenic and commensal, infections with *E. dispar* are characteristically asymptomatic. Recently, however, there have been reports of patients infected with *E. dispar* experiencing gastrointestinal symptoms (Fotedar et al., 2007).

11.3 Cryptosporidiosis

In cryptosporidiosis caused by *Cryptosporidium,* immunocompetent individuals experience acute watery diarrhoea, which is usually self-limited and accompanied by non-specific symptoms such as abdominal pain, nausea and fatigue. In immunocompromised hosts, however, clinical manifestations of cryptosporidiosis vary with the level of immunosuppression. For instance, in case of low levels of CD4 helper T cells, immunocompromised patients could have persistent diarrhoea due to cryptosporidiosis (Brink et al., 2002). *Cryptosporidium* is an apicomplexan protozoan affecting humans and many animals. Molecular divergence between the two *C. parvum* variants, which were shown to have differences in epidemiological and clinical features, was discovered by using numerous techniques. These variants are now known as *C. parvum* in humans and in animals, and *C. hominis* in humans (Morgan-Ryan et al., 2002). A further important advance in the understanding of this protozoan is the publication of the *C. parvum* and *C. hominis* genome sequences. However, it has been suggested that there exist differences in the genetic make-up of *Cryptosporidium* populations, indicating variation in their infectivity for humans (Jex et al., 2008). In addition to genotypic differences, phenotypic differences have also been demonstrated suggesting that additional genetic pleomorphisms within the known genotypes exist. Monoxenous life cycle has an asexual stage, or sporozoites, and a sexual stage, or oocysts, and is completed within the small intestine. Sporulated thin-walled oocysts are autoinfective. Thick-walled oocysts that transmit the cryptosporidial infection from one host to another are resistant forms, even in chlorinated water, upon being excreted (Currrent and Garcia, 1991). Cryptosporidial oocysts can be excreted for weeks after the diarrhoea subsides. *Cryptosporidium* can survive in source waters for a long period of time. Cryptosporidial infection is transmitted by drinking contaminated water or eating contaminated food, and by animal-to-human or faecal-oral routes. The infective dose is low. In healthy, immunocompetent people, ingestion of as few as up to 30 *Cryptosporidium* oocysts can cause infection, whereas in immunocompromised patients even fewer oocysts are required (DuPont et al., 1995).

11.4 Isosporiasis

Isosporiasis, a diarrhoeal illness that is caused by *Isospora belli,* generally causes watery diarrhoea and non-specific gastrointestinal symptoms such as cramps and abdominal pain. In immunocompetent individuals, isosporiasis is usually transient; however, immunocompromised patients can experience persistent diarrhoea resembling the cryptosporidial diarrhoea mentioned above (Mudholar & Namey, 2010). *I. belli* is a coccidian protozoan. Although ubiquitous, *I. belli* is more frequently encountered in the tropical and subtropical countries. Humans are the sole identified reservoir for *I. belli* infection. Transmission has not yet been elucidated, even though *I. belli* has been suggested to be transmitted through contaminated water. Similar to *Cryptosporidium,* the *I. belli* life cycle has an asexual stage and a sexual stage in the intestine. Oocysts are immature and incapable of infecting the human host after excretion. The large oocysts mature outside the body and become sporulated and infective within a two to three day period.

11.5 Cyclosporiasis

Cyclosporiasis, a diarrhoeal disease caused by *Cyclospora,* is generally the cause of self-limited diarrhoea accompanied by cramping, abdominal pain, nausea and other non-specific symptoms (Türk et al., 2004). Immunocompromised hosts, however, may experience prolonged diarrhoea that may become quite serious if left untreated (Türk et al., 2004). *C. cayetanensis* is a coccidian protozoan that has been associated with diarrhoea in the developing world. It is considered an obligatory intracellular parasite found in jejunum. *Cyclospora* reservoirs are yet to be defined, even though humans appear to be the only reservoir for *Cyclospora,* similar to *I. belli* (Ortega & Sanchez, 2010). It has been proposed that this coccidian protozoan parasite may be transmitted via contaminated water and food. In order to become infective, very large *Cyclospora* oocysts, which resemble those of *Cryptosporidium* but are roughly twice the size, need sporulation outside the body, in the environment: in this they are dissimilar to *Cryptosporidium* but similar to *I. belli.*

11.6 Microsporidiosis

Microsporidiosis is commonly found in immunosuppressed individuals (Matthis et al., 2005). Among the numerous microsporidian species, only *Enterocytozoon bieneusi* and *Encephalitozoon intestinalis* are associated with intestinal infection in humans worldwide. Therefore, infection with *E. bieneusi* or *E. intestinalis* should be considered in cases of chronic diarrhoea. Microsporidia are small, obligatory, intracellular organisms that infect vertebrate and invertebrate hosts. Although it has been proposed that they belong to the protist group of archezoa, microsporidia have molecularly been re-classified from protozoa to fungi or a sister group of fungi (Parfrey et al., 2006). Microsporidia have specialized polar tubes, asexually reproduce within the cell, and form thick-walled spores that are capable of surviving in the environment for a long period of time.

11.7 Dientamoebiasis

Recently, *Dientamoeba fragilis* has been regarded as a pathogenic organism (Katz & Taylor, 2001). Most patients with dientamoebiasis report frequent unformed stools and abdominal pain. Mucus in the stool is sporadically observed. In about 30 percent of patients with dientamoebiasis, diarrhoea is persistent and may turn into the chronic form, which lasts more than four weeks, with abdominal pain being the predominant symptom (Stark et al., 2005). *D. fragilis* is one of the smaller parasites that can live in the human large intestine. Unlike other intestinal protozoa that are mainly detected in the developing world, *D. fragilis* is often seen in developed countries with high levels of hygiene. Once classified as an amoeba, it has been demonstrated to be a close relative of the trichomonads (Johnson et al., 2004). It is considered to be a non-flagellated trichomonad. It is worthwhile mentioning that *D. fragilis* has no apparent cyst-like forms (in this it is dissimilar to other intestinal protozoa). Although it still remains unclear (Barratt et al., 2011), it has been proposed that infection between humans occurs during the trophozoite stage. Our as-yet-unpublished results corroborate the possibility of intrafamily transmission (Stark et al., 2009).

11.8 Blastocystosis

Once thought to be a harmless inhabitant of the human gut, *Blastocystis* is now considered a potential pathogen. Immunocompromised or debilitated individuals seem more prone to getting a diarrhoea attributable to blastocystosis (Vassalos et al., 2008). *Blastocystis* sp. is a ubiquitous anaerobic protozoan parasite that lives in the intestine of humans, other animals and arthropods. *Blastocystis* isolates have been separated into at least 10 subtypes according to phylogenetic trees that have been constructed from sequences of the small subunit ribosomal RNA (Stensvold et al., 2009). Subtype 3 has been found to be the most common genotype (Tan, 2008). The protozoan is more frequently encountered in tropical and subtropical countries. *Blastocystis* is polymorphic. It has various morphological forms, including vacuolar, granular, amoeboid, cyst, multivacuolar and avacuolar forms, with the vacuolar form being the most commonly detected in stool examination. Amoeboid forms are predominantly seen in isolates from symptomatic patients (Tan, 2008). *Blastocystis* vacuolar forms could transit to *Blastocystis* cysts and vice versa. Thus, faecal–oral transmission has been proposed. Also, it is transmitted by contaminated water or by human-to human and animal-to-human routes.

11.9 Mechanisms of diarrhoea production

Diarrhoea caused by *Giardia* is mediated by increased rates of transit of small intestine origin as well as enhanced chloride secretion (Cotton et al., 2011). Yet the mechanisms of pathogenesis are poorly understood (Buret, 2007). However, host and parasite factors seem to contribute to the pathogenesis of *Giardia* infection. Increase in rates of enterocyte apoptosis and disruption of epithelial tight junctions lead to dysfunction in the small intestinal barrier resulting in activation of CD8 cytotoxic T-lymphocytes. CD8 lymphocytes may induce brush border microvilli injury and enterocyte malfunction that leads to malabsorption and maldigestion of small intestine origin (Buret, 2005). *Cryptosporidium* is localized within a unique intracellular but extracytoplasmic niche (Tzipori & Ward, 2002). The coccidian parasite is found attached to brush border microvilli of epithelial cells of the small intestine where it can cause damage that leads to the death of enterocytes. To replace the damaged cells, cell division is triggered in the crypt region resulting for instance in hyperplasia. The absorptive function of the villar tips is impaired and chloride secretion by the crypt cells increases, thus leading to an overall enhancement of intestinal secretion. Under this proposed mechanism, *Cryptosporidium*-induced diarrhoea is classified as osmotic (Sears & Guerrant, 1994). The host immune system is likely to reduce the number of thin-walled oocysts in an attempt to prevent autoinfection, which tends to perpetuate cryptosporidial infection in the host. In principle, the mechanism of diarrhoea production appears to follow the same pattern as seen in isosporiasis and cyclosporiasis.

E. histolytica has been suggested to produce several potential virulence factors such as adhesins that enable adherence to the host cell, amoebapores that are capable of forming a hole in a target cell; and cysteine proteinases that can degrade extracellular matrix components. Intestinal inflamation, killing of mucosal cells and invasion of protozoan are the combined effects of these virulence factors (Padilla-Vaca & Anaya-Velázquez, 2010). Lysis of host neutrophils may also contribute to the cell damage. In a host-parasite interplay, however, it is quite possible that the virulence may reflect how much control the host is capable of exercising over invasion and replication of *Entamoeba* trophozoites (Galván-Moroyoqui et al., 2008). Invasion of intestinal epithelium by *Entamoeba* trophozoites can result in the development of dysentery, ulcers, or an amoeboma (Suriptiastuti, 2010). Dysenteric syndrome is characterized by the production of small volumes of bloody, mucoid stools without faecal leukocytes. Amoebic 'flask-shaped' ulcers can be observed in sections of the gastrointestinal tract. Amoeboma is the formation of amoebic granuloma in the intestinal wall. If entroinvasive illness turns into chronic amoebic colitis, the disease mimics inflammatory bowel disease. *D. fragilis* is considered to cause non-invasive, superficial irritation of the colonic mucosa, along with an eosinophilic inflammatory response (Johnson et al., 2004). *Blastocystis* is also considered to be the cause of non-invasive mucosal inflammation. Our published results have shown that *Blastocystis* subtype 3 might be pathogenic, only when amoeboid forms of *Blastocystis* are present (Katsarou-Katsari et al, 2008), and suggest that there are intra-specific differences within *Blastocystis* subtypes that contribute to the protozoan parasite's pathogenicity (Vassalos et al., 2010). The host immune status seems to play some role on the development of blastocystosis. Immunocompromised patients will suffer from diarrhoeal disease as the potential pathogenic forms of *Blastocystis* thrive when host defences are weakened. Interplay with intestinal microbiota may differ between pathogenic and non-pathogenic forms of *Blastocystis* (Vassalos et al., 2008). *E. bieneusi* clusters have been found in intestinal and biliary tract cells, whereas *E. intestinalis* infects the intestinal tract and may also disseminate to the mesenteric nodes and kidney. In the context of host-parasite relationship, microsporidia seem to be highly sophisticated parasites. Not only is proteome complexity reduced in the microsporidia but also several eukaryotic pathways are pared down to what appears to be minimal functional units so that host cell manipulation can be achieved (Williams, 2009).

11.10 Routine diagnostic arsenal

The challenge is to identify the likely intestinal protozoal agent involved in diarrhoeal disease as fast and accurately as possible so that therapeutic management can start.

Conventional ova and parasite testing that involves light microscopic examination of stool samples is employed for the low cost detection of intestinal protozoal diarrhoeal disease. The method, however, is a labour intensive and time consuming process, and requires an experienced microscopist. On the other hand, antigen detection assays are considered to be rapid and reliable methods for detecting enteric protozoan parasites, without the need for skilled microscopy. Direct fluorescent antibody, enzyme-linked immunosorbent assay (ELISA), and rapid dipstick-like tests are the diagnostic procedures in use for antigen detection in diagnosis of protozoa of the intestine.

Giardial infection can be diagnosed by identification of cysts and trophozoites in the stool; wet mount preparations and trichrome stained smears of stool specimens are the recommended procedures. *Entamoeba* cysts and trophozoites can also be observed by examining a fresh stool and by using trichrome stain. *Cryptosporidium* oocysts can be visualized with a modified acid fast stain. Similarly, identification of *Isospora* oocysts requires acid fast staining. To detect *Cyclospora*, however, Safranin stain is used. *Cyclospora* can also be identified in stool samples, since the protozoan is able to autofluoresce at 330 to 380 nm under ultraviolet microscopy. Microsporidial infection can be diagnosed by identification of free and intracytoplasmic spores with Giemsa and modified trichrome, or with fluorochrome stains such as calcofluor and Uvitex 2B, stains that have an affinity for chitin. Morphological differences between *E. bieneusi* and *E. intestinalis* can be made out in small intestine biopsy specimens by electron microscopy.

It is possible to detect *Giardia* by using direct immunofluorescence or ELISA. *Cryptosporidium* oocysts can be detected by using monoclonal antibody-based direct immunofluorescence assay or ELISA. Newly developed stool antigen detection methods, i.e. ELISA, capable of discriminating between *E. histolytica* and *E. dispar* may also prove particularly useful. For laboratory diagnosis of the enteric protozoans *G. intestinalis, E. histolytica,* and *Cryptosporidium* spp., diagnostic kits using immunochromatography are now commercially available. To detect microsporidia, free and intracytoplasmic spores can be examined using an indirect immunofluorescent assay with monoclonal antibodies.

PCR-based methods are also increasingly used for the detection of intestinal protozoa in case of diarrhoea. Inexpensive in-house PCR protocols can be adapted to detect intestinal protozoa. Furthermore, the trend has been moving from the detection of a single intestinal protozoal agent involved in diarrhoeal disease to a multiplex approach, thus allowing simultaneous identification of multiple protozoan parasites in order not to loose valuable time (Stark et al., 2011). In our laboratory, nested multiplex PCR is routinely used to differentiate *E. histolytica* from the non-pathogenic *E. dispar* (Evangelopoulos et al., 2000). As for the differentiation of intestinal protozoa other than *Entamoeba* spp. at the inter- or intra-specific level, further refinements are required in PCR-based methods. Thus, outbreaks of intestinal protozoal diarrhoeal disease could be readily investigated and research in molecular epidemiology could be made possible. Polymerase chain reaction techniques, such as real time PCR based on SYBR-Green fluorescence, can also be used to simultaneousley identify microsporidial species (Polley et al. 2011). In diarrhoeal patients with dientamoebiasis, highly variable intermittent shedding of *D. fragilis* trophozoites has been shown to confound diagnosis when methods such as microscopy, culture or conventional PCR are used to detect the protozoan. However, intermittent shedding does not seem to interfere with the diagnosis of dientamoebiasis in cases where real time PCR, which demonstrates high sensitivity, is employed. This is thus being seen as the method of choice (Stark et al., 2010).

11.11 Treatment and management

The agents that are used for the treatment of intestinal protozoal diarrhoeal diseases are set out in Table 5. Concerning the treatment of giardiasis, there are several drugs including the 5-nitroimidazole and benzimidazole derivatives, quinacrine, furazolidone, paromomycin, and nitazoxanide that have been proved effective and approved. Metronidazole is considered the antiprotozoal agent of choice for the treatment of giardial infection; however, decreased susceptibility to metronidazole has been reported. Therefore, albendazole can alternatively be administered. Combination therapy may also be used when first line drugs fail, nitazoxanide is not available, or co-infection with other parasites occurs (Lopez-Velez et al., 2010).

Where cysts are detected in an asymptomatic *Entamoeba* carrier, a luminal agent, such as diloxanide or paromomycin, should be given to treat intraluminal infection and clear amoebic cysts (Stanley, 2003). In enteroinvasive disease, i.e. severe colitis due to *E. histolytica,* tissue penetrating metronidazole should be administered against invasive trophozoites and then a luminal amoebicide should be given to kill any remaining cysts. Using *in vivo* models, metronidazole was found to be the most effective (Becker et al., 2011). However, if metronidazole tolerance occurs, tinidazole may alternatively be used (Gonzales et al., 2009). Cryptosporidial infection is self-limited and immunocompetent hosts may only need to be treated supportively. In immunocompromised patients with cryptosporidiosis, the most commonly used agents are paromomycin, and azithromycin, which are partially effective. Nitazoxanide, a thiazoline compound, has been shown to be effective in immunocompetent individuals. However, nitazoxanide could be effective in case immune response is appropriate (Gargala, 2008). Consequently, in immunocompromised patients, it is necessary to combine treatment against cryptosporidial infection with a therapy for restoring immunity (Cabada & White, 2010).

In cases of symptomatic *Isospora* or *Cyclospora* infections, trimethoprim-sulfamethoxazole, a sulfonamid antibiotic, is administered. In immunocompromised patients experiencing recurrent diarrhoeal disease, secondary prophylaxis with trimethoprim-sulfamethoxazole attempts to treat *Isospora* or *Cyclospora* infection, and thus prevent relapses. Nitazoxanide is also in use for the treatment of isosporiasis and cyclosporiasis in patients with sulfa allergy (Zimmer et al., 2007).

Microsporidial infection of immunocompetent individuals is self-limited and does not require antiparasite treatment. Many agents have been tested in the treatment of microsporidia infection. However, the results have shown variable therapeutic success in the treatment of microsporidiosis in humans. Albendazole has been demonstrated to be effective against *Encephalitozoon* spp. such as *E. intestinalis* but not against *Enterocytozoon bieneusi.* Fumagillin, an irreversible inhibitor of methionine aminopeptidase-2, has been demonstrated to be effective for eradicating *E. bieneusi,* despite its side effects. In renal transplant recipients, fumagillin shows acceptable safety when monitoring immunosuppressive therapy (Champion et al., 2010).

Currently, there is no consensus for the treatment of symptomatic dientamoebiasis (Johnson et al., 2004). The therapeutic agents commonly used to treat *D. fragilis* infection are metronidazole, paromomycin, newer nitroimidazole derivatives such as secnidazole and ornidazole, tetracycline, or a combination therapy.

Concerning *Blastocystis* infections, the treating agents that are currently in use have been considered to be generally effective. However, decreased susceptibility to metronidazole has

Protozoa	Drug(s) of choice	Alternative drug(s)
Giardia intestinalis	Metronidazole 250 mg t.i.d. × 5 days Tinidazole 2 g × 1 day	Albendazole 400 mg q.d. × 5 days Quinacrine 100 mg t.i.d. × 5 days Paromomycin 25 – 30 mg kg^{-1} per day in 3 doses × 7 days
Entamoeba histolytica	*Asymptomatic carriers (cysts)* Paromomycin 500 mg t.i.d. × 10 days Diloxanide furoate 500 mg t.i.d. × 10 days *Symptomatic patients (trophozoites)* Metronidazole 750 mg t.i.d. × 5 days or Tinidazole 2 g × 3 days followed by paromomycin 500 mg t.i.d. × 10 days or diloxanide furoate 500 mg t.i.d. × 10 days	Diloxanide furoate 500 mg t.i.d. × 10 days plus Tetracycline 250 mg q.i.d. × 10 days followed Chloroquine 500 mg q.i.d. × 7 days
Cryptosporidium.	Nitazoxanide 500 mg b.i.d. × 3- 14 days	Albendazole 400 mg b.i.d.x 7-14 days Paromomycin 500 mg t.i.d. × 14 days
Isospora belli	Trimethoprim- Sulfamethoxazole (160mg/800mg) b.i.d. × 10days	Ciprofloxacin 500mg b.i.d. × 7 days Pyrimethamine 75 mg q.d. plus folinic acid 10 mg q.d. × 10 days
Cyclospora cayatensis	Trimethoprim- Sulfamethoxazole (160mg/800mg) q.i.d. ×10days	Nitazoxanide 500 mg b.i.d. × 3- 14 days
Encephalitozoon intestinalis	Albendazole 400 mg b.i.d. × 14-28 days	
Enterocytozoon bieneusi	Albendazole 400 mg b.i.d. × 28 days	Fumagillin 60 mg q.d. × 14 days
Dientamoeba fragilis	Tetracycline 500 mf q.i.d. × 10 days	Paromomycin 25 – 30 mg kg^{-1} per day in 3 doses × 7 days Metronidazole 750 mg t.i.d. × 5- 10 days
Blastocystis sp.	Nitazoxanide 500 mg b.i.d. × 3 days	Metronidazole 750 mg t.i.d. × 5- 10 days Trimethoprim- Sulfamethoxazole (160mg/800mg) b.i.d. × 7 days

Table 5. Treatment of diarrhoeal disease due to intestinal protozoa: drugs of choice and alternative drugs.

been described. An asymptomatic *Blastocystis* carrier should be followed up so that a thorough examination could be ordered in case symptoms become evident. The use of broad spectrum antimicrobial should be restrained, being used only in cases of symptomatic *Blastocystis* infections. Thus, the emergence of resistant *Blastocystis* strains should be prevented (Vassalos et al., 2008).

12. Conclusion

Since the mid-1950s when the term 'emporiatrics' was coined by Waters and Kean, substantial progress has been made in dealing with traveller's diarrhoea. Rather than being seen as an unavoidable scourge for the hapless tourist, traveller's diarrhoea has been considered an illness that requires further investigation and fuller action. Currently, an increasing number of pathogens likely to be responsible for traveller's diarrhoea have been identified (Jiang et al., 2010). Concerning classical enteropathogens, such as ETEC, the mode of action and regulation by host factors is known. Also, progress in prophylaxis has been dramatic. Old, but still good, advice for sound eating and drinking habits can now be coupled with drug administration.

When taking only chemoprophylaxis, travellers may be at a lower risk of contracting traveller's diarrhoea but they are not 100 percent immune from a variety of pathogens likely to be responsible for the illness. Travellers would be thus in error if they assume that they are safe and pay no attention to hygiene and sanitation rules (Wagner & Wiedermann, 2009). There has been sustained research effort for a vaccine that would be effective against ETEC, the leading cause of traveller's diarrhoea, and reduce the duration and severity of the symptoms. A vaccine, which combines cholera toxin subunit B with killed whole cell (W/rBS), is currently being assessed in clinical trials (Svennerholm, 2010).

Concerning traveller's diarrhoea treatment, the emergence of resistance against antibiotics has led to research for novel drugs or therapeutic regimens. In the United States, rifaximin has now been approved for the treatment of traveller's diarrhoea attributable to non-invasive *E. coli*. Rifaximin is still being evaluated for the prevention of traveller's diarrhoea (Armstrong et al., 2010).

In any such cases, prompt management is currently recommended, since it has been proved that induced intestinal irritation may lead to temporary or prolonged functional disorders, as is the case with persistent traveller's diarrhoea that is mainly of parasitic origin (Connor, 2011). Intestinal protozoa found in travellers complaining of persistent diarrhoea upon their return home from exotic destinations have practically been the sole enteric protozoa detected in the industrialized countries. Owing to high levels of hygiene and food safety, there has been a dramatic decline in infections caused by intestinal protozoa in the developed countries. In the last decades, however, intestinal infections due to opportunistic protozoa have emerged because of a marked increase in the number of immunocompromised individuals from a range of causes. Also, immigration from and adventurous travel to developing tropical countries with low hygienic level and a high prevalence of ubiquitous enteric protozoa have recently increased. Therefore, lately, cases of intestinal protozoal diarrhoeal disease have been increasing in the developed world.

This re-emergence has rekindled interest in research on intestinal protozoa. Inter- or intra-specific genotype differences may help explain variations in phenotypic features, various pathogenic mechanisms, and the presence of virulence factors of enteric protozoa. For *E. histolytica*, the parasite lifestyle was examined at the whole-genome level so that new genes encoding virulence factors along with signaling pathways and processes could be identified (Lorenzi et al. 2010; Weedal & Neil Hall, 2011). Ongoing research on host and parasite factors likely to contribute to the pathogenesis of giardiasis may elucidate assemblage-specific pathogenic mechanisms (Cotton et al., 2011). New potential drug targets have been discovered in an attempt to develop the next generation of antiprotozoals. Researchers test novel promising drugs that target unique proteins and metabolic pathways of the protozoan *G. intestinalis* (Lale et al. 2010). Others continue to attempt to develop an antiprotozoal agent that would be effective against the coccidian *Cryptosporidium*. Nitazoxanide, which was discovered in the 1980s, has routinely been considered an alternative treatment option in case of diarrhoeal disease due to *Giardia, Entamoeba, Isospora* and *Cyclospora*. In immunocompromised hosts, however, nitazoxanide fails to treat cryptosporidiosis unless it is combined with antiretroviral therapy, perhaps because of partial antiparasitic effect of protease inhibitors (Cabada & White, 2010). Despite its side effects, fumagillin is used for treating microsporidia infections. Fumagillin analogs have recently been shown to be active against *E. histolytica* (Arico-Muendel et al., 2009). Concerning dientamoebiasis and blastocystosis, the ambiguity that surrounds the mode of transmission of *D. fragilis* (Barratt et al., 2011) and the pathogenic stage of *Blastocystis* (Vassalos et al., 2008; Tan, 2008) complicates the management of these intestinal infections. Likewise, the role of interplay between host defence mechanisms and intestinal protozoan survival strategies is complex. Further investigation of host-parasite relationship is of critical importance in the design and implementation of new vaccines and candidate drugs.

13. Acknowledgement

Firstly, we would like to offer our heartfelt thanks to Dr Michael Vassalos, Professor Emeritus of National School of Public Health, Athens, Greece, for his encouragement, critical reading and helpful suggestions. Our thanks are also due to Dr Nicholas Vakalis, Professor of Parasitology, Entomology and Tropical Diseases at the National School of Public Health, Athens, Greece for his support and guidance. We express our thanks to Dr Donicrt G. Evely for thorough manuscript editing as a native English speaker and expert. We would like to thank the staff of the Department of Parasitology, Entomology and Tropical Diseases at the National School of Public School, Athens, Greece for technical assistance. Also, we thank Ms Chrysoula Salamanou for help in preparing the manuscript.

14. References

Adachi, J.A.; Mathewson, J.J.; Jiang, Z.D.; Ericsson, C.D. & DuPont, H.L. (2002). Enteric pathogens in Mexican sauces of popular restaurants in Guadalajara, Mexico, and Houston, Texas. *Annals of Internal Medicine* Vol.136, No.12, (June 2002), pp. 884–88, ISSN 0003-4819

Ajami, N.; Koo, H.; Darkoh, C.; Atmar, R.L.; Okhuyesen, P.C.; Jiang, Z.-D.; Flores, J. & DuPont, H.L. (2010). Characterization of norovirus-associated traveler's diarrhea. *Clinical Infectious Diseases*, Vol.51, No.2, (July 2010), pp. 123-130, ISSN 1058-4838

Alon, D.; Shitrit, P.& Chowers, M. (2010). Risk behaviors and spectrum of diseases among elderly travelers: a comparison of younger and older adults. *Journal of Travel Medicine*, Vol.17, No.4, (July-August 2010), pp. 250-255, ISSN 1195-1982

Anderson, E.J. & Weber, S.G. (2004). Rotavirus infection in adults. *The Lancet Infectious Diseases*, Vol.4, No.2, (February 2004), pp. 91-99, ISSN 1473-3099

Apelt, N.; Hartberger, C.; Campe, H. & Löscher, T. (2010). The prevalence of norovirus in returning international travelers with diarrhea. *BMC Infecioust Diseases*, Vol.10, No.131, (May 2010), pp. 1-6, ISSN 1471-2334 (Electronic)

Arico-Muendel, C.; Centrella, P.A.; Contonio, B.D.; Morgan, B.A.; O'Donovan, G.; Paradise, C.L.; Skinner, S.R.; Sluboski, B.; Svendsen, J.L.; White, K.F.; Debnath, A.; Gut, J.; Wilson, N.; McKerrow, J.H.; DeRisi, J.L.; Rosenthal, P.J. & Chiang, P.K. (2009). Antiparasitic activities of novel, orally available fumagillin analogs. *Bioorganic and Medicinal Chemistry Letters*, Vol.19, No.17, (September 2009), pp. 5128-5131. ISSN 0960-894X

Armstrong, A.W.; Ulukan, S.; Weiner, M.; Mostafa, M.; Shaheen, H.; Nakhla, I.; Tribble, D.R. & Riddle, M.S. (2010). A randomized, double-blind, placebo-controlled study evaluating the efficacy and safety of rifaximin for the prevention of travelers' diarrhea in US military personnel deployed to Incirlik Air Base, Incirlik, Turkey. *Journal of Travel Medicine*, Vol.17, No.6, (November-December 2010), pp. 392-394. ISSN 1195-1982

Attar, A.; Flourié, B.; Rambaud, J.C.; Franchisseur, C.; Ruszniewski, P. & Bouhnik, Y. (1999). Antibiotic efficacy in small intestinal bacterial overgrowth-related chronic diarrhea: A crossover, randomized trial. *Gastroenterology*, Vol.117, No.4, (October 1999), pp. 794 – 820, ISSN 0016-5085

Bandres, J.C.; Mathewson, J.J. & DuPont, H.L. (1998). Heat susceptibility of bacterial enteropathogens. Implicationsfor the prevention of travelers' diarrhea. *Archives of Internal Medicine*, Vol.148, No.19, (October 1988), pp. 2261–2263, ISSN 003-0026

Bao, R. (2006). Bismuth. In, *Goldfrank's Toxicologic Emergencies*. N. Flomenbaum, L.W. Goldfrank, R. Hoffman, M.A. Howland, N. Lewin & L. Nelson (Ed.), McGraw-Hill Companies, Inc. , 1269- 1273, ISBN 0-07-147914-7, New York, USA

Barratt, J.L.; Harkness, J.; Marriott, D.; Ellis, J.T. & Stark, D. (2011). The ambiguous life of *Dientamoeba fragilis*: the need to investigate current hypotheses on transmission. *Parasitology*, Vol.138, No.5, (April 2011), pp.557-572. ISSN 0031-1820

Becker, S.; Hoffman, P. & Houpt, E.R. (2011). Efficacy of antiamebic drugs in a mouse model. *The American Journal of Tropical Medicine and Hygiene*, Vol.84, No.4, (April 2011), pp. 581-586, ISSN 0002-9637

Borg, M. (2007). Food hygiene and gastroenteritis. In, *IFIC Basic Concepts of Infection Control*, C. Friedman & W. Newsom (Eds.), International Federation of Infection Control, 163-170, ISBN 978-0-9555861-0-1, Portadown, UK

Brink, A.K.; Mahe, C.; Watera C.; Lugada E.; Gilks, C.; Whitworth, J. & French, N. (2002). Diarrhea, CD4 counts and enteric infections in a community-based cohort of HIV-infected adults in Uganda. *The Journal of Infection*, Vol.45, No.2, (August 2002), pp. 99-106. ISSN: 0163-4453

Buret, A.G. (2005). Immunopathology of giardiasis: the role of lymphocytes in intestinal epithelial injury and malfunction. *Memórias do Instituto Oswaldo Cruz*, Vol.100, Suppl.1, (March 2005), pp. 185-190. ISSN 0074-0276

Buret, A.G. (2007). Mechanisms of epithelial dysfunction in giardiasis. *Gut*, Vol.56, No.3, (March 2007), pp. 316-317. ISSN 0017-5749

Cabada, M.M. & White, A.C. Jr. (2010). Treatment of cryptosporidiosis: do we know what we think we know? *Current Opinion in Infectious Diseases*, Vol.23, No.5, (October 2010), pp.494-499, ISSN 0951-7375

Cailhol, J. & Bouchaud, O. (2007). [Turista: traveler's diarrhea]. *Presse Medicale* , Vol.36, No.4-C2, (April 2007), pp. 717-722, ISSN 0075-4982

Chapin, A.R.; Carpenter, C.M.; Dudley, W.C.; Gibson, L.C.; Pratdesaba, R.; Torres, O.; Sanchez, D.; Belkind-Gerson, J.; Nyquist, I.; Kärnell, A.; Gustafsson, B.; Halpern, J.L.; Bourgeois, A.L. & Schwab, K.J. (2005). Prevalence of norovirus among visitors from the United States to Mexico and Guatemala who experience traveler's diarrhea. *Journal of Clinical Microbiology*, Vol.43, No.3, (March 2005), pp. 1112-1117, ISSN 0095-1137

Champion, L.; Durrbach, A.; Lang P; Delahousse, M.; Chauvet, C.; Sarfati, C.; Glotz, D. & Molina, J.M. (2010). Fumagillin for treatment of intestianl microsporidiosis in reanl transplant recipients. *American Journal of Transplantation*, Vol.10, No.8, (August 2010), pp. 1925-1930, ISSN 1600-6135

Clark, C.G. (2004). *Entamoeba histolytica* and *Entamoeba dispar*, the non-identical twins, In, *The Pathogenic Enteric Protozoa:* Giardia, Entamoeba, Cryptosporidium *and* Cyclospora, C.R. Sterling & R.D. Adam (Eds), 15-26, Kluwer Academic Publishers, ISBN 1-4020-7794-7, Boston MA, USA

Clemens, J.D.; Sack, D.A.; Harris, J.R.; Chakraborty, J.; Neogy, P.K.; Stanton, B.; Huda, N.; Khan, M.U.; Kay, B.A. & Khan, M.R. (1988). Cross-protection by B subunitwhole cell cholera vaccine against diarrhea associated with heat-labile toxinproducing enterotoxigenic *Escherichia coli*: results of a large-scale field trial. *The Journal of Infectious Diseases*, Vol.158, No.2, (August 1988), pp. 372-377, ISSN 0022-1899

Connor, B.A. (2011). Persistent travelers' diarrhea, In: *CDC Health Information for International Travel 2012*, G. W. Brunette (Ed.), 537-549, Oxford University Press, ISBN 978-0-19-976901-8, New York, USA

Cotton, J.A.; Beatty, J.K. & Buret, A.G. (2011). Host parasite interactions and pathophysiology in *Giardia* infections. *International Journal of Parasitology*, (June 2011), doi:10.1016/j.ijpara.2011.05.002, ISSN 0029-7519

Current, W.L. & Garcia, L.S. (1991). Cryptosporidiosis. *Clinical Microbiology Reviews*, Vol.3, No.4, (June 1991), pp. 325-358, ISSN 0893-8512

Diemert, D.J. (2006). Prevention and self-treatment of traveler's diarrhea. *Clinical Microbiology Reviews*, Vol.19, No.3, (July 2006), pp. 583-594, ISSN 0893-8512

Domènech-Sánchez, A.; Juan, C.; Rullan, A.J.; Pérez, J.L. & Berrocal, C.I. (2009). Gastroenteritis outbreaks in 2 tourist resorts, Dominican Republic. *Emerging Infectious Diseases*, Vol.15, No.11, (November 2009), pp. 1877-1878, ISSN 1080-6040

DuPont, H.L. (2008) Systematic review: prevention of travellers'diarrhoea. *Alimentary Pharmacology and Therapeutics*, Vol.27, No.9, (May 2008), pp. 741–751, ISSN 0269-281

DuPont, H.L. & Ericsson, C.D .(1993). Prevention and treatment of traveler ' s diarrhea . *The New England Journal of Medicine*, Vol.328, No.25, (June24, 1993), pp. 1821 – 1827, ISSN 0028-4793

DuPont, H.L. & Khan, F.M. (1994). Travelers' diarrhea: Epidemiology, microbiology, prevention, and therapy. *Journal of Travel Medicine*, Vol.1, No.2, (June 1994) pp. 84-93, ISSN 1708-8305

DuPont, H.L.; Ericsson, C.D. & DuPont, M.W. (1986). Emporiatric enteritis: lessons learned from U.S. students in Mexico. *Transactions of the American Clinical and Climatological Association.* Vol. 97, pp. 32–42, ISSN 0065-7778

DuPont, H.L.; Chappell, C.L.; Sterling, C.R.; Okhuysen, P.C.; Rose, J.B. & Jakubowski, W. (1995). The infectivity of *Cryptosporidium parvum* in healthy volunteers. *The New England Journal of Medicine,* Vol.180, No.332, (March 1995), pp. 855-859, ISSN 0028-4793

DuPont, H.L.; Jiang, Z.D.; Okhuysen, P.C.; Ericsson, C.D.; de la Cabada, F.J.; Ke, S.; DuPont, M.W. & Martinez-Sandoval, F. (2005). A randomized, blind, placebo-controlled trial of rifaxin to prevent traveler's diarrea. *Annals of Internal Medicine,* Vol.142, No.3, (May 2005), pp. 805-812, ISSN 0003-4819

DuPont, H.L.; Ericsson, C.D.; Farthing, M.J.; Gorbach, S.; Pichering, L.K.; Rombo, L.; Steffen, R. & Weinke, T. (2009a). Expert review of the evidence base for prevention of travelers' diarrhea. *Journal of Travel Medicine,* Vol.16, No.3, (May-June 2009), pp. 149-160, ISSN 1195-1982

DuPont, H.L.; Ericsson, C.D.; Farthing, M.J.; Gorbach, S.; Pichering, L.K.; Rombo, L.; Steffen, R. & Weinke, T. (2009b). Expert review of the evidence base for self-therapy of travelers' diarrhea. *Journal of Travel Medicine,* Vol. 16, No. 3, (May-June 2009), pp. 161–171, ISSN 1195-1982

DuPont, H.L.; Galler, G.; Garcia-Torres, F.; Dupont, A.W.; Greisinger, A. & Jiang, Z.D. (2010). Travel and travelers' diarrhea in patients with irritable bowel syndrome. *The American Journal of Tropical Medicine and Hygiene,* Vol.82, No.2, (February 2010), pp. 301-305, ISSN 0002-9637

El-Ganayni, G.A.; Attia, R.A; & Motawea, S.M. (1994). The relation between ABO blood groups, HLA typing and giardiasis in children. *Journal of the Egyptian Society of Parasitolology,* Vol.24, No.2, (August 1994), pp. 407-412, ISSN 0253-5890

Ericsson, C.D. (2005).Nonantimicrobial agents in the prevention and treatment of traveler´s diarrhea. *Clinical Infectious Diseases,* Vol.41, Suppl.8, (December 2005), pp. S557-S563, ISSN 1058-4838

Ericsson, C.D.; DuPont, H.L.; Okhuysen, P.C.; Jiang, Z.D.& DuPont, M.W. (2007). Loperamide plus azithromycin more effectively treats travelers' diarrhea in Mexico than azithromycin alone. *Journal of Travel Medicine,* Vol.14, No.5, (September-October 2007), pp. 312-319, ISSN 1195-1982

Ericsson, C.D.; DuPont, H.L. & Steffen, R. (2008). *Travelers' Diarrhea.* BC Decker Inc, ISBN 998-1-55009-371-1, Hamilton , Ontario.

Evangelopoulos, A.; Spanakos, G.; Patsoula, E.; Vakalis, N. & Legakis, N. (2000). A nested, multiplex, PCR assay for the simultaneous detection and differentiation of *Entamoeba histolytica* and *Entamoeba dispar* in faeces. *Annals of Tropical Medicine and Parasitology,* Vol.94, No.3, (April 2000), pp. 233-240, ISSN 0003-4983

Flores, J.; DuPont, H.L.; Lee, S.A.; Belkind-Gerson, J.; Paredes, M.; Mohamed, J.A.; Armitige, L.Y.; Guo, D.C.; & Okhuysen, P.C. (2008) . Influence of host interleukin-10 polymorphisms on development of traveler's diarrhea due to heat-labile enterotoxin- producing Escherichia coli in travelers from the United States who are visiting Mexico. *Clinical and Vaccine Immunology.* Vol.15, No.8, (August 2008), pp. 1194–1198, ISSN 1556-6811

Fotedar, R.; Stark, D.; Beebe, N.; Marriott, D.; Ellis, J. & Harkness, J. (2007). Laboratory diagnostic techniques for *Entamoeba* species. *Clinical Microbiology Reviews*, Vol.20, No.3, (July 2007), pp. 511-532, ISSN 0893-8512

Fowler, B.A. & Sexton, M.J. (2007). Bismuth. In, *Handbook on the Toxicology of Metals,Third Edition*, G.F. Nordberg; B.A., Fowler; M. Nordberg & L., Friberg (Eds), 117, Academic Press/Elsevier B.V., ISBN 978-0-12-369413-3, Burlington MA, San Diego CA, London UK

Frachtman, R.L.; Ericsson, C.D. & DuPont, H.L. (1982). Seroconversion to *Entamoeba histolytica* among short-term travelers to Mexico. *Archives of Internal Medicine*, Vol.142, No.7, (July 1982), pp. 1299. ISSN 0003-9926

Franzén, O.; Jerlström-Hultqvist, J.; Castro, E.; Sherwood, E.; Ankarklev, J.; Reiner, D.S.; Palm, D.; Andersson, J.O.; Andersson, B. & Svärd, S.G. (2009). Draft genome sequencing of *Giardia intestinalis* assemblage B isolate GS: Is human giardiasis caused by two different species? *PLoS Pathogens*, Vol.5, No.8, (August 2009), e1000560. ISSN 1553-7366

Frech, S.A.; DuPont H.L.; Bourgeois, A.L.; McKenzie, R.; Belkind-Gerson, J.; Figueroa, J.F.; Okhuysen, P.C.; Guerrero, N.H.; Martinez-Sandoval, F.G.; Meléndez-Romero, J.H.; Jiang, Z.D.; Asturias, E.J.; Halpern, J.; Torres, O.R.; Hoffman, A.S.; Villar, C.P.; Kassern, R.N.; Flyer, D.C.; Andersen, B.H.; Kazempour, K.; Breich, S.A.& Glenn, G.M..(2008). Use of a patch containing heat-labile toxin from Escherichia coli against travellers' diarrhoea: a phase II, randomised, double-blind, placebo-controlled field trial. *The Lancet*, Vol. 71, No.9629, (June 14, 2008), pp. 2019–2025, ISSN 0140-6736

Freedmann, D.O.; Weld, L.H.; Kozarsky, P.E.; Fisk, T.; Robins, R.; von Sonnenburg F.; Keystone, J.S.; Pandey, P.; Cetron, M.S. & Geosentinel Surveillance Network (2006). Spectrum of disease and relation to place of exposure among ill returned travelers. *The New England Journal of Medicine*, Vol.354, No 2, (January 2006), pp. 119–130, ISSN 0028-4793

Gallelli, L.; Colosimo, M.; Tolotta G.A.; Falcone, D.; Luberto, L.; Curto, L.S.; Rende, P.; Mazzei, F.; Marigliano, N.M.; De Sarro, G. & Cucchiara, S. (2010). Prospective randomized double-blind trial of racecadotril compared with loperamide in elderly people with gastroenteritis living in nursing homes. *European Journal of Clinical Pharmacology*, Vol.66, No.2, (February 2010), pp. 137-44. ISSN 0031-6970

Galván-Moroyoqui, J.M.; Del Carmen Dominguez-Robles, M. & Meza, I. (2008). The interplay between *Entamoeba* and enteropathogenic bacteria modulates epithelial cell damage. *PloS Neglected Tropical Diseases*, Vol.2, No.7, (July 2008), e266. ISSN 1935-2727

Gargala, G. (2008). Drug treatment and novel drug target against *Cryptosporidium*. *Parasite*, Vol.15, No.3, (September 2008), pp. 275-281, ISSN 1252-607X

Gonzales, M.L.; Dans, L.F. & Martinez, E.G. (2009). Antiamoebic drugs for treating amoebic colitis. *Cochrane Database for Systematic Reviews*, Vol.15, No.2, (April 2009), CD006085. ISSN 1469-493X

Goodgame, R. (2003). Emerging Causes of Traveler's Diarrhea: Cryptosporidium, Cyclospora, Isospora, and Microsporidia. *Current Infectious Disease Reports*, Vol.5, No 5, (February 2003), pp. 66-73, ISSN 1523-3847

Gottlieb, T & Heather, C.S. (2011). Diarrhoea in adults (acute). *Clinical Evidence [Electronic Resource]*, Vol.pii, No.0901, (February 2011), ISSN 1752-8526

Harris, J.B.; Khan. A.J.; LaRosque, R.C.; Dorer, D.J.; Chowdhury, F.; Faruque, A.S.; Sack, D.A.; Ryan, E.T.; Qardi, F. & Caldewood, S.B.. (2005). Blood group, immunity, and risk of infection with Vibrio cholerae in an area of endemicity. *Infection and Immunity*, Vol.73, No.11, (November 2005), pp. 7422-7427, ISSN 1098-5522

Hill, D.R (2000). Occurrence and self-treatment of diarrhea in a large cohort of Americans traveling to developing countries. . *The American Journal of Tropical Medicine and Hygiene*, Vol.62, No.5, (May 2000), pp. 585-589, ISSN 0002-9637

Hill, D.R.; Ford, L. & Lalloo, D.G. (2006). Oral cholera vaccines: use in clinical practice.*The Lancet Infectious Diseases*, Vol.6, No 6, (June 2006), pp. 361–373, ISSN 1473-3099

Hill, D.R. & Beeching, N.J. (2010). Travelers' diarrhea. *Current Opinion in Infectious Diseases*, Vol.23, No.5, (October 2010), pp.481-487, ISSN 0951-7375

Hilton, E.; Kolakowski, P.; Singer, C. & Smith, M. (1997) Effi cacy of *Lactobacillus* GG as a diarrheal preventive in travelers. *Journal of Travel Medicine*, Vol.4, No.1, (March 1997), pp. 41–43, ISSN 1195-1982

Houf, K. & Stephan, R.(2007). Isolation and characterization of the emerging foodborn pathogen *Arcobacter* from human stool. *Journal of Microbiological Methods*, Vol. 68, No. 2, (February 2007), pp. 408-413, ISSN 0167-7012

Huang, P.; Farkas, T.; Marionneau, S.; Zhong, W. ; Ruvoën-Clouet, N. ; Morrow, A.L.; Altaye, M.; Pickering, L.K.; Newburg, D.S.; LePendu, J & Jiang, X..(2003). Noroviruses bind to human ABO, Lewis, and secretor histo-blood group antigens: identification of 4 distinct strainspecific patterns. *The Journal of Infectious Diseases*, Vol.188, No.1, (July 2003), pp. 19-31, ISSN 0022-1899

Huang, D.B.; Awasthi, M.; Le B.M.; Leve, M.E.; DuPont, M.W.; DuPont, H.L. & Ericsson, C.D. (2004). The role of diet in the treatment of travelers' diarrhea: A pilot study. *Clinical Infectious Diseases*, Vol.39, No.4, (August 2004), pp. 468-471, ISSN 1058-4838

Hutson ,A.M.; Atmar, R.L.; Graham, D.Y. & Estes, M.K. (2002). Norwalk virus infection and disease is associated with ABO histo-blood group type. *The Journal of Infectious Diseases*. Vol.185, No.9. (May 2002), pp. 1335-1337, ISSN 0022-1899

Jex, A.R.; Pangasa, A.; Campbell, B.E.; Whipp, M.; Hogg, G.; Sinclair, M.I.; Stevens, M. & Gasser, R.B. (2008). Classification of *Cryptosporidium* species from patients with sporadic cryptosporidiosis by use of sequence-based multilocus analysis following mutation scanning. *Journal of Clinical Microbiology*, Vol.46, No.7, (July 2008), pp. 2252-2262, ISSN 0095-1137

Jiang, Z.D.; Okhuysen, P.C.; Guo, D.C.; He, R.; King, T.M.; DuPont, H.L. & Milewicz, D.M. (2003). Genetic susceptibility to enteroaggregative Escherichia coli diarrhea: polymorphism in the interleukin-8 promotor region.*The Journal of Infectious Diseases*, Vol.188, No.4, (15 August 2003), pp. 506-511, ISSN 0022-1899

Jiang, Z.D.; DuPont, H.L.; Brown, E.L.; Nandy, R.K.; Ramamurthy, T.; Sinha, A.; Ghosh, S.; Guin, S.; Gurleen, K.; Rodrigues, S.; Chen, J.J.; McKenzie, R. & Steffen, R. (2010). Microbial etiology of travelers' diarrhea in Mexico, Guatemala, and India: importance of enterotoxigenic *Bacteroides fragilis* and *Arcobacter* species. *Journal of Clinical Microbiology*, Vol.48, No.4, (April 2010), pp. 1417-1419, ISSN 0095-1137

Johnson, E.H.; Windsor, J.J. & Clark, C.G. (2004). Emerging from Obscurity: Biological, Clinical, and Diagnostic Aspects of *Dientamoeba fragilis*. *Clinical Microbiology Reviews*, Vol.17, No.3, (July 2004), pp. 553-570, ISSN 0893-8512

Johnson, P.C.; Ericsson, C.D.; DuPont, H.L.; Morgan, D.R.; Bitsura, J.A & Wood, L.V. (1986). Comparison of loperamide with bismuth subsalicylate for the treatment of acute travelers' diarrhea. *JAMA: the Journal of the American Medical Association*, Vol.255, No.6, (14 February 1986), pp. 757–760, ISSN 1538-3598

Kansouzidou, A.; Charitidou, C.; Varnis, T.; Vavatsi, N, & Kamaria, F. (2004). Cyclospora cayetanensis in a patient with travelers' diarrhea: case report and review. *Journal of Travel Medicine*, Vol.11, No.1, (January-February 2004), pp. 61-63, ISSN 1195-1982

Karst, S.M. (2010). Pathogenesis of noroviruses, emeging RNA viruses. *Viruses*, Vol.2, No.3, (2010), ISSN 1999-4915

Katsarou-Katsari, A.; Vassalos, C.M.; Tzanetou, K.; Spanakos, G.; Papadopoulou, C & Vakalis, N. (2008). Acute urticaria associated with amoeboid forms of *Blastocystis* sp. subtype 3. *Acta Dermato-venereologica*, Vol.88, No.1, (January 2008), pp. 80-81, ISSN 0001-5555

Katz, D.E. & Taylor, D.N. (2001). Parasitic infections of the gastrointestinal tract. *Gastroenterology Clinics of North America*, Vol.30, No.3, (September 2001), pp. 797-815, ISSN 0889-8553

Koo, D., Maloney, K. & Tauxe, R. (1996). Epidemioplogyof diarrheal disease outbreaks on cruise ships, 1986 through 1993. *JAMA: the Journal of the American Medical Association*, Vol. 275, No. 7, (Februar 1996), pp, 545-547, ISSN 1538-3598

Koo, H.L., Jiang, Z.D., Brown, E., Garcia, C., Qi ,H.& DuPont, H.L. (2008). Coliform contamination of vegetables obtained from popular restaurants in Guadalajara, Mexico, and Houston, Texas. *Clinical Infectious Diseases*, Vol.47, No.2, (July 2008), pp. 218–221, ISSN 1-58-4838

Koo, H.L. & DuPont, H.L. (2010). Rifaximin: a unique gastrointestinal-selective antibiotic for enteric diseases. *Current Opinion in Gastroenterology*, Vol.26, No.1, (January 2010), pp. 17–25, ISSN 0267-1379

Kornylo, K.; Kim, D.K.; Widdowson, M.A.; Turabelidze, G. & Averhoff, F.M. (2009). Risk of norovirus transmission during air travel. *Journal of Travel Medicine*, Vol.16, No.5, (September-October 2009), pp. 349-351, ISSN 1195-1982

Kuschner, R.A.; Trofa, A.F; Thomas, R.J.; Hoge, C.W.; Pitarangsi, C.; Amato, S.; Olafson, R.P.; Echeverria, P.; Sadoff, J.C. & Taylor, D.N. (1998). Use of azitromicyn for the treatment of Campylobacter enteritis in travelers to Thailand, an area where ciprofloxacin resistance is prevalent. *Clinical Infectious Diseases*, Vol.21, No.3, (September 1998), pp.341-345, ISSN 1058-4838

Lalle, M. (2010). Giardiasis in the post genomic era: treatment, drug resistance and novel therapeutic perspectives. *Infectious Disorders Drug Targets*, Vol.10. No.4, (August 2010), pp. 283-294. ISSN 1871-5265

Lama, J.R.; Seas, C.R.; León-Barúa, R.; Gotuzzo, E. & Sack, R.B. (2004). Environmental temperature, cholera, and acute diarrhoea in adults in Lima, Peru. *Journal of Health, Population and Nutrition*, Vol.22, No.4, (December 2004), pp. 399-403, ISSN 1606-0997

Lasek-Nesselquist, E.; Welch, D.M. & Sogin, M.L. (2010). The identification of a new *Giardia duodenalis* assemblage in marine vertebrates and a preliminary analysis of *G.*

duodenalis population biology in marine systems. *International Journal of Parasitology*, Vol.40, No.9, (August 2010), pp. 1063-1074, ISSN 0029-7519

Lauerman, J.F. (2001). Weathering diarrheal illness effects of El Niño in the South Pacific. Environmental Health Perspectives, Vol.109, No.2, (February 2001), pp. A84–A85, ISSN 0091-6765

Lauwaet, T.; Davids, B.J.; Reiner, D.S. & Gillin, F.D. (2007). Encystation of *Giardia lamblia*: a model for other parasites. *Current Opinion in Microbiology*, Vol.10, No.6, (December 2007), pp.554-559, ISSN 1369-5274

Leder K.(2009). Intestinal Protozoa: *Giardia, Amebiasis, Cyclospora, Blastocystis hominis, Dientamoeba fragilis*, and *Cryptosporidium parvum*. In, *Tropical Diseases in Travelers*, E. Schwartz (Ed), 294-302, Blackwell Publishing, ISBN 978-1-4051-8441-0, The Atrium, Southern Gate, Chichester, West Sussex, UK

Lever, D.S. & Soffer, E. (2009). Acute diarrhea. In, *Current Clinical Medicine 2009/ Cleveland Clinic*, W.D. Carey, (Ed). Saunders Elsevier Inc., 474-478, ISBN 978-1-4160-6643-9, Philadelphia, USA

Li, S.T.; Grossman, D.C. & Cummings, P. (2007). Loperamide therapy for acute diarrhea in children: systematic review and meta-analysis. *PLoS Medicine*, Vol. 4, No.3, (March 2007), e98. ISSN 1549-1277

Lindenbaum, J. (1965). Malabsorption during and after recovery from acute intestinal infection . *BMJ* , Vol.2, No.5457, (August 1965), pp. 326 – 329, ISSN 0007-1447

Lindgren, M.M.; Kotilainen, P.; Huovinen, P.; Hurme, S.; Lukinmaa, S.; Webber, M.A.; Piddock, L.J.; Siitonen, A.; & Hakanen, A.J. (2009) Reduced fl uoroquinolone susceptibilityin *Salmonella enterica* isolates from travelers, Finland. *Emerging Infectious Diseases*, Vol. 5, No.5, (May 2009), pp. 809–812, ISSN 1080-6059

Lopez-Velez, R.; Batle, C.; Jiménez, C.; Navarro, M.;Norman, F. & Perez-Molina, J. (2010). Short Course Combination Therapy for Giardiasis after Nitroimidazole Failure. *The American Journal of Tropical Medicine and Hygiene*, Vol.83, No.1, (July 2010), pp. 171-173, ISSN 0002-9637

Lorenzi, H.A.; Puiu, D.; Miller, J.R.; Brinkac, L.M.; Amedeo, P.; Hall, N. & Caler, E.V. (2010). New assembly, reannotation and analysis of the *Entamoeba histolytica* genome reveal new genomic features and protein content information. *PloS Neglected Tropical Diseases*, Vol.4, No.6, (June 2010), e716, ISSN 1935-2727

Lorrot, M. & Vasseur, M. (2007). How do the rotavirus NSP4 and bacterial enterotoxins lead differently to diarrhea? Virology Journal, Vol.4, (March 2007), pp.1-6, ISSN 1743-422X

Marionneau, S.; Airaud, F.; Bovin, N.V.; Pendu ,J.L. & Ruvoen-Clouet, N. (2005). Influence of the combined ABO, FUT2, and FUT3 polymorphism on susceptibility to Norwalk virus attachment. *The Journal of Infectious Diseases*, Vol.192, No.6, (September 2005), pp. 1071-1077, ISSN 0022-1899

Marshall, J.A. (2002). Mixed infections of intestinal viruses and bacteria in humans. In, *Polymicrobial diseases*, K.A. Brogden & J.A. Guthmiller (Eds.), ASM Press, 299-316, ISBN 1-55581-244-9, Washington, USA

Mathis, A.; Weber, R. & and Deplazes, P. (2005). Zoonotic potential of the microsporidia. *Clinical Microbiology Reviews*, Vol.18, No.3, (July 2005), pp. 423-445, ISSN 0893-8512

Mattila, L.; Siitonen, A.; Kyronseppa, H.; Simula, I.; Oksanen, P.; Stenvik, M,; Salo, P.& Peltola, H..(1992). Seasonal variation in etiology of traveler's diarrhea. Finnish-

Moroccan Study Group. *The Journal of Infectious Diseases*, Vol.165, No.2, (February 1992), pp. 385-388, ISSN 0022-1899

McFarland, L.V. (2007). Meta-analysis of probiotics for the prevention of traveler's diarrhea. *Travel Medicine and Infectious Disease*, Vol.5, No.2, (March 2007), pp. 97–105, ISSN 1873-0442

Mensa, L.; Marco, F.; Vila, J.; Gascon, J. & Ruiz, J. (2008) Quinolone resistance among *Shigella* spp. isolated from travellers returning from India. *Clinical Microbiology and Infection*, Vol.14, No.3, (March 2008), pp. 279–281 , ISSN 1469-0691

Meraz, I.M.; Jiang, Z.D.; Ericsson, C.D.; Bourgeois, A.L.; Steffen, R.; Taylor, D.N.;Hernandez, N. & DuPont, H.L. (2008).Enterotoxigenic *Escherichia coli* and diffusely adherent *E. coli* as likely causes of a proportion of pathogen-negative travelers' diarrhea—a PCR-based study. *Journal of Travel Medicine*, Vol.15, No.6, (November- December 2008), pp. 412-418, ISSN 1195-1982

Mohamed, J.A.; DuPont, H.L.; Jiang, Z.D.; Belkind-Gerson, J.; Figueroa, J.F.; Armitige, L.Y.; Tsai, A.; Nair, P.;Martinez-Sandoval, F.J.; Guo, D.C.; Hayes, P. & Okhuysen, P.C. (2007). A novel single-nucleotide polymorphism in the lactoferrin gene is associated with susceptibility to diarrhea in North American travelers to Mexico. *Clinical Infectious Diseases*, Vol.44, No.7, (April 2007), pp. 945–952, ISSN 1058-4838

Mohamed, J.A.; DuPont, H.L.; Jiang, Z.D.; Flores, J.; Carlin, L.G.;Belkind-Gerson, J.; Martinez-Sandoval, F.G.; Guo, D.; White, A.C. Jr & Okhuysen, P.C. (2009). A single-nucleotide polymorphism in the gene encoding osteoprotegerin, an anti-inflammatory protein produced in response to infection with diarrheagenic Escherichia coli, is associated with an increased risk of nonsecretory bacterial diarrhea in North American travelers to Mexico. *The Journal of Infectious Diseases*, Vol.199, No.4, (February 2009), pp. 477–485, ISSN 0022-1899

Morgan-Ryan, U.M.; Fall, A.; Ward, L.A.; Hihjjawi, N.; Sulaiman, I.; Fayer, R.; Thompson, R.C.; Olson, M.; Lal, A. & Xiao, L. (2002). *Cryptosporidium hominis* n. sp. (Apicomplexa: Cryptosporidiidae) from *Homo sapiens*. *The Journal of Eukaryotic Microbiology*, Vol.49, No.6, (November-December 2002), pp. 433-440, ISSN 1066-5234

Mudholkar, V.G. & Namey, R.D. (2010). Heavy infestation of *Isospora belli* causing severe watery diarrhea. *Indian Journal of Pathology & Microbiology*, Vol.53, No.4, (October-December 2010), pp. 824-825, ISSN 0377-4929

Müller, A.; Bialek, R.; Kämper, A.; Fätkenheuer, G.; Salzberger, B. & Franzén. C.(2001). Detection of micosporidia in travelers with diarrhea. *Journal of Clinical Microbiology*, Vol.39, No.4, (April 2001), pp. 1630-1632, ISSN 0095-1137

Navaneethan, U. & Giannella, R.A. (2008). Mechanisms of infectious diarrhea. *National Clinical Practice. Gastroenterology and Hepatology*, Vol.5, No.11, (November 2008), pp. 637-647, ISSN 1743-4378

Norman, F.F.; Pérez-Molina, J.; Pérez de Ayala, A.; Jiménez, B.C.; Navarro, M. & López-Vélez R. (2008). Clostridium difficile-associated diarrhea after antibiotic treatment for traveler's diarhea. *Clinical Infectious Diseases*, Vol.46, No.7, (April 2008), pp. 1060-1063, ISSN 1058-4838

Okhuysen, P.C. (2001). Traveler's diarrhea due to intestinal protozoa. *Clinical Infectious Diseases*, Vol.33, No.1, (July 1, 2001), pp. 110–114, ISSN 1058-4838

Okhuysen, P.C. (2005). Current concepts in traveler´s diarrhea: epidemiology, antimicrobial resistance and treatment. *Current Opinion in Infectious Diseases*, Vol.18, No.6, (December 2005), pp.522-526, ISSN 0951-7375

Okyuysen, P.C.; Jiang, Z.D.; Carlin, L.; Forbes, C. & DuPont, H.L. (2004). Postdiarrhea chronic intestinal symptoms and irritable bowel syndrome in North American travelers to Mexico. *The American Journal of Gastroenterology*, Vol.99, No.9, (September 2004), pp. 1774–1778, ISSN 0002-9270

Ortega, Y.R. & Sanchez, R. (2010). Update on *Cyclospora cayetanensis*, a food-borne and waterborne parasite. *Clinical Microbiology Reviews*, Vol.23, No.1, (January 2010), pp. 218-234, ISSN 0893-8512

Ostrosky-Zeichner, L. & Ericsson, C.D. (2001). Travelers' diarrhea. In: *Travel Medicine*, J.N. Zuckerman (Ed.), 153-164, John Wiley & Sons, Ltd, ISBN 0-471-49079-2, Chichester, UK

Padilla-Vaca, F. & Anaya-Velázquez , F. (2010). Insights into *Entamoeba histolytica* virulence modulation. *Infectious Disorders Drug Targets*, Vol.4, No.10, (August 2010), pp.242-250, ISSN 1871-5265

Paredes-Paredes, M.: Okhuysen, P.C.; Flores, J.; Mohamed, J.A.; Padda, R.S.; Gonzalez-Estrada, A.; Haley, C.A.; Carlin, L.G.; Nair, P. & DuPont, H.L. (2011). Seasonality of diarrheagenic *Escherichia coli* pathotypes in the US students acquiring diarrhea in Mexico. *Journal of Travel Medicine*, Vol.18, No.2, (March-April 2011), pp. 121-125, ISSN 1195-1982

Parfrey, L.W.; Barbero, E.; Lasser, E.; Dunthorn, M.; Bhattacharya, D.; Patterson, D.J. & Katz, L.A. (2006). Evaluating support for the current classification of eukaryotic diversity. *PloS Genetics*, Vol.2, No.12, (December 2006), e220. ISSN 1553-7390

Peñaranda, M.E.; Cubitt, W.D.;Sinarachatanant, P.; Taylor, D.N.; Likanonsakul, S.; Saif, L. & Glass, R.I. (1989). Group C rotavirus infections in patients with diarrhea in Thailand, Nepal, and England. *Journal of Infectious Diseases*, Vol.160, No.3, (September 1989), pp. 392-397, ISSN 0022-1899

Pitzinger, B.; Steffen, R. & Tschopp, A.(1991). Incidence and clinical features of traveler's diarrhea in infants and children. *The Pediatric Infectious Disease Journal*, Vol.10, No.10. (October 1991), pp. 719-723, ISSN 0891-3668

Piyaphanee, W.; Kusolsuk. T.; Kittitrakul, C.; Suttithym, W.; Ponam, T. & Wilairatana, P. (2011). Incidence and impact of travelers' diarrhea among foreign backpackers in Southeast Asia: a result from Khao San road, Bangkok. *Journal of Travel Medicine.* Vol.18, No.2, (March-April 2011), pp. 109-114, ISSN 1195-1982

Polley, S.D.; Boadi, S.; Watson, J.; Curry, A. & Chiodini P.L. (2011). Detection and species identification of microsporidial infections using SYBR Green real-time PCR. *Journal of Medical Microbiology*, Vol.60, Pt4, (April 2011), pp. 459-466, ISSN 0022-2615

Rose, S.R.; Keystone, J.S. & Hackett, P. (2010). Travelers' Diarrhea. In, *International Travel Health Guide. Updated Online Edition, 2010,* Chapter 6, Travel Medicine, Inc., Northampton MA, (March 14, 2010), Retrieved from http://www.travmed.com/health_guide.htm

Sanders, J.W.; Riddle, M.S.; Brewster, S.J. & Taylor, D.N. (2008). Epidemiology of traveler's diarrhea. In, *Travel Medicine*, J.S. Keystone; P.E. Kozarsky; D.O. Freedman; H.D. Nothdurft & B.A. Connor (Eds.), Chapter 16, Mosby Elsevier, 2008, ISBN 0323034535, Maryland Heights, USA

Sari Kovats, R.; Buma, M.J.; Hajat, S.; Worrall, E. & Haines, A. (2003). El Nino and health. *The Lancet*, Vol.362, No.9394, (November 2003), pp. 1481-1489, ISSN 0140-6736

Sears, C.L. & Guerrant, R.L. (1994). Cryptosporiodiosis: the complexity of intestinal pathophysiology. *Gastroenterology*, Vol.106, No.1, (January 1994), pp. 252–254, ISSN 0016-5085

Shah, N.; DuPont, H.L. & Ramsey, D.J. (2009). Global etiology of travelers' diarrhea: systematic review from 1973 to the present. *The American Journal of Tropical Medicine and Hygiene*, Vol.80, No.4, (April 2009), pp. 609-614, ISSN 0002-9637

Sheridan, J.F.; Aurelian. L.; Barbour, G.; Santosham, M.; Sack, R.B. & Ryder, R.W. (1981). Traveler's diarrhea associated with rotavirus infection: analysis of virus-specific immunoglobulin classes. *Infection and Immunity*, Vol.31, No.1, (January1981), pp. 419-429, ISSN 0019-9567

Stanley, S.L. Jr. (2003). Amoebiasis. *The Lancet*, Vol.361, No.9362 (March 2003), pp. 1025-1034, ISSN 0140-6736

Stark, D.; Al-Qassab, S.E.; Barratt, J.L.; Stanley, K.; Roberts, T.; Marriott, D.; Harkness, J. & Ellis, J.T. (2011). Evaluation of multiplex tandem real-time PCR for detection of *Cryptosporidium* spp., *Dientamoeba fragilis*, *Entamoeba histolytica*, and *Giardia intestinalis* in clinical stool samples. *Journal of Clinical Microbiology*, 2011 Jan;Vol.49, No.1, (January 2011), pp. 257-262, ISSN 0095-1137

Stark, D.; Barratt, J.; Ellis, J.; Harkness, J & Marriott, D. (2009). Repeated *Dientamoeba fragilis* infections: a case report of two families from Sydney, Australia. *Infectious Diseases Reports*, Vol.1, e4, (November 2009). ISSN 20367430

Stark, D.; Barratt, J.; Roberts, T.; Marriott, D.; Harkness, J. & Ellis, J. (2010). Comparison of microscopy, two xenic culture techniques, conventional and real-time PCR for the detection of *Dientamoeba fragilis* in clinical stool samples. *European Journal of Clinical Microbiology and Infectious Disease*, Vol.29, No.4, (April 2010), pp. 411-416. ISSN 0934-9723

Stark, D.; Beebe, N.; Marriott, D.; Ellis, J. & Harkness, J. (2005). Prospective study of the prevalence, genotyping, and clinical relevance of *Dientamoeba fragilis* infections in an Australian population. *Journal of Clinical Microbiology*, Vol.43, No.6, (June 2005), pp. 2718-2723, ISSN 0095-1137

Steffen, R.; van der Linde, F.; Gyr. K. & Schär, M. (1983). Epidemiology of diarrhea in travelers. *JAMA: the Journal of the American Medical Association*, Vol.249, No.9, (March 1983), pp. 1176-1180, ISSN 1538-3598

Steffen, R.; Rickenbach, M.; Wilhelm, U.; Helminger, A. & Schär, M. (1987). Health problems after travel to developing countries. *The Journal of Infectious Diseases*, Vol.156, No.1, (July 1987), pp. 84-91, ISSN 0022-1899

Steffen, R.; Collard, F.; Tornieporth, N.; Campbell-Forrester, S.; Ashley, D., Thompson, S.; Mathewson, J.J.; Maes, E.; Stephenson, B.; DuPont, H.L. & von Sonnenburg, F. (1999). Epidemiology, etiology, and impact of traveler's diarrhea in Jamaica. *JAMA: the Journal of the American Medical Association*, Vol.281, No.9, (March 1999), pp. 811-817, ISSN 1538-3598

Steffen, R. (2005). Epidemiology of traveler's diarrhea. *Clinical Infectious Diseases*. Vol. 41, Suppl. 8,(December 2005), pp. S536–S540, ISSN 1058-4838.

Stensvold, C.R.; Alfellani, M.A.; Nørskov-Lauritsen, S.; Prip, K.; Victory, E.L.; Maddox, C.; Nielsen, H.V. & Clark, C.G. (2009). Subtype distribution of Blastocystis isolates from synanthropic and zoo animals and identification of a new subtype. *International Journal of Parasitology*, Vol.39, No.4, (March 2009), pp.473-479, ISSN 0029-7519

Stermer, E; Lubezky, A.; Potasman, I.; Paster, E. & Lavy, A. (2006).Is traveler's diarrhea a significant risk factor for the development of irritable bowel syndrome? A prospective study. *Clinical Infectious Diseases*, Vol.43, No.7, (October 2006), pp. 898-901, ISSN 1058-4838

Suriptiastuti, M.S. (2010). Host-parasite interactions and mechanisms of infections in amebiasis. *Universa Medicina*, Vol.29, No.2, (May-August 2010), pp. 104-113, ISSN 1907-3062

Svennerholm, A.M. (2011). From cholera to enterotoxigenic *Escherichia coli* (ETEC) vaccine development. *The Indian Journal of Medical Research*, Vol.133, No,2, (February 2011), pp. 188-196. ISSN:0971-5916

Synder, J.D. & Blake, P.A. (1982). Is cholera a problem a problem for US travelers? *JAMA: the Journal of the American Medical Association*, Vol.247, No.16, (23 April), pp. 2268-2269, ISSN 1538-3598

Tan, K.S. (2008). New insights on classification, identification, and clinical relevance of *Blastocystis* spp. *Clinical Microbiology Reviews*, Vol.21, No.4, (October 2008), pp. 639-665, ISSN 0893-8512

Taylor, D.N. & Echeverria, P. (1986). Etiology and epidemiology of traveler's diarrhea in Asia. *Review of Infectious Diseases*, Suppl.2, (May-June 1986), pp. S136-141, ISSN 0162-0886

Taylor, D.N.; Houston, R.; Shlim, D.R.; Bhaibulaya, M.; Ungar, B.L. & Echeverria, P. (1988). Etiology of diarrhea among travelers and foreign residents in Nepal. *JAMA: the Journal of the American Medical Association*, Vol.260, No.9, (September 1988), pp. 1245–1248, ISSN 1538-3598

Taylor, D.N.; McKenzie, R.; Durbin, A.; Carpenter, C.; Haake, R. & Bourgeois, A.L. (2008). Systemic pharmacokinetics of rifaximin in volunteers with shigellosis. *Antimicrobial Agents and Chemotherapy*, Vol.52, No.3, (March 2008), pp. 1179–1181, ISSN 0066-4804

Teague, N.S.; Srijan, A.; Wongstitwilairoong, B.; Poramathikul, K.; Champathai, T.; Ruksasiri, S.; Pavlin, J. & Mason, C.J. (2010). Enteric pathogen sampling of tourist restaurants in Bangkok, Thailand. *Journal of Travel Medicine*, Vol.17, No.2, (March-April 2010), pp. 118-123, ISSN 1195-1982

Tjoa, W.S.; DuPont, H.L.; Sullivan, P.; Pickering, L.K.; Holguin, A.H.; Olarte, J.; Evans, D.G.; Evans, D.J. Jr. (1977). Location of food consumption and travelers' diarrhea. *Amercan Journal of Epidemiology*, Vol.106, No.1, (July 1977), pp. 61-66, ISSN 0002-9262

Topazian, M. & Bia, F.J. (1994). New parasites on the block: emerging intestinal protozoa. *Gastroenterologist*, Vol.2, No.2, (June 1994), pp. 147-159, ISSN 1065-2477

Tribble, D.R.; Sanders. J.W.; Pang, L.W.; Mason.; C; Pitarangsi, C.; Baqar, S.; Armstrong, A.; Hshieh, P.; Fox, A.; Maley, E.A.; Lebron, C.; Faix, D.J., Lawler, J.V.; Nayak., G., Lewis, M., Bodhidatta, L. & Scott, D.A. (2007). Traveler's diarrhea in Thailand: randomized, double-blind trial comparing single-dose and 3-day azithromycinbased regimens with a 3-day levofloxacin regimen. *Clinical Infectious Diseases*, Vol.44, No.3, (February 2007), pp. 338–346, ISSN 1058-4838

Türk M.; Türker, M.; Ak, M.; Karaayak, B. & Kaya, T. (2004). Cyclosporiasis associated with diarrhoea in an immunocompetent patient in Turkey. *Journal of Medical Microbiology*, Vol.58, No.3, (March 2004), pp. 255-257, ISSN 0022-2615

Tuteja, A.K.; Taley, N.J.; Gelman,S.S.; Alder. S.C.; Thompson, C.; Tolman, K. & Hale, D.C. (2008). Development of functional diarrhea, constipation, irritable bowel syndrome, and dyspepsia during and after traveling outside the USA. *Digestive Diseases and Sciences*, Vol.53, No.1, (January 2008), pp. ; 271-276, ISSN 0163-2116

Tzipori, S. & Ward, H. (2002). Cryptosporidiosis: biology, pathogenesis and disease. *Microbes and Infection*, Vol.4, No.10, (August 2002), pp. 1047-1058, ISSN 1286-4579

Vassalos, C.M.; Spanakos, G.; Vassalou, E.; Papadopoulou, C. & Vakalis, N. (2010). Differences in clinical significance and morphologic features of *Blastocystis* sp. subtype 3. (2010). *American Journal of Clinical Pathology*, Vol.133, No.2, (February 2010), pp.251-258, ISSN 0002-9173

Vassalos, C.M.; Vakalis, N. & Papadopoulou, C. (2008). *Blastocystis* and its pathogenic potential: latest aspect. *Reviews in Medical Microbiology*, Vol.19, No.4, (October 2008), pp. 87-97, ISSN 0954-139X

Vassalos, C.M.; Vassalou, E.; Sofos, N. & Vakalis, N. Health Problems of Spiritual/Heritage Tourists and Christian "Hajji" Pilgrims Upon Returning from the Middle East. *CISTM12 Abstracts – Poster Presentations*, Poster No.06.14, Bosron, USA, (May 2011), p.58

Vassalou, E.; Vassalos, C. M.; Piperaki, E.-T. & Vakalis, N. (2010). To notice the unnoticed (Studying overlooked intestinal protozoa in Greece). *"Research in Progress 2010: Shorts Presentations and Posters"*, The Royal Society of Tropical Medicine & Hygiene, London, UK, (December 2010), Poster No.24

Vollet, J.J.; Ericsson, C.D.; Gibson, G.; Pickering, L.K.; DuPont, H.L.; Kohl, S. & Conklin, R.H. (1979). Human rotavirus in an adult population with traveler's diarrhea and its relationship to the location of food consumption. *Journal of Medical Virology*, Vol.4, No.2, (1979), pp. 81-87. ISSN 0146-6615

Wagner, A. & Wiedermann, U. (2009). Travellers' diatthoea-pros and cons of different prophylactic measures. *Wiener klinische Wochenschrift*, Vol.121, Suppl.3, (October 2009), pp. 13-18, ISSN 0043-5325

Weedall, G.D. & Neil Hall, N. (2011). Evolutionary genomics of *Entamoeba*. *Research in Microbiology*, Vol.162, No.6, (July-August 2011), pp. 637-645. ISSN 0923-2508

Widdowson, M.A.; Cramer, E.H.; Hadley, L. & Bresee, J.S. (2002). Outbreaks of acute gastroenteritis on cruise ships and on land: identification of a predominant circulating strain of norovirus-United States, 2002. *Journal of Infectious Diseases*, Vol.190, No.1, (December 2004), pp. 27-36, ISSN 0022-1899

Williams, B.A. (2009). Unique physiology of host-parasite interactions in microsporidia infections. *Cellular Microbiology*, Vol.11, No.11, (November 2009), pp. 1551-1560, ISSN 1462-5814

Yates, J. (2005). Traveler's diarrhea. *American Family Physician*, Vol.71, No.11, (July 2005), pp. 2095-2100, 2107-2108,ISSN 0002-838X

Zimmer, S. M.; Schuetz A. N. & C. Franco-Paredes, C. (2007) . Efficacy of nitazoxanide for cyclosporiasis in patients with sulfa allergy. *Clinical Infectious Diseases*, Vol.44, No.3, (February 2007), pp. 466-467, ISSN 1058-4838

Part 3

Appendicitis

8

Alvarado Score Between 4 and 6, the Place of the CT Scan

S. Loudjedi[1], M. Bensenane[2], N. Meziane[1], F. Ghirane[1] and M. Kherbouche[1]
[1]*Department of Surgery B,*
[2]*Department of Radiology,*
University of Abu-Bakr Belkaid, Tlemcen,
Algeria

1. Introduction

The appendicitis is the inflammation of the appendix. The appendix is a small tube like pouch that is part of the large intestine. The appendix has no known function, but it can become diseased.
Symptoms vary widely. It can affect all ages and both sexes.
The exact cause is unknown. The appendix may be blocked with faeces from the intestinal tract, which leads to infection. When infected, the appendix becomes swollen, inflamed and filled with pus.
Curable with surgery, people can live a normal life without their appendix.
About 8% of the population may develop acute appendicitis during their lifetime. The clinical diagnosis is evident in 80% of cases, but in the remaining cases the lack of parallelism anatomoclinical sometimes makes the diagnosis very difficult. Since 1986, the clinical and biological Alvarado score is a test used in clinical practice in surgery dealing with pain in the right iliac fossa. We sought to identify the role of computed tomography (CT) in the diagnosis of acute appendicitis in patients with a score of 4 to 6 Alvarado. In this view, it would be disposed to negative laparotomy, which represents between 15% and 30% and also prevents progression to such complications as acute peritonitis. [1]

2. Historical evolution of its diagnosis and treatment

Since the middle Ages, physicians have recognised a clinical entity associated with severe inflammation of the cecal region. Termed "typhlitis" or "paratyphlitis"(from the Greek *typhlos,* meaning "blind" and referring to the anatomy of the first part of the cecum). The disease was for hundreds of years considered fatal. In 1886, Professor Reginald Fitz at Harvard Medical School gave the first clear, logical description of the clinical and pathologic features of the disease by using the term appendicitis. [2]
In 1889, the New York surgeon Charles McBurney advocated prompt diagnosis and early appendectomy and so led the medical profession towards the modern treatment of the disease. [3]

Subsequently, surgical results in patients with an acutely inflamed, non-perforated appendix were satisfactory, but rates of postoperative morbidity and mortality were high among patients for whom delayed diagnosis led to a perforated appendix with peritonitis. [3] Endless debate raged about types of drainage, the best choice of irrigation fluids, the question of whether irrigation of the peritoneal cavity dilutes or spreads infection, and safe offered a way to treat complicated appendicitis and promised to make these ways to clean the contaminated abdominal wound. The development of antibiotic agents questions unnecessary and reduce morbidity and mortality from complicated appendicitis to a rate closer to that of non-perforated appendicitis. The article by Drs Henley and Haugen was an early attempt to understand the benefits of the new drugs.

Five of the fifty-one patients described in the article were treated by the conservative Ochsner method with the addition of sulpha drugs. Results were good : no mortality occurred and the mean length of hospitalisation was 14 days (one patient remained hospitalised for 37 days, but this data point was the sole outlier). Four patients returned for interval appendectomy before recurrence, and one patient was unavailable for follow-up.

The other patients described by Drs Henley and Haugen were treated with surgery when the diagnosis was made. The infection was treated by a sulfathiazole emulsion placed both in the abdominal cavity and in the layers of the wound. Sulfadiazine was given postoperatively, first intravenously and then by mouth. One patient received no sulphonamide, and three patients received sulphonamide only locally to the wound. The 46 patients in the series had 21 septic complications (at a total septic complication rate of about 50%) and a mean postoperative hospital stay of 15 days. This finding should be compared with those that were usual in the pre-antibiotic era: a 75% rate of wound infection in addition to intra-abdominal and chest infections when peritonitis or a gangrenous appendix was found at operation. [3] To the surgeons' and to sulphonamide's credit, no mortality occurred among the patients in the series. Sulphonamide administered at this dosage would thus seem helpful - but not a complete success - in eliminating morbidity from sepsis. Recognising this likelihood, the authors reported that subsequent cases were being treated to raise levels of the drug in the blood. The technique used by the authors for retrograde removal of the retrocecal appendix is described near the end of the article and is still being used regularly to good effect at the KP Oakland Medical Centre.

3. Modern developments

Many antibiotic schedules have been explored in the 57 years that have ensued since the publication of the article by Drs Henley and Haugen, and clinicians have had considerable success in reducing sepsis in patients with complicated appendicitis. Current practice usually includes a regimen of multiple antibiotics begun preoperatively and directed at aerobic and anaerobic bacteria. Use of the drugs is discontinued after several doses if the disease is found to be uncomplicated; if the peritoneum is soiled, the drug regimen is continued as long as clinically appropriate. Adequate preoperative levels of antibiotic agents in the blood help protect against wound infection and the development of peritonitis. Secondary closure of the wound on the second or third postoperative day may prevent infection.

With use of modern antibiotic agents, sepsis nonetheless develops in 5% to 20% of patients with complicated appendicitis. [2] Modern antibiotic regimens have thus reduced – but have not eliminated - the high cost of treating mixed bacterial infections in the abdominal cavity and surgical wound. In England and Wales, during the pre-antibiotic era, 3000 deaths from appendicitis were reported each year; by 1985, the mortality rate was reduced to 147 deaths per year and is now less than 1%. [2][3]

Modern abdominal imaging and nuclear medicine have led to immeasurably improved treatment of the complications of appendicitis, but the diagnosis of early appendicitis has not been improved since 1944 despite advances in abdominal imaging and laboratory techniques. Diagnosis still depends on a carefully assembled medical history, skilled physical examination and routine laboratory testing. Even when a highly capable physician has made the diagnosis, a normal appendix is found in about 15% of operations. [4] Laparoscopic surgery is well-accepted as the primary operation and is especially beneficial when a normal appendix is found and the rest of the abdomen must be searched so as to establish the postoperative diagnosis.

More than one hundred years have passed since McBurney reported his study of acute appendicitis in eight patients.

Acute appendicitis is the most common cause of acute abdominal pain in young adults. This is one of the most common surgical emergencies, with a lifetime prevalence of about 1 to 7.1 1.5-1.9/1000. Its incidence is for men. [5]

Surgery for acute appendicitis is the most frequently performed operation (10% of all emergency abdominal operations). [6]

The diagnosis of acute appendicitis is based purely on the history of the disease, clinical examination and few laboratory tests (white blood cell count). The morphological examinations were not of great interest for the diagnosis. Definitive diagnosis is obtained only after histological examination of the part of appendicitis. [7] A negative appendectomy rate of 20-40% was reported in the literature[6] and many surgeons accept a rate of 30.6%, as the removal of a healthy appendix is an economic burden on both patients and health resources. Errors or delays in surgery can cause complications such as perforation and finally peritonitis. [8]

Difficulties in diagnosis occur in the very young, elderly women of childbearing age and pregnant women because they generally have an unusual array. [9] Although there is a lot of progress in gastroenterology, there has been no major improvement in the diagnostic accuracy of acute appendicitis, which varies between 25-90% with an optimal rate is 80% (which is lower in women than in men). A number of scoring systems have been advocated to minimise the number of unnecessary interventions performed in emergencies. These rating systems are valuable tools and valid for the discrimination between acute appendicitis and a clear atypical feature. [9] At present many rating systems for the diagnosis of acute appendicitis are available. The Alvarado scoring system is one of these and is based purely on the patient's history, clinical examination and laboratory tests and so is very easy to apply. [10] The Alvarado score includes the left shift of the decision of mature neutrophils.

4. Alvarado score

The Alvarado score is a rating system used in the clinical diagnosis of appendicitis. The score was 6 for clinical and laboratory measurements, with a total of 10 points. Elements of the patient's history, physical examination and laboratory tests are considered:

- Abdominal pain that migrates to the right iliac fossa.
- Anorexia (loss of appetite) or ketones in the urine.
- Nausea or vomiting.
- Pain in the form of pressure in the right iliac fossa.
- Rebound tenderness.
- Fever of 37.3 ° C or more.
- Leukocytosis, with more than 10 000 white cells per microlitre in serum.
- Neutrophilia (or an increase in the percentage of neutrophils in the count of white blood serum).

The two most important defences in the lower right quadrant and leukocytosis are assigned two points, and six other factors are assigned one point each for a possible ten points.
A score of 5 or 6 is compatible with the diagnosis of acute appendicitis. A score of 7 or 8 indicates a probable appendicitis, and a score of 9 or 10 indicates a very probable acute appendicitis.
Between 4 and 6 the diagnosis of appendicitis leads to problems. The aims of our study is how to introduce the role for a CT scan in this situation?
A popular mnemonic used to remember the score factors is MANTRELS: Alvarado - migration to the right iliac fossa, anorexia, nausea/vomiting, tenderness in the right iliac fossa, rebound pain, high temperature (fever), leukocytosis and the movement of leukocytes to the left (factors listed in the same order as presented above). Due to the popularity of this symbol, the score is sometimes called the Alvarado score MANTRELS Alvarado describes the original score of a possible 10 points, but medical facilities who are unable to perform a white blood cell count use a modified Alvarado score with a total of nine points and which might not be as accurate as the original score. A high score of diagnosis was confirmed in a number of studies around the world. The consensus is that the Alvarado score is a non-invasive, safe diagnostic method that is simple, reliable and reproducible and able to guide the clinician in the management of the case.

Migratory right iliac fossa pain 1
Nausea / vomiting 1
Anorexia 1
Signs
Tenderness in right iliac fossa 2
Rebound tenderness in the right iliac fossa 1
High temperatures 1
Laboratory results
Leukocytosis 2
Passage to the left of neutrophils 1
Total 10

Table 1. Symptoms Alvarado scoring system a score

5. Appendicitis and CT scan

Computed tomography (CT) is becoming the preferred imaging modality for suspected acute appendicitis, particularly in adults. CT is more accurate in the diagnosis of acute appendicitis since it is less operator-dependent than ultrasonography (US). [11]

Therefore, the use of CT has been advocated, so far, in the minority of patients with acute appendicitis that present with atypical clinical features.

Although in most cases the diagnosis of acute appendicitis is usually clear on the basis of clinical features, there is a significant negative laparotomy rate. Therefore, some authorities now recommend CT for all patients with suspected acute appendicitis or for those with equivocal acute appendicitis. CT may also be helpful in the preoperative evaluation of patients undergoing laparoscopic appendectomy. [12]

CT seems to be more sensitive (96% vs. 76%) and accurate (94% vs. 91%) than US in diagnosing acute appendicitis, whereas they are almost equal when it comes to specificity (89% vs. 91%). CT imaging tailored to evaluate acute appendicitis has proven to be particularly successful, with a sensitivity of 100%, a specificity of 95%, a positive predictive value of 97%, a negative predictive value of 100%, and accuracy of 98%. [5][6]

Multidetector-row CT (MDCT) currently has an important role in the diagnosis of acute appendicitis and its severity. Some authors suggest that they can diagnose acute appendicitis with an accuracy of 99%. It is also possible to reconstruct the entire form and position of appendices from successive CT findings because of high-resolution thin-slice MDCT images. [13]

CT examination protocol

The patient is prepared with 800–1000 ml of oral contrast medium for bowel opacification 60–90 min prior to scanning. The scan is performed with the patient in the supine position, following an intravenous injection of 100–120 ml of iodinated contrast medium at a rate of 3 ml/s and a scan delay of approximately 60 s. The combination of oral and intravenous contrast medium provides the most information about the inflamed appendix and the surrounding tissues. [14]

It was reported that oral administration of up to 800 ml of the contrast medium at least 1 h before CT scanning enables opacification of both the small bowel and the right colon in most patients. [15]

CT appearance of appendicitis

The appearance of appendicitis on CT depends on the extent and severity of inflammation and the presence or absence of complications. Inflammation of the appendix results from obstruction of its lumen from fecaliths, foreign bodies, lymphoid hyperplasia, parasites or tumours (primary or metastatic). A prompt and accurate diagnosis of acute appendicitis significantly decreases morbidity and mortality. Although in most cases clinical symptoms and signs may strongly suggest a diagnosis of acute appendicitis, the clinical presentation is atypical in 20% of cases, while in another 20% the condition is misdiagnosed. The clinical features in children are often atypical, with generalised rather than localised abdominal pain, whereas in the elderly there is a wider range of differential diagnosis than in the younger population because of the frequency of age-related diseases, such as diverticulitis. The diagnosis may also be delayed in the elderly as they complain less of pain than younger patients do and clinical signs are less pronounced. There is also an increased risk of misdiagnosis in young females because gynaecological diseases can mimic acute appendicitis. Women suspected of having appendicitis benefit mostly from preoperative CT or US, and they have a significantly lower negative appendectomy rate than do women who do not undergo preoperative imaging. [12]

For some female patients, clinicians order pelvic US to be performed within 24 h of a CT study. The diagnosis of acute appendicitis is usually based on clinical symptoms and laboratory tests; however, one third of patients with acute appendicitis show atypical clinical symptoms and physical findings. In this group of patients radiological imaging can play an important clinical role. The inflamed appendix shows a variable degree of distension, has a diameter measuring 6–40 mm and a wall thickness of 1–3 mm. The wall is usually asymmetrically thickened and enhances with an intravenous contrast medium. [16] As the disease progresses, a periappendiceal inflammatory mass called phlegmon may develop.

Thickening and enhancement with an intravenous contrast medium may also be observed in the adjacent wall of the cecum or ileum if they are involved in the inflammatory process. Progression of the inflammatory process may lead to the findings ranging from a sealed abscess to widespread incidence of abdominal inflammatory seeding with multiple abscesses. An abscess with a well-defined border usually indicates chronicity, and the presence of air bubbles or air fluid levels inside indicates the presence of gas-forming organisms or the communication of the abscess with the bowel. If periappendiceal fat is involved in the inflammatory process then it shows an increased haziness, streaky densities and/or fluid collection. In 30% of appendicitis cases the arrowhead sign is present and it has 100% specificity. It describes focal thickening of the cecal wall around the root of the appendix, which funnels toward the point of obstruction of the appendiceal lumen. [17]

6. Patients and methods

We conducted a study that was conducted on 100 consecutive patients admitted to the emergency department of Tlemcen with a clinical diagnosis of suspected acute appendicitis during the period from March to July 2011. Patients of all ages and both sexes presenting to the emergency room with pain in the lower right quadrant of the abdomen were included in the study. Patients with signs of urological, gynaecological and surgical procedures other than appendicitis, particularly patients with right iliac fossa mass, were excluded from the study.

All enrolled patients were hospitalised and first evaluated by surgeons: clinical examination, blood count, urine microscopy and a routine examination, and the abdomen without preparation were all performed. Next, a case was completed for each patient by a student in surgery. These files recorded general information about patients using more than eight variables based on the Alvarado scoring system. From the calculation of the Alvarado score for each patient, stratification was stable and the patients were divided into three groups.

1. An Alvarado between 7-10 (emergency surgery group): these patients were prepared and all underwent an emergency appendectomy.
2. Alvarado between 4-6 (observation group): these patients were admitted and randomly placed into two groups: one group was subjected to repeated clinical examinations for 24 hours and the other to a CT scan. For the first group, the patients were kept under observation for 24 hours with frequent reassessment of the clinical data. The condition of some patients has improved within an hour, as represented by a decrease in the score and - therefore - they came out with instructions that they should return if symptoms persist or increased in intensity.

3. An Alvarado between 1-4: these patients, after being given initial symptomatic treatment, were released and sent home with instructions to return if symptoms persisted or their condition worsened.

The diagnosis of acute appendicitis was confirmed by the operative findings and the histopathological evaluation of the specimen appendectomy.

Finally, the reliability of the Alvarado ratings was assessed by calculating the negative appendectomy rate (the proportion of surgical patients with a normal appendix), which was 19.

7. Results

We conducted our study on patients with clinical features suggestive of acute appendicitis. A total of 100 patients were enrolled in this study. All patients who received conservative treatment were excluded from the study. In addition, five patients with a mass at the appendix , were also excluded from the study.

Of the 100 patients, 59 were female (59%) and 41 were male (41%) (the ratio of men to women was 1:1.4). The average age was 33.5 years (range 3-64 years). Most patients were younger.

The group results were good, as follows : we received 25 patients (25%) with a score of 1-4 Alvarado (Among whom 10 were female and 15 were male). All were released after the initial evaluation and symptomatic treatment. 3 patients were readmitted for a recurrence of pain with a typical picture of acute appendicitis and a score of 7 or more in 48 hours. They were admitted and underwent an appendectomy. Histopathological examination of part of appendicitis revealed in all patients an acute inflammation of the appendix and operative findings and histopathological reports have shown that all 3 patients had confirmed inflamed appendices.

51 patients (51%) had a score of 4-6. In the group of patients undergoing a CT scan, the morphological diagnosis of acute appendicitis was made in all cases (i.e. in 12 patients). In the second group subjected to repeated clinical examination, 5 patients progressed to acute appendicitis and were admitted to the operating room (appendicitis was confirmed by histopathology); 7 patients have had regression of the clinical picture and were released with symptomatic treatment.

8. Discussion and conclusions

A healthy appendix on appendectomy should no longer exist given the sensitivity of the scanner before the critical period of suspected appendicitis. The Alvarado score was an artefact of size which serves to give greater assistance with diagnosis, especially among young surgeons.

The history, physical examination, temperature scanning of the complete blood count and abdominal defence are useful for achieving a more accurate diagnosis. In developed countries, advanced technology such as CT scans and laparoscopy are available and are useful in establishing a treatment regimen, but in less developed facilities such reviews are not so readily available in most hospitals and are also costly to do, especially if we advocate a careful and repeated clinical examination of 24 to 48 hours by experienced clinicians for patients with scores of 4 to 6. In fact, we cannot rely on a single survey (which counts as low level evidence), but rather must rely on a combination of complete physical examination and routine laboratory tests, such as complete blood count. The Alvarado score helped the medical decision-making for both senior surgeons and beginners.

The abdominal CT scan is the best way to test for acute appendicitis when the score is between 4 and 6. However, cost, feasibility and availability of this review still leave room for repeated examination, which requires hospitalization for 24 to 48 hours

9. References

[1] Stephens PL, Mazzucco JJ. Comparison of ultrasound and the Alvarado score for the diagnosis of acute appendicitis. Conn Med 1999;63:137-40.
[2] Lally KP, Cox CS, Andrassy RJ. Appendix. In: Townsend CM, Beauchamp RD, Evers BM, Mattox KL, editors. Sabiston textbook of surgery: the biological basis of modern surgical practice. 16th ed. Philadelphia: WB Saunders; 2001. p 917-28.
[3] Ellis H, Nathanson LK. Appendix and appendectomy. In: Zinner MJ, Schwartz SI, Ellis H, editors. Maingot's abdominal operations. 10th ed. Stamford, CT: Appleton & Lange; 1997. p 1191-1227.
[4] Hale DA, Molloy M, Pearl RH, Schutt DC, Jaques DP. Appendectomy: a contemporary appraisal. Ann Surg 1997 Mar;225(3):252-61.
[5] Cuschieri A. The small intestine and vermiform appendix; In: Cuscheri A, G R, A R Mossa.(ed). Essential surgical practice. 3rd ed. London: Butter worth Heinman. 1995;1325-8
[6] Pal KM, Khan A. Appendicitis, a continuing challenge. J Pak Med Assoc 1998;48:189-92.
[7] Kumar V, Cotran RS, Robbins SL. Appendix; In Robbin's Basic Pathology. 5th ed. London:W.B Saunders 1992; 520
[8] Dado G, Anania G, Baccarani U, Marcotti E, Donini A, Risaliti A et al. Application of a clinical score for the diagnosis of acute appendicitis in childhood. J Pediatr Surg 2000;35:1320-2. group. Diagnostic scores for acute appendicitis. Eur J Surg 1995;161:273-81
[9] Fenyo G, Lindberg G, Blind P, Enochsson L, Oberg A. Diagnostic decision support in suspected acute appendicitis: validation of a simplified scoring system. Eur J Surg 1997;163;831-8.
[10] Alverado A. A practical score for the early diagnosis of acute appendicitis. Ann Emerg Med 1986;15:557-65.
[11] Bursali A, Arac M, Oner YA, Celik H, Eksioglu S, Gumus T. Evaluation of the normal appendix at low -dose non-enhanced spiral CT. Diagn Interv Radiol 2005;11:45–50.
[12] Ghiatas AA, Chopra S, Chintapalli KN. Computed tomography of the normal appendix and acute appendicitis. Eur Radiol 1997; 7:1043–1047.
[13] Miki T, Ogata S, Uto M. Enhanced multidetector- row computed tomography (MDCT) in the diagnosis of acute appendicitis and its severity. Radiat Med 2005; 23:242–255.
[14] Rao PM, Rhea JT, Novelline RA. Helical CT technique for the diagnosis of appendicitis: prospective evaluation of a focused appendix CT examination. Radiology 1997; 202:139–144.
[15] Wijetunga R, Tan B, Rouse J. Diagnostic accuracy of focused appendiceal CT in clinically equivocal cases of acute appendicitis. Radiology 2001; 221:747–753.
[16] Rao PM, Rhea JT, Novelline RA. Helical CT combined with contrast material administered only through the colon for imaging of suspected appendicitis. AJR Am J Roentgenol 1997; 169:1275–1280.
[17] Oliak D, Yamini D, Udami VM. Nonoperative management of perforated appendicitis without periappendiceal mass. Am J Surg 2000; 179:177–181.

9

Perforated Appendicitis

Ali Akbar Salari
Shahid Sadoughi University of Medical Sciense, Yazd, Iran

1. Introduction

1.1 General consideration

All physicians should have a thorough knowledge of appendicitis. Although most patients with acute appendicitis can be easily diagnosed, there are many in whom the signs and symptoms are quite variable, and a firm clinical diagnosis may be difficult to establish. It is for this reason that the diagnosis is made rather liberally, with the full expectation that some patients will be operated on and found to have a normal appendix. It is preferable to maintain broad indications, as this tends to include the group of patients with indefinite signs and symptoms who actually have the disease but do not fulfill the classic criteria for the diagnosis. Following this course, patients who might proceed to perforation of the appendix, with a host of possible secondary complications, are spared that fate. Therefore, it is generally agreed that 10% to 15% of patients having a diagnosis of acute appendicitis by acceptable standards in most hospitals will actually be found at operation to have a normal appendix.

2. Anatomy

The vermiform appendix is located in the right lower quadrant, arises from the cecum, and is generally 6 to 10 cm in length. It has a separate mesoappendix with an appendicular artery and vein that are branches of the ileocolic vessels. The appendix is lined with colonic epithelium characterized by many lymph follicles numbering approximately 200, with the highest number occurring in the 10- to 20-year-old age group. After the age of 30, the number of lymph follicles is reduced to a trace, with total absence of lymphoid tissue occurring after the age of 60. The appendix may lie in a number of locations, essentially at any position on a clock wise rotation from the base of the cecum. It is important to emphasize that the *anatomic* position of the appendix determines the symptoms and the site of the muscular spasm and tenderness when the appendix becomes inflamed (Fig. 1)

2.1 Pathophysiology

It is widely accepted that the inciting event in most instances of appendicitis is obstruction of the appendiceal lumen. This may be due to lymphoid hyperplasia, inspissated stool (a fecalith), or some other foreign body. Given the correlation with the incidence of appendicitis by age and the size and distribution of the lymphoid tissue, it is likely that lymphoid obstruction or partial obstruction of the lumen is a common cause. Obstruction of

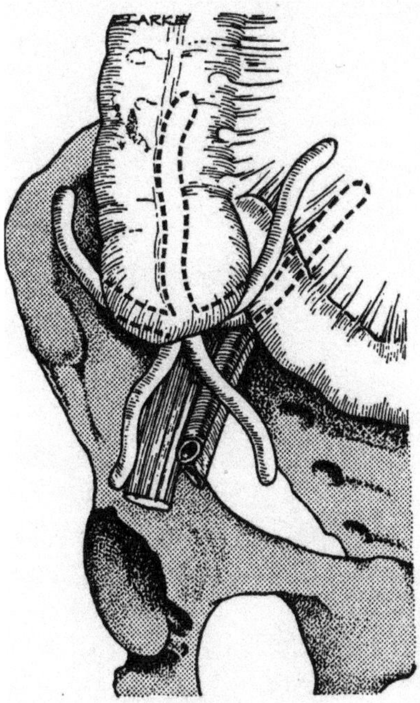

Fig. 1. The various possible positions of the appendix vermiformis

the lumen leads to bacterial overgrowth as well as continued mucous secretion. This causes distention of the lumen, and the intraluminal pressure increases. This may lead to lymphatic and then venous obstruction. With bacterial overgrowth and edema, an acute inflammatory response ensues. The appendix then becomes more edematous and ischemic. Necrosis of the appendiceal wall subsequently occurs along with translocation of bacteria through the ischemic wall. This is gangrenous appendicitis. Without intervention, the gangrenous appendix will perforate with spillage of the appendiceal contents into the peritoneal cavity. If this sequence of events occurs slowly, the appendix is contained by the inflammatory response and the omentum, leading to localized peritonitis and everntually an appendiceal abscess. If the body does not wall off the process, the patient may develop diffuse peritonitis.

2.2 Bacteriology

The flora in the noninflamed appendix is similar to the colon with a variety of facultative aerobic and anaerobic bacteria found; hence, the bacteria involved in appendicitis are the same as for other colonic disease. The incidence of obtaining positive cultures from the peritoneal cavity depends on the stage of appendicitis found. In patients with acute, nonperforated appendicitis, peritoneal fluid will culture bacteria in fewer than half of the patients. However, Peritoneal cultures will be positive in more than 85% of patients with gangrenous or perforated appendicitis. The number of bacterial species that can be cultured depends on how vigorously the investigators attempt to isolate them, with some investigators showing an average of more than nine different species. In 1938, Altemeier clearly demonstrated the polymicrobial nature of perforated appendicitis, and for practical purposes little has changed.

The usefulness of routine peritoneal cultures in patients with perforated appendicitis has been questioned. The flora are generally known, the results are not available for several days, and many times, no change in treatment plan is made despite culture results. It appears reasonable to avoid routine cultures and to obtain them only in patients with persisting infection or surgical site infection.

3. Clinical diagnosis

The diagnosis of acute appendicitis is made primarily on the basis of the history and the physical findings, with additional assistance from laboratory examinations. The *typical* history is one of onset of generalized abdominal pain followed by anorexia and nausea. The pain then becomes most prominent in the epigastrium and gradually moves toward the umbilicus, finally localizing in the right lower quadrant. Vomiting may occur during this time. Examination of the abdomen usually shows diminished bowel sounds, with direct tenderness and spasm in the right lower quadrant. As the process continues, the amount of spasm increases, with the appearance of rebound tenderness. The temperature is usually mildly elevated (approximately 38° C.) and usually rises to higher levels in the event of perforation. Direct tenderness is usually present in the right lower quadrant and may involve other parts of the abdomen, particularly if perforation has occurred. The appendix is usually situated at or around McBurney's point (a point one third of the way on a line drawn from the anterior superior spine to the umbilicus). However, it must be emphasized that the exact *anatomic location* of the appendix can be at any point on a 360-degree circle surrounding the base of the cecum, as shown in (Figure 1) This is the site where the pain and tenderness are usually maximal, and the exact site may vary from patient to patient.

Rovsing's sign, elicited when pressure applied in the left lower quadrant reflects pain to the right lower quadrant, is often present. The psoas sign may be positive and is elicited by extension of the right thigh with the patient lying on the left side. As the examiner extends the right thigh with stretching of the muscle, pain suggests the presence of an inflamed appendix overlying the psoas muscle. The obturator sign can be elicited with the patient in the supine position with passive rotation of the flexed right thigh. Pain with this maneuver indicates a positive sign. Rectal examination generally elicits tenderness at the site of the inflamed appendix in the right lower quadrant. If the appendix ruptures, abdominal pain becomes intense and more diffuse, the muscular spasm increases, and there is a simultaneous increase in the heart rate above 100, with a rise in temperature to 39° or 40° C. At this time, the patient appears toxic, and it becomes obvious that the clinical situation has deteriorated.

Olivier Monneuse and colleague, in France from 2002-2005 review of 326 patients, this study was designed to quantify the proportion of patients with a preoperative diagnosis of acute appendicitis that had isolated right lower quadrant pain without biological inflammatory sign's and then to determine which imaging examination led to the determination of the diagnosis.

The diagnosis acute appendicitis can not be excluded when an adult patient present with isolated rebound tenderness in the right lower quadrant evwen without fever and biological inflammatory signs.

Author's study of total 465 patients with abdominal pains referred to the two main hospitals Yazd Iran during 10 months 400 cases confirmed appendicitis 335 patients had anorexia.

Anorexia increases probability of appendicitis but its absences can not rule out diagnosis of acute appendicitis.

3.1 Imaging studies

Abdominal radiographs obtained in the evaluation of patients with acute abdominal pain typically include the flat and upright abdominal radiograph, as well as a chest radiograph. This sequence of studies may be useful in patients with atypical presenting symptoms and physical signs. However, plain abdominal radiographs should not be considered "routine" or "mandatory" components of the evaluation of patients with acute abdominal pain. Pneumoperitoneum on an upright abdominal radiograph suggests a diagnosis other than appendicitis. Rarely does a perforated appendix present with pneumoperitoneum (1 to 2%). Abdominal radiographs may demonstrate a fecalith, localized ileus, or loss of the peritoneal fat stripe. Gas in the appendix is not a sign specific for appendicitis and should not mandate laparotomy for appendicitis.

3.2 Computed Tomography

Recent improvements in CT technology have improved image resolution to the 0.5- to 1.0-cm range, thus improving the accuracy of CT scanning. Typically, CT has been reserved for patients with an equivocal history and physical and laboratory findings. CT is useful in patients with an observed inflammatory abdominal process, and the presentation is atypical for appendicitis. The accuracy of CT is greatest when a deliberate effort is made to visualize the appendix. Although some reports discount the use of intravenous contrast agent and only limited enteric contrast agent, the optimal technique requires complete small bowel opacification. The terminal ileum and cecum must be filled with contrast agent to improve the recognition of the normal or abnormal appendix and to avoid confusing unopacified ileal loops with the appendix. Unless contraindicated, intravenous contrast agent should be used as well. Specific, fine (5-mm) image intervals should be obtained in the region of the appendix.

In general, CT findings of appendicitis increase with the severity of the disease. The normal appendix appears as a thin tubular structure in the right lower quadrant that may or may not opacity with contrast. Appendicoliths appear as ring like homogeneous calcifications and are seen in approximately 25% of the population.

Classically, a CT diagnosis of acute appendicitis includes an abnormal appendix with periappendiceal inflammation. The appendix is considered abnormal when it is distended or thickened and greater than approximately 5 to 7 mm in size. The wall of the inflamed appendix is circumferentially thickened and may appear as a "halo" or "target." CT findings of periappendiceal inflammation suggest appendicitis; these include periappendiceal abscess, fluid collections, edema, and phlegmon. Periappendiceal inflammation or edema is visualized as clouding of the mesenteric fat ("dirty fat"), local fascial thickening, and ill-defined right lower quadrant soft tissue densities. Intravenous contrast agent-enhanced studies help to define the inflamed appendiceal and periappendiceal tissue. CT is especially useful in distinguishing those patients presenting late in their clinical course (48 to 72 hours) who may have developed a phlegmon or abscess, thus altering potential therapy.

The true sensitivity of CT in diagnosing acute appendicitis is unknown. Retrospective studies, studies of consecutive patients, and studies with debatable inclusion criteria have made the application of CT to individual patients with a truly equivocal presentation (those who have undergone non diagnostic ultrasonography, evaluation by an experienced surgeon, and a brief period of repetitive examination) problematic. A reasonable estimate is that CT is 90% sensitive to the detection of intra-abdominal inflammation, with an 80 to 90% positive predictive value.

3.3 Barium enema

The barium enema has been used as a diagnostic adjunct in evaluating patients with equivocal clinical signs of appendicitis. This study was used primarily in the 1970s and early 1980s before the availability of CT and higher-quality ultrasonography. A positive study may show nonfilling of the appendix with indentation of the cecum, indicative of pericecal inflammation. A false-negative study (partial filling of appendix) can occur in up to 10% of patients. The equivocal study can occur in up to 40% of patients evaluated with this technique, due principally to partial filling of the appendix. Barium enema is no longer routinely used to evaluate patients with suspected acute appendicitis.

3.4 Ultrasound

Ultrasonography is often used as the initial diagnostic imaging study in the majority of patients in whom the clinical diagnosis of appendicitis is equivocal. Ultrasound is noninvasive and rapidly available and avoids radiation exposure. Most studies of graded compression ultrasound demonstrate a sensitivity of more than 85% and a specificity of more than 90%. However, the sonogram for appendicitis is a highly operator-dependent study. Sonographic criteria for the diagnosis of acute appendicitis are the demonstration of a noncompressible appendix of 7 mm or greater in anteroposterior diameter, the presence of an appendicolith, interruption of the continuity of the echogenic submucosa, and periappendiceal fluid or mass. A fecalith in combination with localized right lower quadrant pain is highly diagnostic of appendicitis. False-positive studies can be due to secondary inflammation of the appendix as a result of inflammatory bowel disease, salpingitis, or other causes. False-negative sonograms are usually due to nonvisualization of a retrocecal appendix and a gasfilled cecum, which prevents visualization of the appendix. In addition, perforation significantly decreases the diagnostic accuracy of graded compression of the appendix. Thus, the ultrasonographic diagnosis of perforated appendicitis depends on the secondary findings on periappendiceal fluid, mass, and loss of the integrity of the submucosa layer. Gaseous distention of the right lower quadrant bowel loops or prolonged symptoms suggesting perforation should make CT the preferred imaging study for improved accuracy and potential utility in planning intervention for appendiceal abscess or phlegmon.

In one study the role of diagnosis imaging in the management of patients with a suspicious of appendicitis is controversial. Early report of good result, with a low frequency of negative appendectomies based on ultrasound or CT Scan. Have been followed by other investigators with contradictory results. The encouraging results reported by toorenvliet et al from Leiden, the Netherlands, using routine ultrasonography and limited CT Scan, must therefore be put into perspective.

4. Laboratory finding

The clinical history and physical examination are most important in establishing a diagnosis of acute appendicitis, but laboratory findings may be helpful. The majority of patients with acute appendicitis have an elevated leukocyte count of 10,000 to 20,000. For those in whom the level is normal, there is generally a shift to the left in the differential leukocyte count, indicating acute inflammation. However, it should be emphasized that a number of patients have a *normal* leukocyte count, especially the elderly. Urinary analysis may show a few red cells, indicating some inflammatory contact with the ureter or urinary bladder; a significant number of erythrocytes in the urine indicates a primary disorder of the urinary tract.

4.1 Perforated Appendicitis

The management of perforated or gangrenous appendicitis varies somewhat from that of acute nonperforated disease. In these patients, the appendix has already perforated, so the need for urgent intervention is less obvious. Patients with perforated appendicitis will often have a longer duration of symptoms, high fever, and a higher white blood count. Most of these patients are volume depleted and require several hours or more of fluid resuscitation before operative intervention. It is important to ensure that the patient has been adequately resuscitated before undertaking an operation. Patients with perforated disease have established peritonitis and should receive appropriate broad-spectrum intravenous antibiotic therapy, which should start as soon as the diagnosis is established." The duration of therapy is controversial. Some authors recommend an empiric time of treatment such as 7 or 10 days. Others suggest treatment until the patient is afebrile with a normal white blood cell count.

As with acute appendicitis, there are two possible approaches: an open laparotomy or laparoscopy. There is some controversy about the use of laparoscopy in patients with advanced disease because the incidence of postoperative intra-abdominal abscess formation in some series has been markedly higher with laparoscopy than with an open approach. Our approach to appendicitis is outlined.

Our study is on 500 patients refereed two main hospitals in Yazd Iran from 1998-1999 to appendectomy : 87% of the patients had acute appendicitis 9.5% perforated appendix (the report by Rao and his calleaguses at the Massachusetts general hospital perforation rate of appendix was 14%) and 3.5% normal appendix : which early diagnosis reduced perforated appendicitis.

4.2 Appendicitis in patients with AIDS or HIV Infection

The incidence of acute appendicitis in HIV-infected patients is re-ported to be 0.5%. This is higher than the 0.1 to 0.2% incidence reported for the general population. The presentation of acute appendicitis in HIV-infected patients is similar to that of noninfecied patients. The majority of HIV-infected patients with appendicitis will have fever, periumbilical pain radiating to the right lower quadrant (91%), right lower quadrant tenderness (91%), and rebound tenderness (74%). HIV-infected patients will not manifest an absolute leukocytosis; however, if a baseline leukocyte count is available, nearly all HIV-infected patients with appendicitis will demonstrate a relative leukocytosis.

4.3 Late cases of appendicitis

In late cases of appendicitis that have led to a very diffuse or general peritonitis, or in those cases of a very fulminating type that are associated with a rapid form of spreading peritonitis, it is often impossible to make a certain diagnosis. Distinction has to be made from the following:

- Primary pneumococcal peritonitis
- Secondary general peritonitis due to other causes (rupture of gastric, duodenal, typhoid, stercoral, or carcinomatous ulcer or of a pyosalpinx)
- Thrombosis of mesenteric vessels
- Acute intestinal obstruction
- Acute pancreatitis
- Pylephlebitis
- In finding out the exact cause, the greatest importance attaches to the history.

5. Special features of acute appendicitis

Appendicitis in infants and young children is difficult to diagnose preoperatively, since these patients cannot provide a history. Therefore, it is unusual to make a firm diagnosis in a patient under the age of 1 year unless perforation has , occurred.
Acute appendicitis during pregnancy also presents diagnostic problems, because during the third trimester, the uterus is rapidly enlarging and causes displacement of the cecum and appendix into the right upper abdomen. Thus, acute appendicitis in these patients causes symptoms and signs higher and more lateral during the third trimester.
In one study by Roland E. Anderson form Sweden, sonography more sensitive in first trimester of pregnancy (81.6%) in second trimester in 58..1% and third trimester 57.9%. But CT Scan in first trimester less than 2nd and 3 rd trimester. So abdominal sonography essential diagnosis for lower quadrant pain in pregnant women in pregnancy. If sonography doesn't help, spiral CT Scan for treatment is useful.

5.1 Presentation with a mass or late complicated appendicitis

Two to five percent of patients with appendicitis present with a palpable right lower quadrant mass. This can represent either a discrete abscess or phlegmonous inflammation.(Fig.2) The management of these patients has been somewhat controversial on a number of issues. Historically, this has been fueled by equivocal imaging studies that could not reliably corroborate the physical findings and an inability to reliably drain an abscess percutaneously. There also has been a bias toward early removal of the perforated appendix/appendiceal abscess to "control intra-abdominal sepsis." The preferred approach to the management of the appendiceal mass is percutaneous drainage, which is performed under image guidance (ultrasound or CT) and intravenous antibiotics directed against aerobic gram-negative and anaerobic organisms. Numerous studies have documented the safety and efficacy of this approach. In late, complicated appendicitis, appendectomy can be a hazardous procedure. Surgery at this stage can serve to disseminate a localized inflammatory process; to injure surrounding inflamed or edematous bowel, resulting in fistulas; or to require more extensive procedures, such as cecectomy or right hemicolectomy.
Authors studies Intrabdominal abscess formation after appendectomy may be intrapritoneal and extrapritoneal causes by primary and secondary infection. Abscess well be in different part of abdomen such as subdiaphragmatic, subhepatic, pelvis and midabdomen. Each one has special clinical signs and diagnosis and treatment.
Bradly and Isaacs in 1978 review of 2621 cases of acute appendicitis treated between 1962 and 1976 in Atlanta found that only 2% had an appendix abscess on admission, and has the average duration of symptom was 9 days.

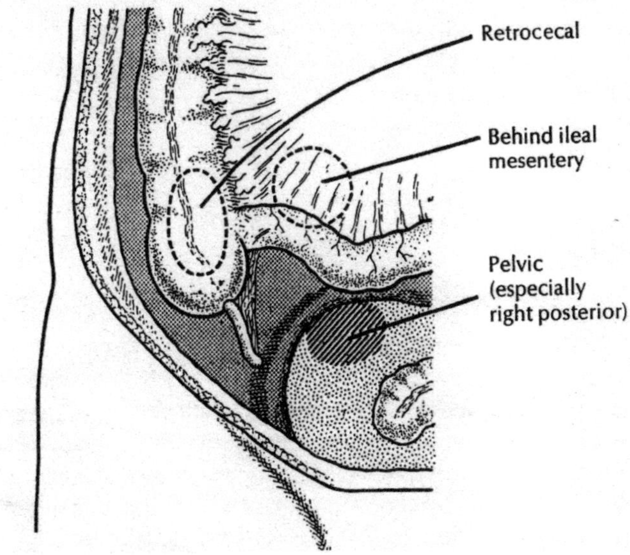

Fig. 2. Those sites where an abscess resulting from Appendicitis may sometimes be overlocked

5.2 Differential diagnosis

There are a number of acute abdominal disorders producing signs and symptoms similar to those of acute appendicitis. These include acute gastroenteritis, cholecystitis, pyelitis, salpingitis, tuboovarian abscess, and ruptured ovarian cyst. Although diarrhea may occur with acute appendicitis, it is much more common with gastroenteritis. In young children, intussusception enters the differential diagnosis. Other less common differential disorders include ureteral stones, cystitis, perforated peptic ulcer, ectopic pregnancy, acute regional enteritis (particularly the first attack), epididymitis, and testicular torsion. If a patient persists in having pain in the right lower quadrant that cannot be explained by some other definitive diagnosis, the patient should be considered to have acute appendicitis and should be operated on or at least carefully observed.

A report of 74 year old female had occasionally experienced right lower abdominal pain in the past. She underwent a barium enema, which revealed a wall irregularity around the appendix, but the appendix itself was not visualized. The patient was referred to hospital for possible appendiceal neoplasm. Colonoscopy revealed a tumor like protrusion with marked redness at the enterance to the appendix. Pathologic analysis of biopsy specimens revealed only inflammatory cells. Differential diagnosis appendiceal crohn's disease or appendiceal neoplasm was made and laparascopic appendectomy was performed. Pathological results appendiceal crohn's disease was made.

6. Treatment

For the vast majority of patients with a diagnosis of acute appendicitis, the appropriate management is appendectomy. For patients with simple acute appendicitis, intravenous fluids should be initiated as well as an antibiotic agent effective against both aerobic and anaerobic organisms. All patients are begun on antibiotics preoperatively and maintained post-operatively as needed. If the appendix is unruptured and not gangrenous, antibiotics can be discontinued after 24 hours. Although many agents are effective, cefoxitin is often the agent of choice on the basis of a multicenter randomized trial of 1735 patients. Half received 2 gm. of cefoxitin preoperatively. Three groups were evaluated: patients with a normal appendix, those with an acutely inflamed appendix, and those with a gangrenous appendix. The incidence of wound infection was significantly lower in all three groups. However, the formation of intra-abdominal abscess was not influenced by preoperative antibiotics. In a recent double-blind controlled study, prophylactic cefotetan was compared with prophylactic cefoxitin in the development of postoperative wound infections in patients with acute nonperforated appendicitis. The results showed that single-dose cefotetan and multiple-dose cefoxitin are equally effective. However, because of the greater convenience and decreased cost, single-dose cefotetan was considered the prophylaxis of choice in appendectomy for nonperforated appendicitis. Clindamycin with an aminoglycoside is indicated when Bacteroides fragilis is present; metronidazole can also be used for this organism.

6.1 Types of treatment

The treatment of appendicitis varies somewhat depending on the stage of the disease. In general, patients should receive fluid resuscitation before surgery, but this may require only 1 or 2 hours in patients with nonperforated disease.

6.2 Acute medical

Patients with acute, non perforated appendicitis should undergo urgent appendectomy. There have been very few studies examining the role of antibiotic therapy alone for appendicitis. Eriksson and Granstrom performed a randomized trial of antibiotic therapy versus surgery for patients with appendicitis. In a small number of patients, the initial success with medical therapy was 95%, but there was a recurrence rate of 35% with short follow-up. Antibiotics alone have been used in rare situations such as with sailors on long submarine tours. Due to the high recurrence rate, the current standard is operative treatment for acute appendicitis. There is a general consensus that prophylactic antibiotics should be administered before the start of the operation, but in acute disease, we use only a single dose. There are a wide number of agents that can be used as long as they provide activity against enteric anaerobics and gram-negative bacteria. We use a single dose of cefoxitin or cefotetan for prophylaxis.

In the past, the incidence of removing a normal appendix was acceptable if it was 20%. However, rates much lower than this have been quoted. An overall negative exploration rate of 20% should not be viewed as an appropriate standard with the availability of ultrasound- and CT-assisted diagnosis. The negative exploration rate in females is still slightly higher than that in males due to the confusion with diseases of the fallopian tubes and ovaries.

Authors study to compare risk of wound infection after appendectomy with and without irrigation after closure of fascia of external oblique muscle and before closure of skin. 200 patients were randomized in two groups: 99 in irrigation group and 101 in control group: irrigation group has significantly lees wound infection after appendectomy.

Clinical trial patients with acute appendicitis are generally in the early stages of disease with inflaming and simple appendicitis. They are not suppurated, gangrene and perforated stages yet; therefore the use of antibiotic prophylaxis can be prevented to save the suffering from antibiotic in a few days as well as the lowering the cost . In our study two groups of patients, one group given antibiotic prophylaxis before operation, other group not given antibiotic. There was a meaningful relation between the experimental group and the contrast one that the cause of reduction can not be related to antibiotic.

6.3 Antibiotic as definitive therapy

Traditional management of acute appendicitis has emphasized emergent surgical management This approach has been based on the\ theory that, over time, simple appendicitis will progress to perforation, with resulting increases in morbidity and mortality. As a result, a relatively high negative appendectomy rate has been accepted to avoid the possibility of progression to perforation. Recent data suggest that acute appendicitis and acute appendicitis with perforation maybe separate disease entities with distinct pathophysiology. A time series analysis performed on a 25-year data set did not find a significant negative relationship between the rates of negative appendectomy and perforation. A study analyzing time to surgery and perforation demonstrated that risk of rupture is minimal within 36 ours of symptom onset. Beyond this point, there is about a 5% risk of rupture in each ensuing 12-hour period. However, in many patients the disease will have an indolent course. In one study 10 of the 18 patients who did not undergo operation for 6 days after their symptoms began did not experience rupture.

One study by Krisna K. Varadhan and Colleagues in Nottingham UK, Antibiotic treatment has been shown to be effective in treating selected patients with acute appendicitis, and three randomized controlled trials (RCTs) have compared the efficacy of antibiotic therapy alone with that of surgery for acute appendicitis. The purpose of this meta analysis of RCTs was to assess the outcome with these two therapeutic modalities. Of the 350 patients randomized to the antibiotic group, 238 (68%) were treated successfully with antibiotics alone and 38 (15%) were readmitted. The remaining 112 (32%) patients randomized to antibiotic therapy crossed over to surgery for a variety of reasons. At 1 year, 200 patients in the antibiotic group remained asymptomatic.

This meta-analysis suggest that although antibiotic may be used as primary treatment for selected patients with suspected uncomplicated at present. Selection bias and crossover to surgery in the RCTs suggest that appendectomy is still the gold standard therapy for acute appendicitis .

6.4 Surgical

There are two approaches to removal of the non perforated appendix: through an open incision, usually a transverse right lower quadrant skin incision (Davis-Rockey) or an oblique version (McArthur-McBurney) with separation of the muscles in the direction of their fibers, or a paramedian incision, but this is not routinely done. The incision is centered on the midclavicular line. Occasionally, where the diagnosis is uncertain, a periumbilical midline incision can be used. Once the peritoneum is entered, the appendix is delivered into the field. This can usually be accomplished with careful digital manipulation of the appendix and cecum. It is important to avoid too extensive of a blind dissection. In difficult cases, extending the incision 1 to 2 cm can greatly simplify the procedure. Once the appendix is delivered into the wound, the mesoappendix is sacrificed between clamps and ties. There are several ways to handle the actual removal of the appendix. Some surgeons simply suture ligate the base of the appendix and excise it. Others place a purse string or Zstitch in the cecum, excise the appendix, and invert the stump into the cecum. We have used both approaches. Once the appendix is removed, the cecum is returned to the abdomen, and the peritoneum is closed. The wound is closed primarily in most patients with non perforated appendicitis because the risk of infection is less than 5%.

Acute appendicitis is one of the commonest of surgical emergencies and appendectomy has become established as the gold standard of therapy. However as the diagnosis of appendicitis in most centers is mainly a clinical one , based on history and examinations diagnostic uncertainly in patients with suspected appendicitis may lead to delay in treatment or negative surgical exploration, adding to the morbidity associated with the condition.

6.5 Laparoscopy

Semm first reported successful laparoscopic appendectomy in, 1983, several years before the first laparoscopic cholecystectomy. However, the widespread use of the laparoscopic approach to appendectomy did not occur until after the success of laparoscopic cholecystectomy. This may be due to the fact that appendectomy, by virtue of its small incision, is already a form of minimal-access surgery.

Laparoscopic appendectomy is performed under general anesthesia. A nasogastric tube and a urinary catheter are placed prior to obtaining a pneumoperitoneum. Laparoscopic appendectomy usually requires the use of three ports. Four ports may occasionally be necessary to mobilize a retrocecal appendix. The surgeon usually stands to the patient's left. One assistant is required to operate the camera.(fig 3) One trocar is placed in the umbilicus

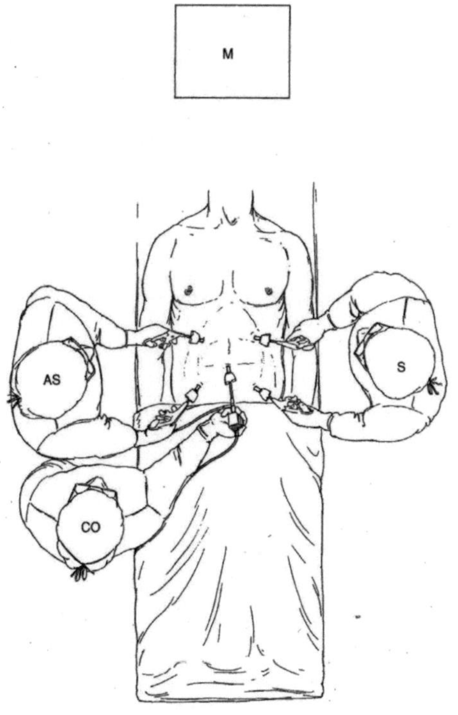

Fig. 3. Diagram of the operating room setup. CO, camera operator AS, assistant surgeon; M. monitor, S, surgeon. Monitor includes VDO, Video cassette recorder, and printer.

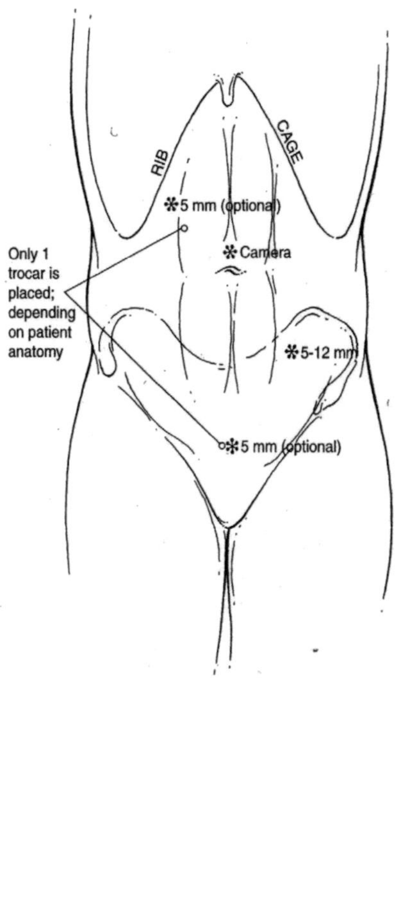

Fig. 4. Port site placement for laparoscopic appendectomy aright upper quadrant or suprapubic trocar is placed depending on patient anatomy

(10 mm), with a second trocar placed in the suprapubic position. Some surgeons will place this second port in the left lower quadrant. The suprapubic trocar is either 10 or 12 mm, depending on whether a linear stapler will be used. The placement of the third trocar (5 mm) is variable and is usually either in the left lower quadrant, epigastrium, or right upper quadrant. Placement is based on location of the appendix and surgeon preference. Initially, the abdomen is thoroughly explored to exclude other pathology. The appendix is identified by following the anterior taeniae to its base. Dissection at the base of the appendix enables the surgeon to create a window between the mesentery and base of the appendix (Fig. 4). The mesentery and base of the appendix are then secured and divided separately. When the mesoappendix is involved with the inflammatory process, it is often best to divide the appendix first with a linear stapler, and then to divide the mesoappendix immediately adjacent to the appendix with clips, electrocautery. Harmonic Scalpel, or staples. he base of the appendix is not inverted. The appendix is removed from the abdominal cavity through a trocar site or within a retrieval bag. The base of the appendix and the mesoappendix should be evaluated for hemostasis. The right lower quadrant should be irrigated. Trocars are removed under direct vision.

6.6 Natural Orifice Transluminal Endoscopic Surgery

Natural orifice transluminal endoscopic surgery (NOTES) is a new surgical procedure using flexible endoscopes in the abdominal cavity. In this procedure, access is gained by way of organs that are reached through a natural, already-existing external orifice. The hope for advantages associated with this method include the reduction of postoperative pain, shorter convalescence, avoidance of wound infection and abdominal-wall hernias, and the absence of scars. The first case of transvaginal removal of a normal appendix has recently been reported. Much work remains to determine if NOTES provides any additional advantages over the laparoscopic approach to appendectomy.

6.7 Outcomes

The mortality rate after appendectomy is less than 1% the morbidity of perforated appendicitis is higher than that of nonperforated cases and is related to increased rates of wound infection, intra-abdominal abscess formation, increased hospital stay, and delayed return to full activity.

Surgical site infections are the most common complications seen after appendectomy. About 5% of patients with uncomplicated appendicitis develop wound infections after open appendectomy. Laparoscopic appendectomy is associated with a lower incidence of wound infections; this difference is magnified among groups of patients with perforated appendicitis (14% versus 26%). Patients with a fever and leukocytosis and a normal appearing wound after appendectomy undergo CT of ultrasonography to exclude an intra abdominal abscess Similarly, if pus emanates from a fascial opening during wound inspection, an imaging study is obtained to identify any undrained intra abdominal fluid collections. In this situation, we place a percutaneous drain into the collection to divert the infected material away from the fascia and facilitate wound healing. For pelvic abscesses that are located in proximity to the rectum or vagina, we prefer ultrasound-guided transrectal or transvaginal drainage, thereby avoiding the discomfort of a percutaneous perineal drain.

7. Tumors

Appendiceal malignancies are extremely rare. Primary appendiceal cancer is diagnosed in 0.9 to 1.4% of appendectomy specimens. These tumors are only rarely suspected preoperatively. Additionally, less than 50% of cases are diagnosed at operation. Most series report that carcinoid is the most common appendiceal malignancy, representing more than 50% of the primary lesions of the appendix. However, a recent review from The National Cancer Institute's Surveillance, Epidemiology, and End Results program found the age-adjusted incidence of appendiceal malignancies to be 0.12 cases per 1,000,000 people per year, and identified mucinous adenocarcinoma as the most frequent histologic diagnosis with 37% of total reported cases. Carcinoid was the second most frequent histologic diagnosis, comprising 33% of total cases.

7.1 Carcinoid

The finding of a firm, yellow, bulbar mass in the appendix should raise the suspicion of an appendiceal carcinoid. The appendix is the most common site of gastrointestinal carcinoid, followed by the small bowel and then rectum. Carcinoid syndrome is rarely associated with appendiceal carcinoid unless widespread metastases are present, which occur in 2.9% of cases. Symptoms attributable directly to the carcinoid are rare, although the tumor can occasionally obstruct the appendiceal lumen much like a fecalith and result in acute appendicitis.

The majority of carcinoids are located in the tip of the appendix. Malignant potential is related to size, with tumors less than 1 cm rarely resulting in extension outside of the appendix or adjacent to the mass. In one report, 78% of appendiceal carcinoids were less than 1 cm, 17% were 1 to 2 cm, and only 5% were greater than 2 cm.94 Treatment rarely requires more than simple appendectomy. For tumors smaller than 1 cm with extension into the mesoappendix, and for all tumors larger than 1.5 cm, a right hemicolectomy should be performed.

One study by Claudio F Feo in Italy on 10 patients with primary of the appendix treated at University of Sasari Italy from 1998 to 2005. There were 5 women and 5 man with a meaning of 59.1 years. Laparatomy was performed in 4 cases : When as the other 6 cases undervent laparascopic exploration: Three operations were completed laparascopically and three were converted to laparatomy. Six tumors were malignant and the remaining were benign. Proportion of preoperative and late mortality were both 10%. Two of four patients with benign tumors died from causes unrelated to the appendical neoplasm. The 6 patients with malignant tumor and the other 2 with benign disease were alive and disease free after a mean follow up of 43 months despite of rarity of appendical primary tumor, surgeons should be aware of these neoplasm for making correct treatment decisions.

8. References

[1] Beauchamp RD, Evers BM, Mattox KL, Sabiston Textbook of Surgery, 16th ed. Philadelphia, W.B.Saunders Company. 2001. P. 919.

[2] Sabiston DC, Lyerly HK, Sabiston Textbook of Surgery, 15th ed. Philadelphia, W.B.Saunders Company. 1997. P. 964.

[3] Brunicardi FC, Anderson DK, Billiar TR, Dunn DL, Hunter JG, Pollock RE. Schwartz's Principles of Surgery. 8th ed , New York , McGraw Hill, 2010. P. 1080.

[4] Salari AA. Intra abdominal abscess. NABZ. Iranian Journal. 1994; 3 : 34-38.

[5] Salari AA. Peritonitis and Intraabdominal abscess. Yazd, Tebgostar, Shahid Sadoghi University of Medical sciences. Yazd, Iran. 2003. P. 93-110.

[6] Sabiston DC, Lyerly HK, Sabiston Textbook of Surgery, 15th ed. Philadelphia, W.B.Saunders Company. 2001. P. 961-969.

[7] Schwartz SI, Shires GT, Spencer FC. Principles of Surgery. 8th ed , New York , McGraw Hill, 1994. P.1304-1318.

[8] Karl A. Zucker, MD., FACS Surgical Laparascopy. Second edition, New York , London, Lippincott Williams Wilkins 2001. p. 231-232.

[9] Ronald F. Anderson. Routine ultrasound and limited computed tomography for the diagnosis of acute appendicitis : A surgeon perspective. World Journal of Surgery. 2011; 35: 295-296.

[10] Salari AA, MD. Sharifi MR , MD. Effects of Antibiotic prophylaxis and non prophlaxis in appendectomised patients without complications. Journal of Shahid Sadoughi University of Medical sciences Yazd Iran 1998; 6 : 42-47.

[11] Butala P. Greenstein AJ, SUR MD, Mehta N, Sadot E, Divino CM. Special Management of acute right lower Quadrant pain in pregnancy : A prospective cohort study. Journal American college of Surgeons, 2010; 211 : 490-497.

[12] Clausio F. FEO, Alberto Porcu, Antonio M. Scan U, Giorgio C, Ginesu, Alessandro Fancellu. Anlonell Lorettu, Giuseppe Dettori. Primary Appendical Tumors : Report on 10 cases Int Surg 2009, 94 : 224-227.

[13] Tamuro Hayama, Keiji Matsuda, Hajime Shibuay, Takuya Akahane, Atsushi Horiuchi, Ryu Shimada, Yoshiko Aoyagi, Keisuke Nakamura, Hideki Yamasa, Soichiro Ishihara, Keijiro Nozawa, Toshiaki Watanable. A case of appendeceal crohn's disease in children a laparascopic appendectomy ware performd. Int Surg 2010; 95 : 338 -342.

[14] Krishna K. Varadhan. David J. Humes. Keith R. Neal. Dileep N. Lobo. Antibiotic theraphy versus appendectomy for acute appendicitis : A Meta – analysis. Word J Surg 2010; 34: 199-209.

[15] Salari AA., MD. Prevention of wound infection after appendectomy by irrigation of wound plus prophylactic antibiotic versus prophylactic antibiotic. Iranian Journal of Surgery. 2003. 11.53-57.

[16] Salari AA, Zare M. Evaluation of perforated appendicitis in Yazd Iran (Shahid Sadoughi University of Medical Scienses and Health Services Yazd Iran. Word J Surg 2007; 31: 125.

[17] Salari AA. Binesh F. Diagnosis value of anorexia in acute appendicitis. Pak J Med Sci 2007: 23: 68-70.

[18] Silen W, Cop S. Early diagnosis of acute abdomen. 19th edition , New York , Oxford University Press. 1996 : 99-110.

[19] Oliver Monneuse. S. Abdalla. Zf. Pilleul. V. Hervieu. L. Gruner. E. Tissot. X. Barth, Pain as the only consistent sign of acute appendicitis: Lack of inflammatory signs does not exclude the diagnosis. World J Surg 2010; 34: 210-215.

[20] Seymour I.Schwartz, Harold Ellis. Maingut Abdominal Operation, 8th ed. USA. Prentice-Hall. 1985; 1274-1278.

[21] Brunicardi FC, Anderson DK, Billiar TR, Dunn DL, Hunter JG, Pollock RE. Schwartz's Principles of Surgery. 8th ed , New York , McGraw Hill, 2005. P 1121-1134.

Part 4

The Colon Pathologies

10

Colonic Pseudo-Obstruction

Abdulmalik Altaf and Nisar Haider Zaidi
Department of Surgery, King Abdul Aziz University Hospital, K.A.A. University, Jeddah, Saudi Arabia

1. Introduction

Colonic pseudo-obstruction is a condition of distention of colon with signs and symptoms of colonic obstruction in the absence of an actual mechanical cause of obstruction. It is a poorly understood disease that is characterized by functional large bowel obstruction.

Intestinal pseudo-obstruction was described in 1938 by the German surgeon W. Weiss who reported mega-duodenum in 6 persons in 3 generations of a German family and described it as an inherited subset of intestinal pseudo-obstruction[2]. A similar condition of pseudo-obstruction of intestine was described by Ingelfinger in 1943. Colonic pseudo-obstruction, however, was first described by Sir William Heneage Ogilvie in 1948 and named after him as "Ogilvie's Syndrome". His description was based on the findings of two patients who had non-mechanical obstruction due to retroperitoneal involvement of the celiac plexus by malignancy[1]. J. Dunlop in 1949 described a similar condition in men aged 56, 58, and 66 years where large bowel colic was the predominant symptom accompanied by constipation, abdominal distension, and progressive loss of weight, but with no evidence of mechanical obstruction to the intestinal flow[3]. In 1958, Dudley et al used the term pseudo-obstruction to describe the clinical appearance of a mechanical obstruction with no evidence of organic disease during laparotomy[4].

Ogilvie's syndrome commonly occurs in patients who are critically ill, have electrolyte imbalance, or on anticholinergic medications. If left untreated, life threatening complications like bowel ischemia or perforation may occur in up to 15% of cases with a mortality of 50%[5].

2. Epidemiology

The prevalence of colonic pseudo-obstruction is difficult to know but the disorder nearly always occurs in hospitalized patients. It is commonly found in patients undergoing major surgeries, patients with advanced malignancies, and in spinal trauma patients. It is usually associated with surgical procedures which require prolonged bed rest. As such, the development of colonic pseudo-obstruction is common in orthopedic procedures like total hip replacement (up to 1.5% of cases) and after total knee replacement (2.3%)[6]. The incidence is higher in hospitalized mentally-disabled patients reaching up to 18.5%[7].

Middle aged or elderly patients are commonly diagnosed with the disorder. The mean age of affected patients is 56.5 years for males and 59.9 years for females with a male to female ratio of 2:1.

3. Physiology of colonic motility

The rate and extent of colonic motility is the accumulative result of neural siganls that cause intrinsic rhythmic contraction of the smooth muscles of the colon. Hyperpolarizing action potentials coincide with peaks of fluctuating potential difference across the cell membrane and result in contraction of the muscle[8]. The contraction of colonic smooth muscles is integrated by the myenteric plexus whose neurons have vesicles that release neurotransmitters, such as acetylcholine, noradrenaline, 5HT, peptides and purines[9]. The neurotransmitters produce spike potentials and rhythmic contractions that have a fixed maximum rate[10]. Nicotinic cholinergic fibers mediate rapid inhibitory reflex while purinergic fibers mediate excitatory descending pathway[11]. The resulting interdigestive myoelectric complexes [IMC] are propagated by the myenteric plexus at an interval of 15 to 195 min., clearing the intestinal lumen[12]. The IMC are stimulated by the vagus nerve and motilin[13]. It is suppressed by ingestion of meals[14].

4. Pathophysiology

Colonic pseudo-obstruction is a form of colonic dysmotility which is a final common pathway of various physiological, electrolyte and biochemical disturbances. There are primary and secondary pseudo-obstruction. Primary pseudo-obstruction is the familial visceral myopathy or hollow visceral myopathy syndrome, a diffuse motility disorder involving autonomous innervations of the intestinal wall. Secondary pseudo-obstruction is associated with other conditions such as the use of some medications, severe metabolic illness, diabetes, uremia, hyperparathyroidism etc.

Colonic pseudo-obstruction can be neurogenic or myogenic in origin. It is the imbalance between sympathetic and parasympathetic innervations supplying colonic smooth muscle that causes pseudo-obstruction. This enteric nervous system forms a neural network residing in the submucosa and intermuscular layer of the colonic wall. Sympathetic nerve supply arises from lower thoracic and lumbar ganglia. The preganglionic nerves from these ganglia form a synapse in preaortic ganglia. The sympathetic nerves arising from these ganglia supply the colon. The parasympathetic nerve supply comes from the vagus nerve to the right half of colon up to splenic flexure, while the rest of colon is supplied by sacral nerve roots. Functional obstruction of the colon can be caused by increased sympathetic tone or decreased parasympathetic tone [15]. This autonomic dysfunction occurs mainly in postganglionic pathways and controls of the enteric nervous system. Two types of neurotransmitters are secreted by this system which are acetylcholine which increases intestinal secretions and motility and noradrenaline which decreases both intestinal secretions and motility.

Some derangements also occur at the cellular and molecular levels and are thought to be part of the pathophysiology of this disorder. The interstitial cells of Cajal (ICC) are the pacemaker cells of the gastrointestinal tract and are essential for normal motility of the bowel. ICC form extensive network of electrically coupled cells some of which act as a pacemaker while others are involved in the relaxation of smooth muscles. ICC are either deranged or absent in patients of pseudo-obstruction.

Nitric oxide may have a role in the development of pseudo-obstruction. It is involved in muscle relaxation and produced by the oxidation of L-arginine, mediated by increased nitrous oxide synthase activity and deficiency of c-kit cells in the intestine [16].

Migrating motor complexes (MMC) are waves of regular electromechanical activity observed in gastrointestinal smooth muscles and occur during fasting. In patients of pseudo-obstruction, there is uncoordinated intestinal contraction due to abnormal burst of MMC [17]. At the cellular level, there is deficiency of alpha actin in the inner circular layer of small bowel smooth muscle. Myosites are weak and undergo atrophy in myopathies and result in ineffective bowel propulsion. Anti-neuronal and anti-calcium channel antibodies cause enteral neuronal degeneration in patients who, in addition, have auto immune diseases and paraneoplastic conditions[18].

5. Etiology

Multiple disorders are associated with colonic pseudo-obstruction (Table 1). However, there is no single factor responsible for the development of pseudo-obstruction.
In a study that analyzed 400 cases of pseudo-obstruction, Vanek et al found the predisposing conditions associated with acute colonic pseudo-obstruction are: non-operative trauma (11.3%), infection [pneumonia,sepsis] (10%), Cardiac [MI, heart failure] (10%), Obstetric and Gynecological disorders (9.8%), abdominal/pelvic surgery (9.3%), Neurologic (9.3%), Orthopedic Surgery (7.3%), miscellaneous medical conditions [metabolic, cancer, respiratory failure, renal failure] (32%), and miscellaneous surgical conditions [Urology, Thoracic, Neurosurgery] (11.8%)[39].

Disorders associated with colonic pseudo-obstruction	
1.Surgical procedures- 1-Pelvic surgery. 2-Obstetric/gyne surgery. 3-Abdominal Surgery. 4-Hip Surgery. 5-Spinal surgery. 6-Thoracic/Cardiovascular Surgery. 7-Caesarean section. 8-Transplantation-Renal/Liver. 2-Drugs- 1-Opiates. 2-Calcium channel blockers. 3-Antidepressants. 4-Antiparkinson drugs. 5-Anticholinergic. 6-Phenothiazines. 7-Laxative Abuse. 8-Amphetamine. 9-Vincristine. 10-Interleukins. 11-Clonidine. 12-Benzodiazepines.	6-Malignancy- 1-Retroperitoneal cancer. 2-Leukemia. 3-Small cell lung cancer. 4-Pelvic radiotherapy. 5-Desseminated metastasis. 7-Neurologic- 1-Demantia. 2-Parkinson's disease. 3-Multiple sclerosis. 4-Cerebrovascular accident. 5-Nerve root compression. 6-Subarachnoid hemorrhage. 8-Pulmonary- 1-Pneumonia. 2-Mechanical ventilation. 3-COPD. 4-Thoracic surgery. 5-Pulmonary thrombus. 9-Cardiovascular - 1-Myocardial infarction. 2-Congestive Heart failure. 3-Peripheral vascular disease. 4-Cardiovascular surgery.

3-Trauma- 1-Abdominal trauma. 2-Pelvic fracture. 3-Spinal trauma. 4-Femoral fracture. 5-Burns. 4-Metabolic Disorders- 1-Electrolyte abnormalities. 2-Alcohalism. 3-Lead toxicity. 4-Diabetes Mellitus. 5-Uremia. 6-Hepatic failure. 7-Hypothyroidism. 5-Infections- 1-Appendicitis. 2-Pancreatitis. 3-Cholecystitis. 4-Abdominal /pelvic abscess. 5-Sepsis. 6-Pseudomembranous colitis. 7-Herpes zoster.	5-Aortic aneurysm. 10-Obstetric- 1-Post partum. 2-Caesarean section.

Table 1.

5.1 Etiological classification

The disorders linked to the development of colonic pseudo-obstruction can be classified according to the pathophysiological derangement they ensue (Table 2).

i. Dysfunction of nerve supply to the bowel

The nerve supply of the bowel is affected in many diseases such as diabetes mellitus, amylodosis, and porphyria. While the motility of small bowel rarely gets affected, autonomic neuropathy commonly affects gastric emptying in diabetes. Colonic dilatation may be found in patients with severe diabetes [19]. In amyloidosis, amyloid deposition in nerves leads to abnormal response to cholinergic agents [20]. In secondary amyloidosis pseudo-obstruction occurs as a terminal manifestation [21]. Degenerative diseases of the myenteric plexus, such as Fabry's disease, also are associated with pseudo-obstruction [22].

Intestinal motility is inhibited by some drugs and result in acute pseudo-obstruction. These drugs include atropine like drugs, clonidine, tricyclic antidepressants and vincristine[23,24,25,26]. Varicella infection is associated with damage of myenteric plexus [27]. Kawasaki disease and Chaga's disease produce an abnormality of gut motility due to an inflammatory reaction in myenteric plexus [28].

ii. Dysfunction of colonic muscle

Colonic smooth muscle dysfunction has been found in many cases of pseudo-obstruction. Visceral as well as skeletal muscle disorders have been linked with pseudo-obstruction of colon. Hereditary visceral myopathy is a degenerative disease of the longitudinal muscle layer which presents as an autosomal dominant disease[29] . Skeletal muscle disorders, such as dystrophia myotonica and polymyositis, may also result in abnormal gastric and bowel motility[30].

1-Dysfunction of nerve of bowel-
- 1-Metabolic-
  - Diabetes Mellitus.
  - Amylodosis.
  - Porphyria.
  - Paraneoplastic syndrome.
- 2-Toxins-
  - Drugs.
  - Insecticides.
  - Heavy metals.
- 3-Inflammatory-
  - Varicella.
  - Chagas disease.
  - Kawasaki disease.

2-Dysfunction of muscle of bowel-
- 1-Familial visceral myopathy.
- 2-Dystrophia myotonica.
- 3-Polymyositis.

3-Combined nerve and muscle dysfunction of bowel-
- 1-Pregnancy.
- 2-Hypoparathyroidism.
- 3-Myxoedema.
- 4-Pheochromocytoma.
- 5-Trauma.
- 6-Enteroglucagonoma.
- 7-Jejuno-ileal bypass.

4-Disorders of collagen and Interstitium of bowel-
- 1-Radiation.
- 2-Mesenteric Panniculitis.
- 3-Scleroderma.
- 4-Ehlers-Danlos syndrome.
- 5-Sarcoidosis.
- 6-Strongyloidosis.

Table 2. Etiological classification

iii. Combined nerve & muscles dysfunction of bowel

Dysfunction of the intrinsic nervous system of bowel and muscular disorders together have been found in many cases of pseudo-obstruction of colon. There is infrequent IMC and slow intestinal transit during pregnancy. There are reports of pseudo-obstruction following cesarean section[31]. Congenital hypoparathyroidism has been associated with pseudo-obstruction[32]. Myxoedema also produces pseudo-obstruction[33]. Abdominal pain and vomiting is also associated with pseudo-obstruction caused by pheochromocytoma[34]. Blunt abdominal trauma is associated with pseudo-obstruction and often is linked with sepsis[35].

iv. Disorders of colonic collagen and interstitium

Collagen metabolism is disturbed in colonic pseudo-obstruction. Irradiation to gut causes fibrosis which is more severe after pelvic irradiation[36]. Mesenteric panniculitis produces pseudo-obstruction by decreasing bowel wall compliance in addition to neural involvement[37]. Scleroderma produces excess collagen and causes pseudo-obstruction, volvulus, diverticulosis and perforation[38].

6. Clinical features

Patients are typically middle aged who are hospitalized for systemic disease or an unrelated surgical problem. The typical presentation is a picture of large intestinal obstruction. The disease can present as acute or chronic pseudo-obstruction. Acute cases present as mild or severe abdominal distension often causing diaphragmatic splinting and difficulty in breathing and usually occur in elderly patients following surgery. Chronic pseudo-obstruction is associated with features of malabsorption and malnutrition.

In acute pseudo-obstruction, marked abdominal distension is the most consistent clinical finding. Frequent other findings include abdominal pain, nausea, and vomiting. Constipation is a frequent symptom but 40% of patients have diarrhea. The pain is usually colicky but may be dull and constant. Fifty percent of patients show abdominal tenderness mainly in right iliac fossa. Bowel sounds may be hyperactive, high pitched or even normal. Ischemia and perforation are the most feared complications of acute colonic pseudo-obstruction; spontaneous perforation has been reported in 3% to 15% of patients with a mortality rate of 50% or higher [39]. The rate of perforation and/or ischemia rapidly increases with a cecal diameters of >10 to 12 cm and also when the duration of distention exceeds 6 days [40].. Fever may be present in some cases. The digital rectal examination typically reveals an empty rectum. Post operative pseudo-obstruction of the colon has been reported in many series following orthopedic, gynecological, urologic and lumbar spine surgery[41,42,43]

7. Investigations

Diagnosis depends on clinical presentation and the results of investigations. Investigations are needed to exclude mechanical cause of obstruction. Electrolyte disturbance is usually found in majority of patients with hypocalcemia, hyponatremia and hypokalemia being the most common laboratory finding. Leukocytosis is a frequent finding in cases of perforation or necrosis of the colonic wall.

Plain abdominal X-rays (Figures 1, 2) is the initial radiological investigation for patients presenting with colonic obstruction. Distension of the colon, especially the caecum, is a common feature and its diameter measurement is essential (Figure 3). A caecal diameter of more than 12cm has been found to be associated more often with perforation, and at a diameter of 12 to 14cm the rate of perforation rose to 7% and climbed to 23% if caecal dilatation was more than 14cm [44]. Animal and retrospective data suggest a critical thresholds of 9 cm for the transverse colon and 12 cm for the cecum; however, many patients present with dimensions greater than this without sequelae[45]. Colonic haustral and mucosal patterns are often maintained on X-rays. Transition from proximal dilated to decompressed colon is usually seen at the splenic flexure. Distension of colon follows Laplace's law which states that pressure required to stretch the walls of hollow viscus varies inversely with its radius [46]. Laplace's law is $T=P^*R/2$ where T is wall tension, P is transmural pressure and R is radius of bowel. Cecum is more vulnerable to distension and perforation as it is the widest part of the colon. Serial plain abdominal x-rays are useful in cases of chronic pseudo-obstruction as they are less likely to perforate than acute obstruction. Serial x-rays are needed to monitor the progress of conservative therapy and to guide further management.

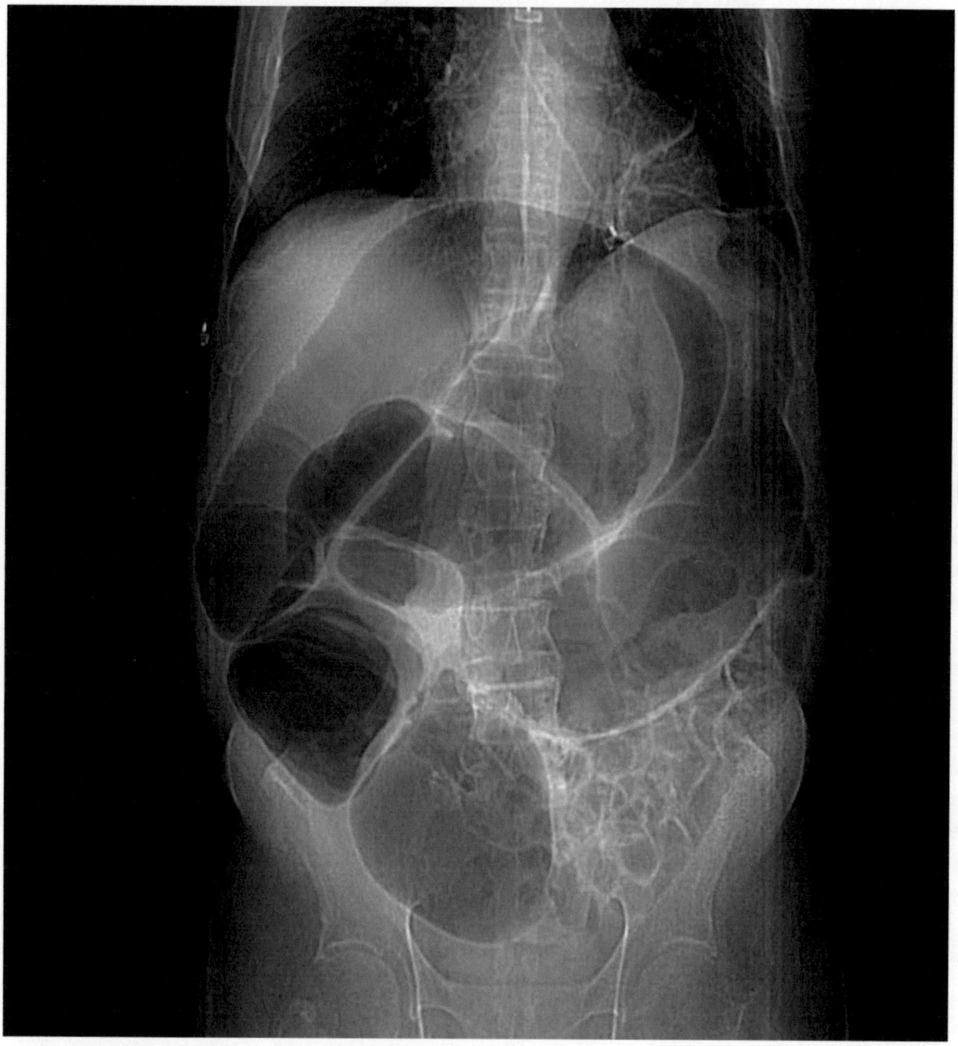

Fig. 1. Distension of colon in pseudo-obstruction

Low et al advised prone lateral view of the rectum to aid in diagnosis. He recommends placing the patient in the right lateral decubitus position for several minutes to allow passage of gas into distal colon. This facilitates the gaseous filling of the rectum when the patient is positioned for a prone lateral view of the pelvis. He found 75% success rate in excluding mechanical obstruction when there was gaseous filling of rectum.

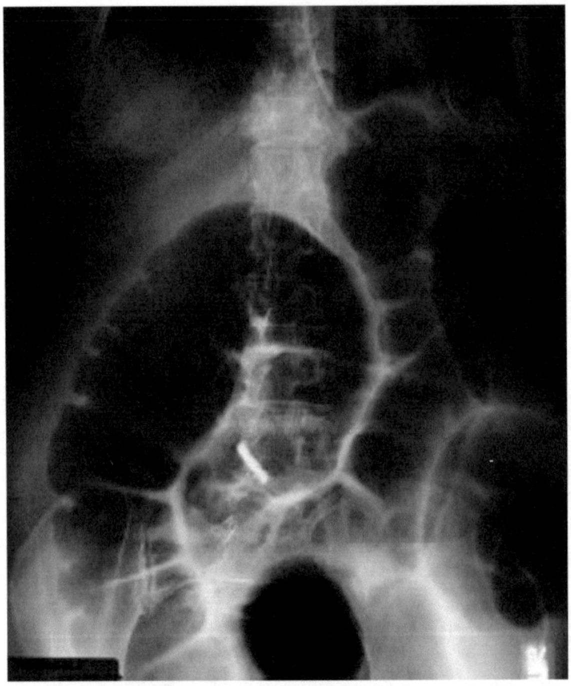

Fig. 2. Transverse colon distension in pseudo-obstruction

Contrast enema is very helpful when pseudo-obstruction of the colon is suspected. It is the investigation of choice to exclude mechanical obstruction and its sequel ,perforation[47]. The contrast material should be introduced under low pressure. There is no need for air to be introduced and the examination should be terminated when dilated colon is reached. Gastrografin is water soluble, clear and can be easily washed at the time of colonoscopy. Because it is hyperosmolar, it causes shift of fluids into lumen and, thus, has a low risk of contaminating the peritoneum when there is a perforation. Gastrografin enema confirms the diagnosis if there is absent, decreased or disorganized motility in any part of colon with decreased haustrations in the absence of any stricture [48].

Computerized tomography [CT] is used to exclude mechanical causes of obstruction and, when intravenous and luminal contrasts are used, the radiologist can comment on the condition of the wall of the colon and luminal pathology. The presence of perforation can be diagnosed when there is extra-luminal leakage of the luminal contrast. CT imaging can also show the presence of other intra-abdominal or retroperitoneal and solid organs pathology.

Colonoscopy is useful if done with caution as these patients may perforate. It can be both diagnostic and therapeutic as it can decompress the distended colon. Capsular endoscopy is not advised in pseudo-obstruction as it can be retained for long time[49].

Manometry and intestinal transit scintigraphy is used commonly in children with Hirschprung's disease. Colonic dysmotility which may be segmental or global may cause massive colonic distension in these patients [50,51].

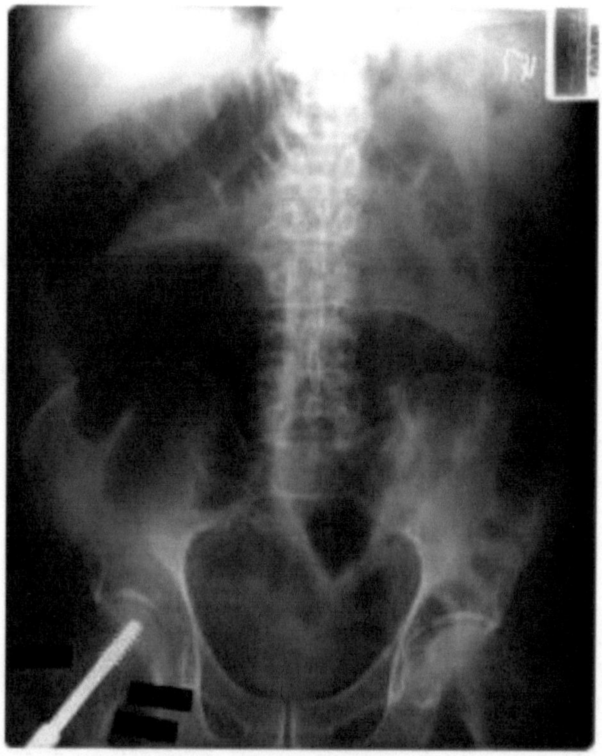

Fig. 3. Distension of the right colon post femoral fracture

8. Differential diagnosis

Colonic pseudo-obstruction must be differentiated from mechanical causes of large bowel obstruction where there is a true physical cause of obstruction including colonic volvulus, strictures and tumors. The differential diagnosis also includes various other causes of mechanical gastrointestinal obstruction as well as functional paralytic ileus and acute gastric distension. The clinical picture of colonic pseudo-obtruction may be confused with other causes of acute abdomen in patients who present late with symptoms and signs of perforation and peritonitis.

8.1 Conservative management

Patients of pseudo-obstruction are managed conservatively initially unless there are signs of mechanical obstruction or perforation. Initial management consists of correction of any precipitating factors that led to the development of pseudo-obstruction. Serial regular clinical examination should be performed for the development of abdominal tenderness or other signs of sepsis/peritonitis and abdominal x-rays should be repeated every twelve hours. Conservative measures can be used alone for 24-48 hours for patients without significant abdominal pain or signs of peritonitis and who have one or more potential underlying factors that are reversible. These patients are kept nil per orally with nasogastric tube suctioning for decompression. Rectal tube insertion has been used to aid in decompressing the distal colon. Body positioning (if feasible) often aid the spontaneous

evacuation of flatus. The patient is placed prone with the hips elevated on a pillow, in the knee-chest position with the hips high, or alternating right and left lateral decubitus position. The use of hyperbaric oxygenation may be effective in the management of chronic idiopathic intestinal pseudo-obstruction due to myopathy[52].
Sloyer et al. reportedsuccessful resolution in 92% of his patients by conservative management, with a mean cecal diameter 11.7 cm and a mean time to resolution of 1.6 days [44]. There was no perforation or death and most patients who responded to the conservative management did so within 3 to 6 days. They recommended invasive therapy only to those who do not respond to this treatment.
Active intervention is indicated for patients who deteriorate despite conservative measures, those with clinical features of ischemia or perforation, and for patients with sepsis (significant pain, fever, leucocytosis), respiratory compromise, or hemodynamic instability.

8.2 Medical treatment

Neostigmine has been used widely for the treatment of colonic pseudo-obstruction. It is an acetylcholinestrase inhibitor which acts in reversible manner. It stimulates muscarinic receptors which in turn increases motor activity of colon and results in propulsion of feces in colon [53]. Its therapeutic effect is because of its parasympathomimetic effect. It increases parasympathetic activity which leads to hyperperistalsis. Neostigmine was first tried by Neely and Catchpole three decades ago in small bowel paralytic ileus[54]. Neostigmine is given intravenously and has a rapid onset [1-20 min] and short duration of action [1-2 hrs][55]. Its half-life is 80 minutes.
A randomized double blinded trial evaluated neostigmine in 11 patients with acute colonic pseudo-obstruction with a cecal diameter of >10 cm and no response to conservative therapy for 24 hrs [55]. The criteria for exclusion were- suspected ischemia or perforation, pregnancy, renal failure, arrhythmias and severe active bronchospasm. Patients were randomized to receive neostigmine 2 mg or saline by intravenous infusion over 3-5 minutes. The primary end point was a clinical response that prompts a decrease in abdominal distension which as determined by physical examination. Secondary end point was the change in abdominal girth and the change in colonic diameter on abdominal radiographs. Patients not responding within 3 hours were eligible for open label neostigmine. A clinical response was observed in 91% of patients randomized to receive neostigmine compared to 0 receiving placebo. The median time to response was 4 minutes. The median reduction in cecal diameter [5 cm vs. 2 cm] and abdominal girth [7 cm vs. 1 cm] were significantly reduced in neostigmine group. Open label neostigmine was given in 8 patients who failed to respond to initial infusion [7 placebo, 1 neostigmine] and all had prompt decompression. The recurrence rate of colonic distension after neostigmine decompression was 11%. Common side effects were mild abdominal cramps and excessive salivation. Symptomatic bradycardia occurred in two patients who required atropine [55]. The side effects of neostigmine are due to excessive parasympathetic activity.
Many other studies also have recommended neostigmine for the treatment of colonic pseudo-obstruction [56, 57, 58, 59]. Neostigmine administration should be done with caution. Patient requires admission to a high dependency unit or cardiac unit for the administration of neostigmine. The medication should be given while the patient is supine on the bed with continuous electro-cardiac monitoring in place. The physician should clinically assess the patient periodically and vital signs measurement should be done every 15-30 minutes. There

are some contraindication for neostigmine use, like mechanical bowel obstruction, suspected bowel ischemia or perforation, uncontrolled cardiac arrhythmias, renal insufficiency and severe bronchospasm.

Neostigmine is a safe, effective and cheap medication in the management of colonic pseudo-obstruction and the current available data recommend its use as the initial therapy of choice for patients not responding to conservative treatment.

Erythromycin is another medication used in the management of colonic pseudo-obstruction. Erythromycin is a motilin receptor agonist that has been shown to decompress the bowel in a few case reports [60]. In one study erythromycin improved gastric emptying and intestinal transit measured by sulphamethizole methods and radio opaque markers, respectively [61]. Side effects include bloating, abdominal pain, nausea and vomiting. Repeated intravenous administration of erythromycin through a peripheral vein may cause phlebitis.

Somatostatin analogue, Octreotide, is used in scleroderma and paraneoplastic syndromes. Its action is independent of motilin. Octreotide increases MMC especially in scleroderma patients by an unknown mechanism. Plasmapheresis may be useful in selected cases of paraneoplastic syndromes where pseudo-obstruction is associated with autoantibodies.Cisaperide and tegaseroid are also used in colonic pseudoobstruction[62,63].

Spinal anaesthesia has resolved some cases of intestinal pseudo-obstruction, which is due to blockade of sympathetic activity.

Hyperbaric oxygen has been used in chronic idiopathic intestinal pseudo-obstruction due to myopathy although the exact mechanism of action is not known.

Antibiotics can be used intermittently to suppress intestinal overgrowth and thus resolve pseudo-obstruction. Common antibiotics used are metronidazole, doxycycline, and ciprofloxacin. Table 3 summarizes the available medical treatment options.

8.3 Colonoscopic treatment

Many patients fail to respond to neostigmine and other conservative methods may need endoscopic decompression. The first use of colonoscopic decompression in cases of pseudo-obstruction was done in 1977 by Kukora et al [64]. These patients have a risk of perforation following bowel ischemia. Colonoscopic decompression is done in these patients to prevent such complications. However, some precautions should be exercised when performing colonoscopy in these patients. Specifically, no oral laxatives or bowel preparation should be given and minimal air insufflation should be used during the procedure. There is no need to attempt to examine whole length of the colon. Suctioning the gas decompresses the colon and mucosal viability is assessed while slowly withdrawing the colonoscope. A per rectal tube for decompression should be left in the colon at the end of the procedure.

The success of colonoscopic decompression has been reported in multiple studies. The initial extent bowel decompression is determined by a reduction in the cecal diameter by radiology. Less than half of the patients benefit from colonoscopic decompression without tube placement[65]. Placement of a tube following colonoscopy is strongly recommended as reported by many studies[66,67,68]. This seems to lower the recurrence rate although its value has not been evaluated in controlled trials. A perforation rate of 3% has been reported following colonic decompression by colonoscopy[69]. Despite of complications colonoscopic decompression in cases of colonic pseudo-obstruction is a useful tool [70]. Colonoscopic decompression of the colon is effective, causing decreased cecal diameter in 73% to 100%of cases[71]. The advantage of endoscopic decompression is that mortality rates for colonoscopic decompression were 1% to 5% compared with 12% to 20% for tube cecostomy[72]. However,

Drug	Dose	Mechanism of action	Advantage	Note
Erythromycin	0.5 g tds or qds	Motilin agonist	Cheap	Less effective if taking opioids
Domperidone	20 mg tds	Blocks dopaminergic receptors	Does not enter BBB	Can cause hyperprolactinemia
Metaclopramide	10 mg tds	Blocks dopaminergic (D2) receptors	Cheap	Can cause extra-pyramidal symptoms
Neostigmine	2 mg IV	Acetylcholinesterase inhibitor	Effective	Needs monitoring in ICU/high dependency

Table 3. Drugs used in the treatment of colonic pseudo-obstruction

Reference	Method used	Success rate (%)
Emmanuel et al	Erythromycin	40
Ponec et al	Neostigmine	91
Perlemuter et al	Octreotide in connective tissue disease	100
Lee et al	Epidural	62
Jetmore et al	Colonoscopic decompression	64

Table 4. Reports of success rate of various methods in pseudo-obstruction

Reference	Method	Recurrence (%)	Morbidity
Farinon et al	Colonoscopy	29	Pain, risk of perforation
Lee et a	Epidural	None	Epidural side effects
Ponec et al	Neostigmine	20	Abdominal pain, cardiac arrhythmia, excess salivation, vomiting
Dalgic et al	Erythromycin	50	Abdominal pain, liver function disturbance,

Table 5. Recurrence of pseudo-obstruction and morbidity associated with each method.

recurrence rates of 10% to 65%have been noted after initial success as documented by increased caecal diameter on radiography[73,74,75].

Recently a randomized trial on the effect of oral Polyethylene Glycol (PEG) electrolyte balanced solution on the relapse of pseudo-obstruction after initial resolution with neostigmine or colonoscopic decompression showed sustained response rate and prevention of such episodes. Patients were randomized to receive PEG (29.5gm) or placebo and monitored for 7 days and it was found that 33% of recurrence rate in the patients who received placebo while none in PEG group. Therapy with PEG also resulted in significant increase in stool and flatus evacuations [76].

8.4 Surgical decompression

Surgery is reserved for those patients who do not respond to nonoperative management and those who present in sepsis, perforation or peritonitis [77]. Early recognition and prompt conservative management of pseudo-obstruction of the colon can minimize complications as well as the need for surgical intervention. Surgical options include percutaneous endoscopic colostomy, cecostomy and colectomy. Cecostomy can be done via the open or laparoscopic methods. Tube cecostomy is useful in acute colonic pseudo-obstruction as it achieves successful decompression with fewer complications. It is also useful in patients of chronic intestinal pseudo-obstruction [78].

Colectomy is performed when there is perforation or gangrene of the colon. Right or left colectomy can be offered depending on the site of gangrene or perforation, often with colostomy or end ileostomy. There is a higher risk of abdominal compartment syndrome post abdominal surgery in these cases due to edema of abdominal viscera. Therefore, if primary closure of abdominal wall is difficult then temporary closure with delayed secondary permanent closure should be considered. In the post operative period, attention should be given to improve the splanchanic circulation as a previously dilated colon is more susceptible to perforation. Complications of surgical intervention include abdominal sepsis, anastomotic dehiscence, fistulas and abdominal compartment syndrome. Surgical site infections are also common with subsequent fascial dehiscence and incisional hernia.

A chart summarizing the management of colonic pseudo-obstruction is shown in Figure 4.

9. Prognosis and prevention

Most of the patients stay hospitalized for less than a week. Increased in morbidity and mortality has been shown when surgical treatment was needed [79]. The mortality rate in medically treated patients is 14% and surgically treated patients is 30%, with a higher mortality in patients with cecal perforation or ischemia [80]. The reported incidence of cecal perforation is 3-40% with an associated mortality of 40-50%. A cecal diameter of greater than 14 cm, a delay in colonic decompression and advanced age are the predictors of colonic perforation.

Colonic pseudo-obstruction is a preventable disease in certain occasions, so emphasis should be on preventing this disease rather than on treatment, whenever possible. This can be done by early mobilization of hospitalized patients, prevention of constipation and the development of new pharmacologic agents which can resolve colonic inertia and help in propulsion of feces.

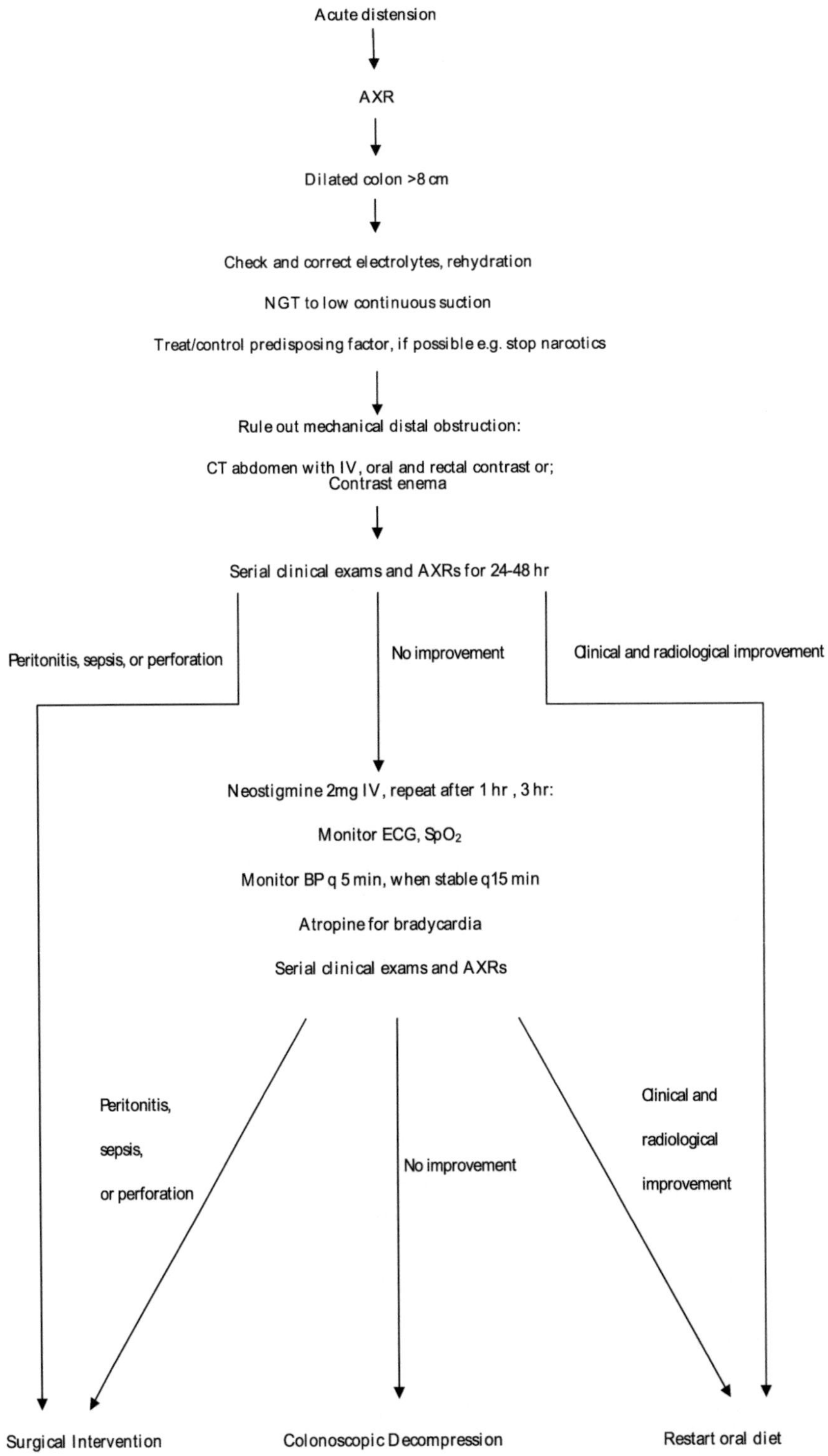

Fig. 4. Management flow chart.

10. References

[1] Ogilvie WH. Large intestine colic due to sympathetic deprivation:a new clinical syndrome. Br Med J 1948;2:671-673.
[2] W. Weiss:Zur Ätiologie des Megaduodenums.Deutsche Zeitschrift für Chirurgie, Leipzig, 1938, 251: 317-330.
[3] J. Dunlop:Ogilvie's syndrome of false colonic obstruction.The British Medical Journal, 1949, 1: 890-891.
[4] H. O. Dudley. I. S.. Sinclair, I. F. McLaren, T. J. McNair, J. E. Newsam:Intestinal pseudo-obstruction.
Journal of the Royal College of Surgeons of Edinburgh, 1958, 3: 206-217.
[5] Eisen GM, Baron TH, Dominitz JA, et al. Acute colonic pseudo-obstruction. *GastrointestEndosc* 2002;56:789-92.
[6] Nelson JD, Urban JA, Salsbury TL, Lowry JK, Garvin KL. Acute colonic pseudo-obstruction (Ogilvie syndrome) after arthroplasty in the lower extremity. J Bone Joint Surg Am 2006; 88:604-10.
[7] Khalid K, Al-Salamah SM. Spectrum of general surgical problems in the developmentally disabled adults. Saudi Med J 2006; 27:70-5.
[8] Brading, A.F. (1979). Smooth muscle. Maintenance of ionic composition. British Medical Bulletin, 35, 227.
[9] Burnstock G. (1982). Studies of autonomic nerves in the gut- past, present and future. Scandinavian Journal of Gastroenterology, 17, suppl. 7, 135..
[10] Duthie, H.L. (1979). Links between basic and clinical studies of gastrointestinal smooth muscle. British Medical Bulletin, 35, 301.FAULK, D.L. (1978).
[11] Hirst, G.D.S. (1979). Mechanisms of peristalsis. British Medical Bulletin, 35, 263.
[12] Sarna, S., Stoddard, C., Belbeck, L. & McWade, D. (1981). Intrinsic nervous control of migrating myoelectric complexes. American Journal of Physiology, 241, G16.
[13] Itoh, Z., Aizawa, I. & Sekiguchi, T. (1981). The interdigestive migrating complex and its significance in man. Clinics in Gastroenterology, 11, 497.
[14] Heppell, J., Becker, J.M., Kelly, K.A. & Zinsmeister, A.R. (1983). Postprandial inhibition of canine enteric interdigestive myoelectric complex. American Journal of Physiology, 244, G160.
[15] Mashour GA, Peterfreund RA. Spinal anesthesia and Ogilvie's syndrome. J Clin Anesth 2005; 17:122-3.
[16] Wang ZQ, Watanabe Y, Toki A, et al. Involvement of endogenous nitric oxide and c-kit-expressing cells in chronic intestinal pseudo-obstruction. J Pediatr Surg 2000; 35:539-44.
[17] Watanabe Y, Ito T, Ando H, Seo T, Nimura Y. Manometric evaluation of gastrointestinal motility in children with chronic intestinal pseudo-obstruction syndrome. J Pediatr Surg 1996; 31:233-8.
[18] Simpson DA, Pawlak AM, Tegmeyer L, Doig C, Cox D. Paraneoplastic intestinal pseudo-obstruction, mononeuritis multiplex, and sensory neuropathy/neuronopathy. J Am Osteopath Assoc 1996; 96:125-8.
[19] Paley, R.G., Mitchell, W. & Watkinson, G. (1961).Terminal colonic dilatation following intractable diarrhea in a diabetic. Gastroenterology, 41, 401.
[20] Battle, W.M., Ruben, M.R., Cohen, S. & Snape, W.J. (1979). Gastrointestinal motility dysfunction in amyloidosis. New England Journal of Medicine, 301, 24.

[21] Legge, D.A., Wollaeger E.F. & Carlson, H.C. (1970).Intestinal pseudo-obstruction in systemic amyloidosis.Gut, 11, 764.
[22] Friedman LS, Kirkham SE, Thistlethwaite JR, Platika D, Kolodny EH, Schuffler MD. 3.;Jejunal diverticulosis with perforation as a complication of Fabry's disease Gastroenterology. 1984 Mar;86(3):558-63.
[23] Bear, R. & Steer, K. (1976). Pseudo-obstruction due to Intestinal pseudo-obstruction 1037 clonidine. British Medical Journal, 1, 197.
[24] Faulk, D.L. (1978). Approach to patients with intestinal pseudo-obstruction. Gastroenterology, 74, 1320.
[25] Faulk, D.L., Anuras, S., Gardner, D., Mitros, F.,Summers, R.W. & Cristensen J. (1978). A familial visceral myopathy. Annals of Internal Medicine, 89, 600.
[26] Sriram, K., Schumer, W., Ehrenpreis, S., Camaty, J.E.& Scheller, L. (1979). Phenothiazine effect on gastrointestinal tract function. American Journal of Surgery, 137,87.
[27] Walsh, T.N. (1982). Pseudo-obstruction of the colon associated with varicella-zoster infection. Irish Journal of Medicine, 151, 318.
[28] Smith, B. (1980). Changes in the myenteric plexus in Chagas' disease. Journal of Pathology and Bacteriology, 94, 642.
[29] Schuffler, M.D. & Pope, C.E. (1977). Studies of idiopathic intestinal pseudo-obstruction. II. Hereditary hollow visceral myopathy: family studies. Gastroenterology, 73, 339.
[30] Patterson, M. & Rios, G. (1959). Disturbed gastrointestinal motility - an unusual manifestation of a systemic muscular disorder: polymyositis or progressive muscular dystrophy. Gastroenterology, 36, 261.
[31] Ravo, B., Pollane M. & Ger, R. (1983). Pseudo-obstruction of the colon following caesarean section. A review.Diseases of the Colon and Rectum, 26, 440.
[32] Cockel, R., Hill, E.E. & Rushton, E.I. (1973). Familial steatorrhoea with calcification of the basal ganglia andmental retardation. Quarterly Journal ofMedicine, 42, 771.
[33] Salerno, N. & Grey, N. (1978). Myxoedema pseudoobstruction.American Journal ofRoentgenology, 130, 175.
[34] Turner, C.E. (1983). Gastrointestinal pseudo-obstruction due to pheochromocytoma. American Journal ofGastroenterology,78, 214
[35] Addison, N.V. (1983). Pseudo-obstruction of the large bowel. Journal of the Royal Society of Medicine, 76, 252.
[36] Lopez, M.J., Memula, N. & Doss, L.L. (1981). Pseudoobstruction of the colon during pelvic radiotherapy.Diseases of the Colon and Rectum, 24, 201
[37] Tytgat, G.N., Roozendaal, K. & Winter, W. (1980).Successful treatment of a patient with retractile mesenteritis with prednisone and azathioprine. Gastroenterology,79, 352.
[38] Krishnamurthy, S., Kelly, M.M., Rohrmann, C.W. & Schuffler, M.D. (1983). Jejunal diverticulosis. Aheterogenous disorder caused by a variety ofabnormalities of smooth muscle or myenteric plexus. Gastroenterology,85, 538.
[39] Vanek VW, Al-Salti M. Acute pseudo-obstruction of the colon (Ogilivie's syndrome): an analysis of 400 cases. Dis Colon Rectum 1986;29:203-10.
[40] Rex DK. Colonoscopy and acute colonic pseudo-obstruction.Gastrointest Endosc Clin N Am 1997;7:499-508.
[41] Johnson C, Rice R, Kelvin F, Foster W, Williford M. The radiographic evaluation of gross cecal distension: emphasis on cecal ileus. AJR Am J Roentgenol 1986;145:1211-7.

[42] Caner H, Bavbeck M, Albayrak A, Calisanellar T, Altinors N.Ogilvie's syndrome as a rare complication of lumbar disc surgery. Can J Neurol Sci 2000;27:77-8.

[43] O'Malley K, Flechner S, Kapoor A, Rhodes RA, Modlin CS,Goldfarb DA, et al. Acute colonic pseudo-obstruction (Ogilvie's syndrome) after renal transplantation. Am J Surg 1999;177:492-6.

[44] Sloyer AF, Panella VS, Demas BE, Shike M, Lightdale CJ,Winawer SJ, et al. Ogilvie's syndrome:successful management without colonoscopy. Dig Dis Sci 1988;33:1391-6.

[45] Chapman AH, McNamara M, Porter G. The acute contrast enema in suspected large bowel obstruction: value and technique. Clin Radiol 1992; 46:273-8.

[46] Slam KD, Calkins S, Cason FD LaPlace's law revisited: cecal perforation as an unusual presentation of pancreatic carcinoma. World J Surg Oncol. 2007 Feb 2;5:14.

[47] Abeyta BJ, Albrecht RM, Schermer CR. Retrospective study of neostigmine for the treatment of acute colonicpseudo-obstruction. Am Surg 2001.

[48] Byrne WJ, Cipel L, Ament ME, Gyepes MT. Chronic idiopathic intestinal pseudo-obstruction syndrome. Radiologic signs in children with emphasis on differentiation from mechanical obstruction. Diagn Imaging 1981; 50:294-304.

[49] Storch I, Barkin JS. Contraindications to capsule endoscopy: do any still exist? Gastrointest Endosc Clin N Am 2006; 16:329-36.

[50] Martin MJ, Steele SR, Mullenix PS, et al. A pilot study using total colonic manometry in the surgical evaluation of pediatric functional colonic obstruction. J Pediatr Surg 2004; 39:352-9.

[51] Panganamamula KV, Parkman HP. Chronic intestinal pseudo-obstruction. Curr Treat Options Gastroenterol 2005;8:3-11.

[52] Yokota T, Suda T, Tsukioka S, et al. The striking effect of hyperbaric oxygenation therapy in the management of chronic idiopathic intestinal pseudo-obstruction. Am J Gastroenterol 2000; 95:285-8.

[53] Law NM, Bharucha AE, Undale AS et al. Cholinergic stimulation enhances colonic motor activity, transit, and sensation in humans. Am J Physiol Gastrointest Liver Physiol 2001;281:G1228–37.

[54] Neely J, Catchpole B. Ileus: The restoration of alimentarytract motility by pharmacologic means. Br J Surg 1971;58:21–8.

[55] Aquilonius SM, Hartvig P. Clinical pharmacokinetics of cholinesterase inhibitors. Clin Pharmacokinet 1986;11:236–49.

[56] Ponec RJ, Saunders MD, Kimmey MB. Neostigmine for the treatment of acute colonic pseudo-obstruction. N Engl JMed 1999;341:137–41.

[57] Loftus CG, Harewood GC, Baron TH. Assessment of predictors of response to neostigmine for acute colonic pseudo-obstruction. Am J Gastroenterol 2002;97:3118–22.

[58] Abeyta BJ, Albrecht RM, Schermer CR. Retrospective study of neostigmine for the treatment of acute colonic pseudoobstruction.Am Surg 2001;67:265–8.

[59] Ponec RJ, Saunders MD, Kimmey MB. Neostigmine for the treatment of acute colonic pseudo-obstruction. N Engl J Med 1999;341:137–41.

[60] Armstrong DN, Ballantyne GH, Modlin IM. Erythromycin for reflex ileus in Ogilvie's syndrome. Lancet 1991;337:378.

[61] Bonacini M, Smith OJ, Pritchard T. Erythromycin as therapy for acute colonic pseudo-obstruction (Ogilvie's syndrome).J Clin Gastroenterol 1991;13:475–6.

[62] MacColl C, MacCannell KL, Baylis B et al. Treatment of acute colonic pseudo-obstruction (Ogilvie's syndrome) with cisapride. Gastroenterology 1990;98:773–6.
[63] Camilleri M. Review article: tegaserod. Aliment Pharmacol Ther 2001;15:277–289.
[64] Kukora JS, Dent TL. Colonic decompression of massive nonobstructive cecal dilation. Arch Surg 1977;112:512–517.
[65] Rex DK. Colonoscopy and acute colonic pseudoobstruction.Gastrointest Endosc Clin North Am 1997;7:499–508.
[66] Nivatvongs S, Vermeulen FD, Fang DT. Colonoscopic decompression of acute pseudo-obstruction of the colon.Ann Surg 1982;196:598–600.
[67] Strodel WE, Nostrant TT, Eckhauser FE et al. Therapeutic and diagnostic colonoscopy in non-obstructive colonic dilatation. Ann Surg 1983;19:416–21.
[68] Bode WE, Beart RW, Spencer RJ et al. Colonoscopic decompression for acute pseudo-obstruction of the colon (Ogilvie's syndrome): report of 22 cases and review of the literature. Am J Surg 1984;147:243–5.
[69] Geller A, Petersen BT, Gostout CJ. Endoscopic decompression for acute colonic pseudo-obstruction. Gastrointest Endosc 1996;44:144–50.
[70] Melange M, Van Gossum A, Houben JJ, de Ronde T, Vanheuverzwyn R,Adler M: Acute dilatation of the colon. Acta Gastroenterol Belg 1991,54:233-6.
[71] Gosche JR, Sharpe JN, Larson GM. Colonoscopic decompression for pseudo-obstruction of the colon. Am Surg 1989;55:111–115
[72] Bode WE, Beart RW, Spencer RJ, Culp CE, Wolff BG,Taylor BM. Colonoscopic decompression for acute pseudoobstruction of the colon (Ogilvie's syndrome). Am J Surg 1984;147:243–245
[73] Nano D, Prindiville T, Pauly M, Chow H, Ross K, Trudeau W. Colonoscopic therapy of acute pseudoobstruction of the colon. Am J Gastroenterol 1987;82:145–148.
[74] Duh QY, Way LW. Diagnostic laparoscopy and laparoscopic cecostomy for colonic pseudo-obstruction. Dis Colon Rectum 1993;36:65-70.
[75] Thompson AR, Pearson T, Ellul J, Simson JN. Percutaneous endoscopic colostomy in patients with chronic intestinal pseudo-obstruction. Gastrointest Endosc 2004; 59:113-5.
[76] Sgouros SN, Vlachogiannakos J, Vassiliadis K, Bergele C, Stefanidis G, et al. Effect of polyethylene glycol electrolyte balanced solution on patients with acute colonic pseudo-obstruction after resolution of colonic dilation: a prospective, randomised, placebo controlled trial. Gut. May 2006;55(5):638-42.
[77] Ramage JI Jr, Baron TH. Percutaneous endoscopic cecostomy: a case series. Gastrointest Endosc 2003; 57:752-5.
[78] Masetti M, Di Benedetto F, Cautero N, et al. Intestinal transplantation for chronic intestinal pseudo-obstruction in adult patients. Am J Transplant 2004; 4:826-9.
[79] Pironi L, Spinucci G, Paganelli F, et al. Italian guidelines for intestinal transplantation: potential candidates among the adult patients managed by a medical referral center for chronic intestinal failure. Transplant Proc 2004; 36:659-61.
[80] Saunders MD, Kimmey MB. Systematic review: acute colonic pseudo-obstruction. Aliment Pharmacol Ther 2005; 22:917-25.

11

Treatment of Colorectal Stricture After Circular Stapling Anastomoses

S. Shimada[1], M. Kuramoto[1], A. Matsuo[1], S. Ikeshima[1],
H. Kuhara[1], K. Eto[1] and H. Baba[2]
[1]*Department of Surgery, Yatsushiro Social Insurance General Hospital,*
[2]*Department of Gastroenterological Surgery, Graduate School of Medical Sciences, Kumamoto University*
Japan

1. Introduction

Performing an end-to-end low rectal anastomosis with the linear single stapling technique was first reported in 1979 (Ravitch & Steichen, 1979). An improved circular stapling technique for anterior resection of the rectum, i.e. double stapling technique, overcoming the problems of insertion of the purse-string on the rectum stump and of disparity in size between the rectum and colon was introduced (Knight & Griffen, 1980). Although conventional double stapling technique is mainly performed for tumors greater than 6 cm from the anal verge (Shrikhande et al., 2007), recent prospective case series have described a variation of double stapling technique for ultra-low anterior resection involving vertical transaction of the rectum followed by an anastomosis with a circular stapler which results in a vertically oriented elliptical anastomotic orifice (Sato et al., 2007). Thus, circular stapling anastomosis of the rectum has been widely used and has been regarded as a safe and quick technique, however, the development of anastomotic strictures is the major post-operative complication of this procedure. (Blamey & Lee, 1982; Cade et al., 1981; Fain et al., 1975; Kumar et al., 2011; Kyzer & Gordon, 1992; Leff et al., 1982; Luchtefeld et al., 1989; Marchena et al., 1997; Smith, 1981; Vezeridis et al., 1982). It has been reported that the circular stapled anastomosis has a higher stricture rate than a handsewn anastomosis in the colon (Brennan et al., 1982; Dziki et al., 1991; MacRae & McLeod, 1998; Polglase et al., 1981) and that the incidence of the stricture after the double stapling technique varies from 0 to 30% (Blamey & Lee, 1982; Cade et al., 1981; Gordon & Vasilevsky, 1984; Kumar et al., 2011; Kyzer & Gordon, 1992; Luchtefeld et al., 1989; Marchena et al., 1997; Smith, 1981).

The complication of anastomotic stricture associated with stapling is harmful and distressing for patients with anterior resection of the rectum. Dilation is the only treatment and is variously used with techniques such as digital, a sigmoidscope, an esophageal dilator, or balloon dilators. (Cade et al., 1981; Leff et al.,1982; Luchtefeld et al., 1989; Moran et al., 1992; Smith, 1981; Verma et al., 1990; Vezeridis et al., 1982; Whitworth et al., 1988). These techniques, however, have their drawbacks, that is, digital or sigmoidscopic dilation has insufficient effects, and esophageal and balloon dilators need fluoroscopy and other optional equipments, and recurrence is common. Dilators can dilate the deformed and

shrunk staple line caused by the thickened circumferential scar formation but hardly split the closed staple line, resulting in reverting to the shape before dilation followed by a re-stricture. Thus, a new device of "staple cutter (STENO-CUTTER™)" was developed to split the circular staple line in the stricture (Shimada et al., 1996).
In the present manuscript, incidence and factors of the stricture, development of this new device of STENO-CUTTER™ for the treatment of the stricture, and the clinical effects and advantages is reviewed. In addition, application of STENO-CUTTER™ for the treatment of intractable stricture caused by anastomotic leakage as well as anastomotic ischemia is described.

2. Incidence and risk factors of stricture after circular stapling anastomoses

With the advance of surgical techniques and the circular staple device, the incidence of leakage of coloproctostomy has been significantly decreasing. On the other hand, the development of anastomotic stricture has become a major post-operative complication (Brower & Freeman, 1984; Knight & Giffen, 1980; Kozarek, 1986; Kumar et al., 2011; Kyzer & Gordon, 1992; Luchtefeld et al., 1989; Marchena et al., 1997). A meta-analysis of 13 randomized controlled trials showed increased stricture rates following stapled anastomosis compared to hand-sewn (MacRae et al., 1998). A previous review of 10 series has reported 6% incidence of strictures with stapled anastomosis (Waxmann et al., 1983). They also noticed a reduced stricture rate with Russian staples, which deliver a single row of staples, compared to the new generation staples, which deliver two rows of staples (Kyzer & Gordon, 1992). In recent series (Kumar et al., 2011), 22.9% developed strictures after stapled anastomosis, which is higher than the 13.3% developed after hand-sewn anastomosis; however, it was not statistically significant.
In our previous study (Shimada et al., 1996), thirty patients with the double stapling coloproctoanastomosis were followed up for six to 24 months in detail and the stricture rate was 30%, suggesting high frequent postoperative complication after coloprostomotic anastomosis by using the double stapling technique. The rectal stricture was defined as the inability to pass a 12.3 mm sigmoidscope (CF-P 20S, OLYMPUS, Tokyo, Japan) through the stenosis. All the patients with stricture had the symptom of frequent bowel movement (Table 1). Among the non-stricture group, temporary frequent defecation was observed in 10 cases (47 %).

Patient No.	Sex	Age	Stage (Dukes)	Resected artery	EEA size (mm)	Distance* (cm)	Cutting** (week)	No. of defecation pre-cut	No. of defecation post-cut	Theraputic success	Repeated cutting	Follow-up (month)
1	F	61	A	SRA	31	4	14	11	3	yes	0	24
2	M	70	B	IMA	31	5	7	12	11	no	0	23
3	F	69	C	IMA	31	4	9	13	4	yes	0	18
4	M	50	B	IMA	31	5	7	14	3	yes	1	15
5	F	53	B	IMA	31	4	6	14	5	yes	0	12
6	F	40	A	SRA	31	4	6	16	4	yes	0	10
7	F	68	B	IMA	31	8	3	12	4	yes	0	10
8	M	73	A	SRA	28	5	14	13	4	yes	1	9
9	M	72	A	SRA	31	6	3	12	5	yes	0	6

* distance from anal verge
** post operative weeks of staple cutting
SRA = superior rectal artery; IMA = inferior messentenic artery; EEA = end-to-end anastomosis staapler.

Table 1. Summary of nine patients with colorectal stricture (Shimada et al., 1996)

It is generally accepted that anastomotic leak results in the high stricture rate, because a leak predispose the patient to intense inflammation and scarring. Regarding risk factors for stricture without postoperative leakage, it has been reported that 103 patients with stapled anastomosis had a 4% stricture rate, and the strictures were more common when a 28 mm diameter stapler was used as compared to one of 31 mm (Miller & Moritz, 1996). In our study (Shimada et al., 1996), however, compared with non-stricture group, there were no significant relationships of sex, age, tumor stage, EEA size, distance of anastomosis from the anal verge, or timing of postoperative diet in the stricture group (Table 2). For one instance of evaluation of blood supply to the anastomosis (Orsay et al., 1995), we compared the incidence of stenosis between devasculization and preservation of the inferior mesenteric artery. However there was no relationship between them.

		stricture (n=9)	non-stricture (n=21)
Sex			
	Male	4	11
	Female	5	10
Age		60.5±11.7	64.0±6.8
Tumor stage			
	Dukes A	4	8
	B	4	6
	C	1	7
Devasculization			
	IMA	5	16
	SRA	4	5
EEA size			
	31 mm	8	20
	28 mm	1	1
Distance from anal verge		4.8±1.3	5.0±0.9
Timing of diet		9.8±2.1	10.8±4.7
Follow up month		15.1±6.0	14.8±5.5

Table 2. Comparison of clinical factors between stricture and non stricture group (Shimada et al., 1996)

3. Development of new device of STENO-CUTTER™ for treatment of the anastomotic stricture

We experienced a case who had been suffering from frequent defecation (more than 10 times a day) for 3 months due to the circular stapling anastomotic stricture after coloproctostomy and was dramatically relieved from the stricture and its symptom after natural loss of the part of the staple ring, and no further recurrence of stricture has been observed. Through this case, we hit on the idea that staple cutting followed by digital dilation might be effective on the anastomotic stenosis caused by a circular stapler. We surmised that the circular stapling anastomoses may have different mechanisms in the formation of stricture from those of handsewn anastomoses. Thus, a new device of "STENO-CUTTER™ (Heiwa Medical Appliance, Yamaguchi, Japan)" was developed to split the circular staple line in the stricture (Shimada et al., 1996). As shown in Fig.1, the staple cutter is so simple and consists of two 5 mm sharp edges and a handle. There are two types of

STENO-CUTTER™ which differ on the total length, i.e., 30.5 cm (STENO-CUTTER-short™) and 30.5 cm (STENO-CUTTER-long™) for treatment of anastomotic stricture due to low and high anterior resection, respectively. The head was made as small as possible to pass the anastomotic stenosis (8 mm wide).

Staple cutting was performed on patients with the stricture of coloproctostomy or colorectostomy with the STENO-CUTTER-short™ or STENO-CUTTER-long™, and dilated digitally or sigmoidscopically, respectively, at the bedside mainly at the outpatient clinic. Using an anoscope (20 mm in diameter, 90 mm in length) (Fig. 1A) or rectoscope (20 mm in diameter, 190 mm in length) (Fig. 1B) with electric light, two feasible sites (usually opposite sites) of the stricture were cut with the staple cutter under direct vision, as shown in Fig. 2.

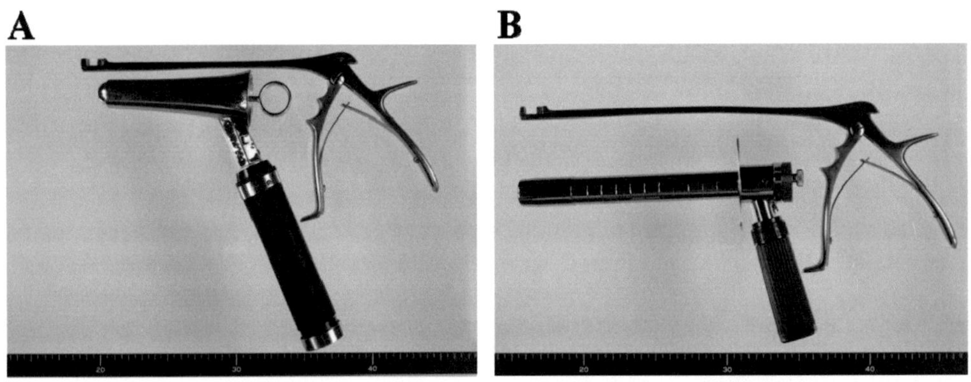

Fig. 1. A new device of "STENO-CUTTER™" (the top of Fig.s) was developed for the treatment of colorectal stenoses after the circular stapling anastomoses by us. The cutter is so simple and consists of two 5 mm sharp edges and a handle. There are two types of STENO-CUTTER™ which differ on the total length, i.e., 26.5 cm (STENO-CUTTER-short™) (A) and 30.5 cm (STENO-CUTTER-long™) (B) for treatment of anastomotic stricture due to low and high anterior resection, assisted by the conventional anoscope (A) and rectoscope (B), respectively. The head was made as small as possible to pass the anastomotic stenosis (8 mm wide).

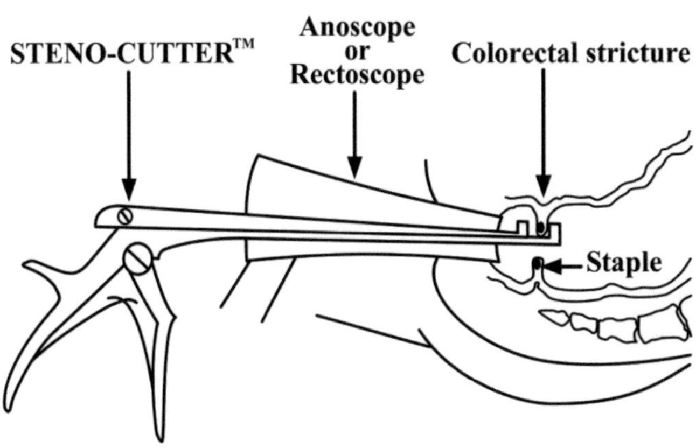

Fig. 2. Presentation of a staple cutting technique by STENO-CUTTER™. The two sites of a colorectal stricture are cut using the assisted by a conventional anoscope or rectoscope.

Successively, complete staple cutting was examined and dilation was performed digitally or sigmoidscopically. The complete staple cutting made dilatation of the stricture digitally or sigmoidscopically very easy. After the treatment of staple cutting and digital or sigmoidscopical dilation, the stricture less than 12.3 mm in diameter expanded more than 20 mm compared with the diameter of an anoscope or sigmoidscopy (Fig. 3). No perforation nor significant bleeding during and/or after the treatment was observed. The first trial was done at 100 post-operative days for fear of causing perforation. However, as each subsequent treatment with staple cutting proved so successful, the post-operative treatment period become more shortened, with the shortest one being done at 23 post-operative days.

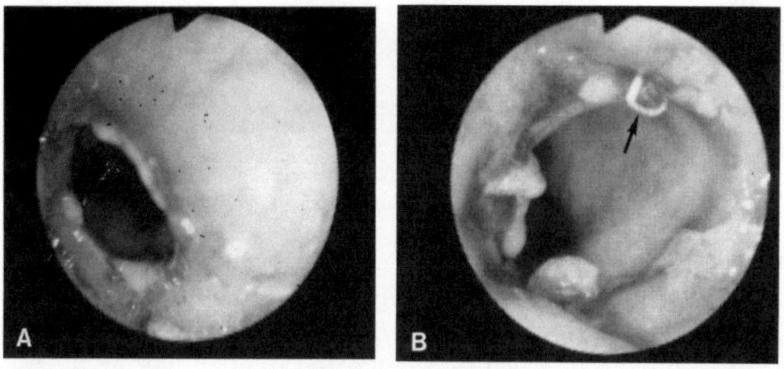

Fig. 3. Endoscopic evaluation of the effect of staple cutting before (A) and after (B) cutting (Shimada et al., 1996). Just two staple cuttings enabled us to dilate easily the stricture to more than 20 mm in diameter compared with anoscope or rectoscope width. The exposed staple (arrow) indicates complete cutting of the staple line.

4. Clinical effects and advantages of the STENO-CUTTER™

Thirty patients with adenocarcinoma of the rectum underwent low anterior resection and low colorectal anastomosis by a double stapling technique using TLH-60 (Johnson & Johnson Co., Ethicon, Cincinnati, OH) and PCEEA (United States Surgical Corporation, Norwalk, CT), and were followed up at least twice a month for more than five years (Shimada et al., 1996). We had no clinically evident anastomotic leaks and no intra-abdominal abscess. There were no significant complications related to surgical techniques. The patients were divided into two groups, stricture and non-stricture group. The rectal stricture was defined as the inability to pass a 12.3 mm sigmoidscope through the stenosis.

Nine out of 30 patients (30 %) had anastomotic stricture with the symptom of distressing frequent bowel movement (Table 1). There was no significant relationship between the clinical factors and the stricture when compared with those of non-stricture patients. Excellent dilation was performed in all of the 9 strictures using the STENO-CUTTER-short™ and the symptom of stricture disappeared dramatically in eight cases (89 %) within one week (Fig. 4). The recurrence of stricture occurred in 2 patients, however it has not been observed after one further use of this treatment. The treatment using STENO-CUTTER-short™ is safe and easy to use even at the bedside, and except for a conventional anoscope or recttoscope no special equipment including fluoroscope was needed.

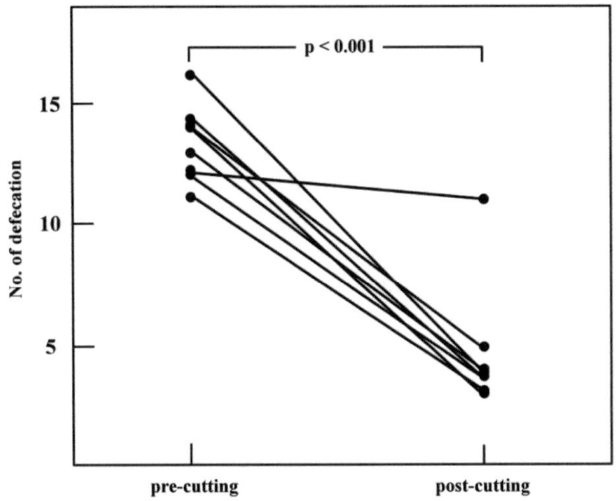

Fig. 4. Clinical effect of the staple cutting (Shimada et al., 1996). The symptom of frequent defecation decreased significantly after the treatment ($p < 0.001$).

In addition, five cases of anastomotic stricture after high anterior resection reconstructed by double stapling technique were treated using STENO-CUTTER-long™ combined with conventional rectoscope (Fig. 1B). Excellent dilation was also performed in all of the 5 strictures and the symptom of stricture disappeared dramatically in all cases within one week. The recurrence of stricture did not occur in all patients. The treatment using STENO-CUTTER-long™ is also safe to use.

5. Application of STENO-CUTTER™ for the treatment of intractable stricture caused by anastomotic leakage

Leakage of colo-rectal anastomosis after low anterior resection reconstructed by a double stapling technique is a relatively rare complication. The incidence of the leakage when using this technique has been reported as from 1.0% to 12.5% (Averbach et al., 1996; Boccola et al., 2010; DuBrow et al., 1995; Griffen et al., 1990; Kumar et al., 2011; Laxamana et al., 1995; Schlegel et al., 2001; Vignali et al., 1997). Once, however, it occurs, granulation tissue followed by firm fibrosis surrounding the anastomosis contributes the formation of severe and long narrowing of the anastomosis. Accordingly, this type of stricture is usually resistant to conventional treatment, resulted in surgical reoperation or the need for permanent stoma (Bailey et al., 2003; Köhler et al., 2000; Ohman & Svenberg, 1983). Recent advances in fluoroscopic and endoscopic modalities enable us to perform an effective, relatively safe, and less invasive treatment such as fluoroscopically guided bougienage, balloon dilation or endoscopic modalities for these patients who experience acute, recurrent, or chronic stricture of the alimentary tract (Garcea et al., 2003; Johansson, 1996; Kozarek, 1986; Lange & Shaffer, 1991; Oz & Forde, 1990; Werre et al., 2000). Good clinical results have been obtained in the simple gastrointestinal anastomotic strictures. These techniques, however, are less helpful for patients with long irregular stricture associated with anastomotic disruption or ischemic injury (Garcea et al., 2003). It is reported that up to 28% of patients have a severe stenosis that can not be cured with these current dilators and require surgical correction with laparotomy (Schlegel et al., 2001).

STENO-CUTTER-short™ was applied in order to evaluate the clinical effects for the treatment of severe rectal stricture associated with anastomotic leakage (Shimada et al., 2007). The details of the cutting procedure using the staple cutter for patients with short strictures have been described as above. Generally, the stricture cutting was performed on patients in lateral position without anesthesia at the bedside mainly at the outpatient clinic. However, in patients with highly severe strictures, before the procedure, intravenous sedation was accomplished with 15 mg of pentazocine and 10 mg of diazepam, and fluoroscopically guided balloon dilatation of an anastomosis with stricture is needed to pass the head of cutter (Fig. 5). Using a conventional anoscope with electric light, the three cuts were made in the right, left and posterior sites of the stricture with the under direct vision, which were considered safer than the anterior part to avoid perforation. Successively, cutting was examined with an endoscope and further dilation was performed digitally (Fig. 6A & 6B).

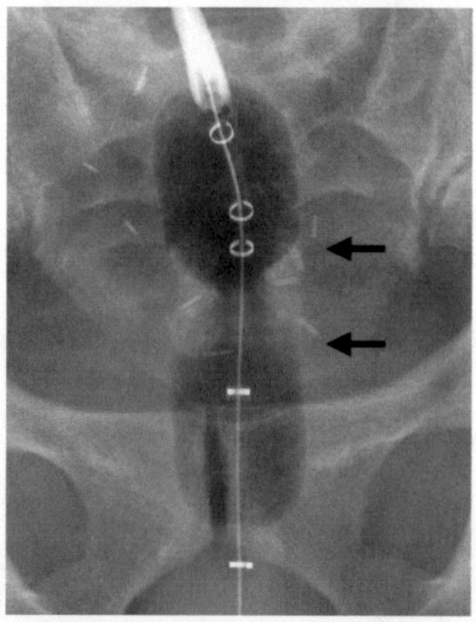

Fig. 5. Fluoroscopic view of the balloon dilation for a stricture associated with leakage (Shimada et al., 2007). The length of the stricture was measured by the length of waist of inflated balloon (arrows). This suggests that balloon dilation is ineffective for strictures caused by anastomotic leakage.

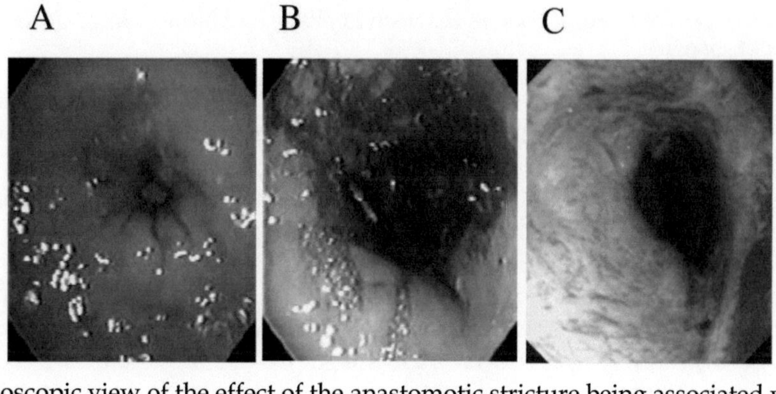

Fig. 6. Endoscopic view of the effect of the anastomotic stricture being associated with leakage by treatment with the STENO-CUTTER™ before (A), just after the surgery (B), and 5 years after treatment (C) (Shimada et al., 2007).

Incidence of leakage after double stapling technique is eleven out of 371 patients (3.0%) (Table 3). Compared with non-leakage group, there were no significant relationships of sex, age, tumor stage, stapler size, or distance of anastomosis from the anal verge in the leakage group. However, the incidence of the subsequent stricture formation in the leakage group (54.5%) was significantly higher than that in the non-leakage group (6.7%) (P < 0.0001) (Table 3). Six out of eleven with leakage had anastomotic stricture with the distressing symptoms of frequent bowel movements and ileus. From the operative records in the stricture cases associated with leaks, it was assumed that the tension at anastomoses caused by absence of mobilization of the splenic flexure of the colon (patients 1, 4 and 5), and contamination of colonic discharge to the anastomosis (patient 2) may affected to the causes of leakage, leading to subsequent severe strictures. A notable feature in the strictures associated with leaks was the progressive narrowing of the anastomoses. Three out of 6 patients (50%) formed almost complete stricture, resulted in the symptom of ileus. All the remaining patients without ileus had the symptom of frequent bowel movements.

	Leakage group	Non-leakage group	*P* value
No. of patients (%)	11 (3)	360 (97)	
Sex			0.903
Male	6	203	
Female	5	157	
Age	62.5±11.9	65.0±7.8	0.475
Tumor stage			0.196
Dukes A	3	138	
B	6	112	
C	2	110	
Devasculization			0.475
IMA	5	126	
SRA	6	234	
EEA size			0.845
33 mm	2	81	
31 mm	8	277	
28 mm	1	2	
Doughnuts			1.000
Complete	11	360	
Incomplete	0	0	
Distance from anal verge	4.9±1.1	5.1±0.8	0.807
Stricture (%)	6/11 (54.5)	24/360 (6.7)	< 0.0001
Follow up month	40.1±17.0	39.8±15.5	0.274

Table 3. Comparison of Clinical Factors between Leakage and Non-leakage Groups (Shimada et al., 2007)

Effects of stricture cutting in the six patients with colorectal stricture associated with leakage were summarized in Table 4. All the six patients had previous treatments: fluoroscopic balloon dilation for cases 1, 2, 4 and 6; esophageal bougie dilation for cases 3 and 5. But, those were little effective in spite of multiple trials. The time of initial treatment by the technique of STENO-CUTTER-short™ ranged from three to seven months (mean ± SD = 5.0 ± 1.4 months) after the multiple conventional dilations. The colorectal strictures thickened with circumferential firm scar formation were observed in all six patients. Furthermore, different from simple strictures without leakage, the strictures formed quite long narrow segments, and the mean length was 1.7 ± 0.4 cm. All the stenoses were biopsied and local recurrences were ruled out. Before the cutting procedure, in such patients with highly severe stricture as patients 1, 2 and 4, fluoroscopically guided balloon dilatation of the anastomosis was needed to pass the head of cutter (Fig. 5). Unlike patients with short strictures without leaks, multiple cuttings were needed for the each site, because the stricture was consisted of a firm fibrosis and formed a long narrow segment as described above. In all six patients, this procedure enabled us to obtain sufficient dilation more than 20 mm in diameter compared with the diameter of the anoscope. In the patients 3 and 5, a single stricture cutting and digital dilation treatment succeeded in significantly decreasing the number of bowel movements within 48 hours, and the occurrence of re-stricture has not been observed. In the patients of 1, 2, 4 and 6, the re-stricture and the symptoms occurred after approximately four weeks from first cutting, although the first treatments were effective in these cases. The patient of 1, 2, 4 and 6 necessitated three, two, two and one more cuttings and digital dilation, respectively. However, the recurrence of stricture has not been occurred in any case in the long follow-up ranged from 17 to 61 months (mean ± SD = 40 ± 17 months). Endoscopic view of Fig. 6C showed lysis of a severe stricture 5 year after the last stenosis cutting for one instance (patient 1). Complications such as perforation and/or significant bleeding were not observed in any case.

Patient No.	Sex	Age	Stage (Dukes)	Resected artery	Stapler size (mm)	Distance* (cm)	Local factor	Previous treatment	Stenosis cutting† (month)	Stenosis length (cm)	No. of defecation Pre-cut	No. of defecation Post-cut	Theraputic success	Repeated cutting	Follow-up month‡
1	F	61	B	IMA	33	6	Tension	Balloon	5	2.4	0 (Ileus)	5	Yes	3	61
2	M	70	B	IMA	33	5	Infection	Balloon	6	2.0	0 (Ileus)	4	Yes	2	55
3	F	69	A	SRA	31	4	None	Bougie	9	1.4	16	4	Yes	0	48
4	M	50	C	IMA	31	5	Tension	Balloon	7	1.8	0 (Ileus)	3	Yes	2	36
5	M	75	B	IMA	31	4	Tension	Bougie	4	1.2	14	5	Yes	0	24
6	F	58	A	SRA	31	4	None	Balloon	6	1.5	16	4	Yes	1	17
Mean±SD		64±9			32±1.0	4.7±0.8			6.2±1.7	1.7±0.4		4.2±0.8		1.3±1.2	40±17

*Distance from anal verge, †Post operative months of stenosis cutting, ‡After the last stenosis cutting
SD = the standard deviation
SRA = superior rectal artery; IMA = inferior messentenic artery; EEA = end-to-end anastomosis staapler.

Table 4. Summary of Six Patients with Colorectal Stricture Associated with Leak

Anastomotic distance from anal verge, pelvic infection, duration of surgery, incomplete doughnuts, and extent of proximal colon resection have been proposed as the factors that may contribute to leakage after a double stapling technique (Averbach et al., 1996; Giffen et al., 1990; Laxamana et al., 1995; Vignali et al., 1997). Our comparison of clinical factors between leakage and non-leakage group could not point out definite factors, with the exception that the leakage was clearly related to the formation of subsequent anastomotic stricture compared with the non-leak group ($P < 0.0001$) (Shimada et al., 2007). It has been emphasized that the leak rate increased progressively with the extent of proximal colon resection (Averbach et al., 1996). Other authors (Giffen et al., 1990; Laxamana et al., 1995; Vignali et al., 1997) also considered that lower rectal anastomosis appeared to increase the clinical leak rate. Our three of six cases (50%) with leakage followed by stricture had tension at the anastomosis caused by the large extent of proximal colon resection. It is generally accepted that a stapled anastomosis is restored by the scar formation according to the secondary wound healing mechanism, whereas a hand-sewn double layer anastomosis is repaired by the primary wound healing mechanism (Buchmann et al., 1983; Graffner et al., 1984; Jansen, 1981). That is, the stapled anastomosis necessitates indirect bridging of the submucosal layer defect by smaller and longer strands of newly synthesized collagen tissue in the outer intestinal layers with a collateral circulation from the submucosal plexus to the arterial plexuses in these layers (Jansen et al., 1981). Therefore, tension at the anastomosis is probably one of the major factors of leakage after the double stapling technique. Because local blood flow of colonic anastomosis is strongly influenced by the tension at the anastomosis. Further, it has been described that the sensitivity of the local microcirculation systems to tension is higher in the colorectum than in the small intestine (Shikata & Shida, 1986). Tension free anastomosis is highly recommended to the low anterior resection (Shimada et al., 2007).

Most of the anastmotic strictures are short narrowings less than 1 cm that can be successfully treated by an esophageal bougie or a balloon dilator (Johansson, 1996; Kozarek, 1986; Lange & Shaffer, 1991; Oz & Forde, 1990; Schlegel et al., 2001; Werre et al., 2000). In our study, all stenoses were irregular, kinked, fixed, and long (mean ± SD = 1.7 ± 0.4 cm). The treatment of stricture caused by disruption and/or ischemic injury is very difficult, since the stricture is usually severe and has a long narrow segment with firm fibrosis (Shimada et al., 2007). Such a stricture may have accelerated effects on the formation of re-stricture, that is, the stricture with hard fibrosis may return to the same condition as was before dilation. Esophageal or balloon dilators can temporary dilate the broad narrow segment caused by the thickened circumferential scar formation but hardly split the hard fibrosis, resulting in reverting to the shape before dilation followed by a re-stricture. These may explain why the current conventional dilations had failed. It has been reported that 27 patients with severe colorectal stenoses resistant to dilation or endoscopic modalities have been treated with surgical resection of strictures followed by reconstruction of new colorectal anastomoses for upper rectal strictures or Soave's procedure for middle or lower rectal strictures (Schlegel et al., 2001). In all cases, intestinal continuity has been restored and the surgical operation has offered satisfactory long-term functional results. If, however, there is a non-surgical technique which is effective, it will be greatly beneficial to patients with severe colorectal strictures as well as to surgeons who want to relieve the quite distressing symptom of his patients. Thus, a device of STENO-CUTTER-short™ was applied to split the stricture formed by the hard fibrosis. This treatment is considered to be a promising option, when current fluoroscopic and endoscopic modalities such as esophageal and balloon dilators failed to relieve the stricture.

6. Application of STENO-CUTTER™ for the treatment of intractable stricture caused by ischemic injury

The resected cervical esophagus is commonly reconstructed by the cervical transposition of a jejunal segment with vascular anastomosis (Chen & Tang, 2000; Fisher et al., 1985; Kasai & Nishihira, 1986; Urayama et al., 1997). However, a major complication of this procedure is disruption and/or ischemic injury of the pharyngo-jejunal anastomosis or the transpositioned jejunal segment, leading to severe stricture, which requires surgical treatment (Fisher et al., 1985; Golshani et al., 1999; Mansour et al., 1997). Because this type of stricture is usually severe and has long narrow segment, it is intractable to dilatation and recurrence is common. Although the STENO-CUTTER™ was initially developed to split a circular stapler line in a colorectal stricture, we considered that the device and technique could be used to cut the severe fibrosis in strictures of pharyngo-jejunal anastomosis after ischemic injury as well as disruption (Shimada et al. 2002).

A 56-year-old Japanese female with cervical esophageal cancer underwent surgery to remove the cervical esophagus after chemo-radiation therapy (chemotherapy: 500 mg/body of 5-fluorouracil and 10 mg/body of cisplatin for 3 weeks; radiation: total of 40 Gy). Reconstruction was done using a jejunal segment with vascular anastomosis. The pharyngo-jejunal anastomosis was performed end-to-side with Albert-Lembert interrupted sutures. Pathological examination revealed that the histological type of the tumor was moderately differentiated adenocarcinoma and that it involved the larynx and thyroid, but there was no lymph node metastasis. Her postoperative course was uneventful and the anastomosis appeared healing well. She was discharged on postoperative day (POD) 27. The patient, however, was readmitted 4 years later with severe dysphagia. An upper gastrointestinal series and endoscopic examination showed a severe stricture in the upper transpositioned jejunal segmant (Fig. 7A and Fig. 9A). Angiography of the cervical arteries suggested ischemic change in the upper part of the transpositioned jejunal segment. Although fluoroscopically guided bougie dilation using a 15-mm bougie was performed twice within 10 days of admission, a radiograph showed minimal improvement of the stricture, and the symptoms of stenosis were unresolved. In the outpatient clinic, multiple bouginages were required for complete dysphagia, every year for the next 3 years, with little improvement each time. Soon after the unsuccessful bouginage, the surgery was performed .

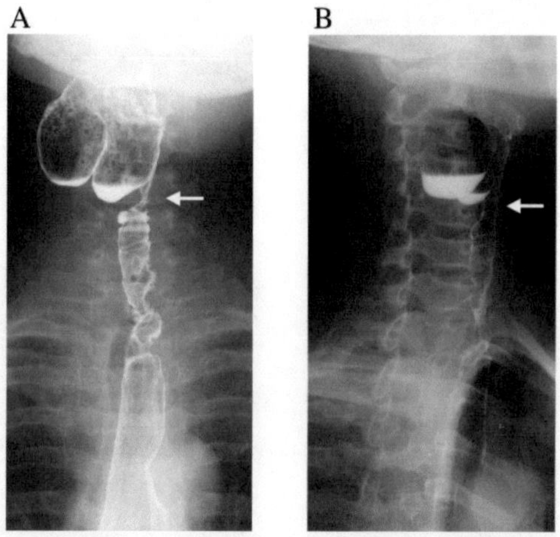

Fig. 7. Upper gastrointestinal series clearly showed the effect of the STENO-CUTTER™ technique, before (A) and after (B) cutting (arrows) (Shimada et al., 2002). This device was initially developed for the treatment of colorectal stenoses after circular stapling anastomoses including the double stapling technique.

With the patient under general anesthesia, we cut the severe stricture in the transpositioned jejunum using a STENO-CUTTER-long™. As shown in Fig. 8A, a conventional rectoscope (19 cm long) was inserted to just in front of the stricture through the patient's mouth, and the stricture was cut by the STENO-CUTTER-long™ under direct vision. The two parts of the stricture were cut so that the severe stenosis was removed (Fig. 8B). The two cuts were made in the right and left anterior sites of the stricture, which were considered safer than the lateral or posterior sites, to avoid injuring the adjacent vessels. The possible complications of the STENO-CUTTER-long™ are bleeding and perforation of the cervical portion, but no substantial bleeding or perforation occurred during or after cutting. After the cutting, a video endoscope (OLYMPUS, GIF-Q200) was inserted to confirm the dilation. The endoscope passed through the anastomosis easily. Histologically, the biopsied specimens showed no malignancy in the stricture. Postoperative recovery was rapid and uneventful, and the patient was discharged without any clinical symptoms. When examined 1 month later, then 6 months later in the outpatient clinic, upper gastrointestinal endoscopy revealed lysis of the stricture in the transpositioned jejunum, and no dysphagia. Complete resolution of the stricture has been maintained without any additional treatment for more than 1 year (Fig. 7B and Fig. 9B).

A B

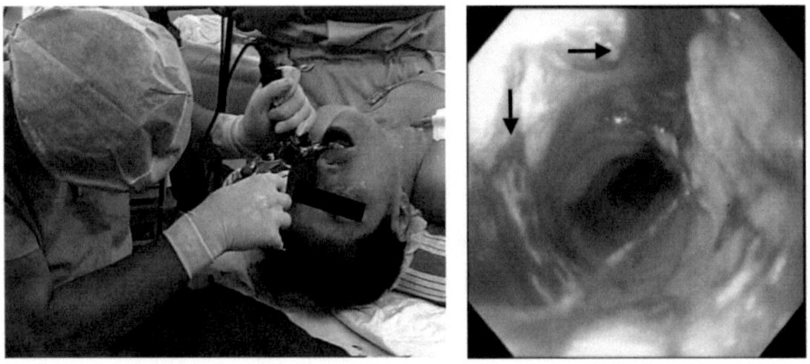

Fig. 8. The technique of cutting with the STENO-CUTTER™ (Shimada et al., 2002). The two sites of the stricture were cut using the cutter assisted by a conventional rectal scope (A). B Endscopic view after cutting (the two arrows indicate the cut sites of stenosis)

A B

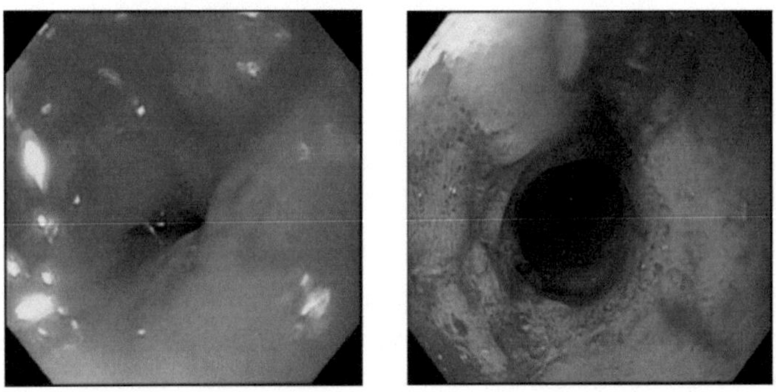

Fig. 9. Endoscopic evaluation of the effect of staple cutting (Shimada et al., 2002). A: before cutting. B: one year after cutting

Severe and recurrent stenosis of a pharyngo-jejunal anastomosis or jejunal segment after reconstruction by transposition of the jejunal segment with a vascular anastomosis is a challenging problem for the surgeon who wants to relieve the patient's distressing symptoms. The treatment of a stricture caused by disruption and/or ischemic injury is very difficult, since it is usually severe and has a long narrow segment with hard fibrosis. This type of stricture may have an accelerated effect on the formation of re-stricture. In other words, a stricture with hard fibrosis may return to the same condition as was before dilation. Esophageal or balloon dilators (Hernandez et al., 2000; Kadakia et al., 1993; Marshall et al., 1996) can temporarily dilate the long narrow segment caused by the thickened circumferential scar formation, but it hardly splits the hard fibrosis. The result is that it reverts to the shape before dilation, followed by a re-stricture. In our patient, repeated esophageal and balloon dilators failed to relieve the symptoms caused by the stricture. A more effective and less invasive therapeutic modality was necessary, and therefore, the STENO-CUTTER™ was used to split the stricture formed by the hard fibrosis.

7. Conclusions

We describe a new method using a STENO-CUTTER™ to successfully treat the patients with colorectal stricture following surgery for rectal cancer. This device is so simple, easy to use under direct vision with the use of a conventional anoscope, and does not need fluoroscope or other special optional equipment. This treatment was generally performed at the bedside even in the outpatient clinic and the significant complications such as bleeding and/or perforation have not been observed. From the excellent efficacy in addition to safe and easy usage, the treatment using the device of STENO-CUTTER™ is highly recommended for the treatment of circular stapling anastomotic stricture of the rectum, even in severe stricture associated with anastomotic leakage or ischemic injury. The positive results achieved in these patients suggest that our new method could represent a promising option of treatment for strictures when conventional modalities fail.

8. References

Averbach, A.M., Chang, D., Koslowe, P. & Sugarbaker, P.H. (1996). Anastomotic leak after double-stapled low colorectal resection. *Diseases of the Colon and Rectum*, Vol.39, No.7, pp. 780-787

Bailey, C.M., Wheeler, J.M., Birks, M. & Farouk, R. (2003). The incidence and causes of permanent stoma after anterior resection. *Colorectal Disease*, Vol.5, No.4, pp. 331-334

Blamey, S.L. & Lee, P.W. (1982). A comparison of circular stapling devices in colorectal anastomoses. *The British Journal of Surgery*, Vol.69, No.1, pp. 19-22

Boccola, M.A., Lin, J., Rozen, W.M. & Ho, Y.H. (2010). Reducing anastomotic leakage in oncologic colorectal surgery: an evidence-based review. *Anticancer Research*, Vol.30, No.2, pp. 601-607

Brennan, S.S., Pickford, I.R., Evans, M. & Pollock, A.V. (1982). Staples or sutures for colonic anastomoses: a controlled clinical trial. *The British Journal of Surgery*, Vol.69, No.12, pp. 722-724

Brower, R.A. & Freeman, L.D. (1984). Balloon catheter dilation of a rectal stricture. *Gastrointestinal Endoscopy*, Vol.30, No.2, pp. 95-97

Buchmann, P., Schneider, K. & Gebbers, J.O. (1983). Fibrosis of experimental colonic anastomosis in dogs after EEA stapling or suturing. *Diseases of the Colon and Rectum*, Vol.26, No.4, pp. 217-220

Cade, D., Gallagher, P., Schofield, P.F. & Turner, L. (1981). Complications of anterior resection of the rectum using the EEA stapling device. *The British Journal of Surgery*, Vol.68, No.5, pp. 339-340

Chen, H.C. & Tang, Y.B. (2000). Microsurgical reconstruction of the esophagus. *Seminars in surgical oncology*, Vol.19, No.3, pp. 235-245

DuBrow, R.A., David, C.L. & Curley, S.A. (1995). Anastomotic leaks after low anterior resection for rectal carcinoma: evaluation with CT and barium enema. *American Journal of Roentgenology*, Vol.165, No.3, pp. 567-571

Dziki, A.J., Duncan, M.D., Harmon, J.W., Saini, N., Malthaner, R.A., Trad, K.S., Fernicola, M.T., Hakki, F. & Ugarte, R.M. (1991). Advantages of handsewn over stapled bowel anastomosis. *Diseases of the Colon and Rectum*, Vol.34, No.6 pp. 442-448

Fain, S.N., Patin, C.S. & Morgenstern, L. (1975). Use of mechanical suturing apparatus in low colorectal anastomosis. *Archives of Surgery*, Vol.110, No.9, pp. 1079-1082

Fisher, S.R., Cole, T.B., Meyers, W.C. & Seigler, H.F. (1985). Pharyngoesophageal reconstruction using free jejunal interposition grafts. *Archves of Otolaryngology*, Vol.111, No.11, pp. 747-752

Garcea, G., Sutton, C.D., Lloyd, T.D., Jameson, J., Scott, A. & Kelly, M.J. (2003). Manegement of Benign Rectal Strictures: a review of present therapeutic procedures. *Diseases of the Colon and Rectum*, Vol.46, No.11, pp. 1451-1460

Golshani, S.D., Lee, C., Cass, D., Thomas, A. & Mandpe, A.H. (1999). Microvascular "supercharged" cervical colon: minimizing ischemia in esophageal reconstruction. *Annals of Plastic Surgery*, Vol.43, No.5, pp. 533-538

Gordon, P.H. & Vasilevsky, C.A. (1984). Experience with stapling in rectal surgery. *The Surgical Clinics of North America*, Vol.64, No.3, pp. 555-566

Graffner, H., Andersson, L., Lowenhielm, P. & Walther, B. (1984). The healing process of anastomoses of the colon. A comparative study using single, double-layer or stapled anastomosis. *Diseases of the colon and rectum*, Vol.27, No.12, pp. 767-771

Griffen, F.D., Knight, C.D. Sr., Whitaker, J.M., Whitaker, J.M. & Knight, C.D. Jr. (1990). The double stapling technique for low anterior resection. Results, modifications, and observations. *Annals of Surgery*, Vol.211, No.6, pp. 745-751

Hernandez, L.J., Jacobson, J.W. & Harris, M.S. (2000). Comparison among the perforation rates of Maloney, balloon, and savary dilation of esophageal strictures. *Gastrointestinal Endoscopy*, Vol.51, pp. 460-462

Jansen, A., Becker, A.E., Brummelkamp, W.H., Keeman, J.N. & Klopper, P.J. (1981). The importance of the apposition of the submucosal intestinal layers for primary wound healing of intestinal anastomosis. *Surgery, Gynecology & Obstetrics*, Vol.152, No.1, pp. 51-58

Johansson, C. (1996). Endoscopic dilation of rectal strictures: a prospective study of 18 cases. *Diseases of the Colon and Rectum*, Vol.39, No.4, pp. 423-428

Kadakia, S.C., Parker, A., Carrougher, J.G. & Shaffer, R.T. (1993). Esophageal dilation with polyvinyl bougies, using a marked guidewire without the aid of fluoroscopy: an update. *The American Journal of Gastroenterology*, Vol.88, No.9, pp. 1381-1386

Kasai, M. & Nishihira, T. (1986). Reconstruction using pedicled jejunal segments after resection for carcinoma of the cervical esophagus. Surgery, *Gynecology & Obstetrics*, Vol.163, No.2, pp. 145-152

Knight, C.D. & Griffen, F.D. (1980). An improved technique for the low anterior resection using the EEA stapler. *Surgery*, Vol.88, No.5, pp. 710-714

Köhler, A., Athanasiadis, S., Ommer, A. & Psarakis, E. (2000). Long-term results of low anterior resection with intersphincteric anastomosis in carcinoma of the lower one-third of the rectum: analysis of 31 patients. *Diseases of the Colon and Rectum*, Vol.43, No.6, pp. 843-850

Kozarek, R.A. (1986). Hydrostatic balloon dilation of gastrointestinal stenoses: a national survey. *Gastrointesttinal Endoscopy*, Vol.32, No.1, pp. 15-19

Kumar, A., Daga, R., Vijayaragavan, P., Prakash, A., Singh, R.K., Behari, A., Kapoor, V.K. & Saxena, R. (2011). Anterior resection for rectal carcinoma - risk factors for anastomotic leaks and strictures. *World Journal of Gastroenterology*, Vol.17, No.11, pp. 1475-1479

Kyzer, S. & Gordon, P.H. (1992). Experience with the use of the circular stapler in rectal surgery. *Diseases of the Colon and Rectum*, Vol.35, No.7, pp. 696-706

Lange, E.E. & Shaffer, H.A. Jr. (1991). Rectal strictures: treatment with fluoroscopically guided balloon dilation. *Radiology*, Vol.178, No.2, pp. 475-479

Laxamana, A., Solomon, M.J., Cohen, Z., Feinberg, S.M., Stern, H.S. & McLeod, R.S. (1995). Long-term results of anterior resection using the double-stapling technique. *Diseases of the Colon and Rectum*, Vol.38, No.12, pp. 1246-1250

Leff, E.I., Hoexter, B., Labow, S.B., Eisenstat, T.E., Rubin, R.J., Salvati, E.P. (1982). The EEA stapler in low colorectal anastomoses: initial experience. *Disesases of the Colon and Rectum*, Vol.25, No.7, pp. 704-707

Luchtefeld, M.A., Milsom, J.W., Senagore, A., Surrell, J.A. & Mazier, W.P. (1989). Colorectal anastomotic stenosis. Results of a survey of the ASCRS membership. *Diseases of the Colon and Rectum*, Vol.32, No.9, pp. 733-736

MacRae, H.M. & McLeod, R.S. (1998). Handsewn vs. stapled anastomoses in colon and rectal surgery: a meta-analysis. *Diseases of the Colon and Rectum*, Vol.41, No.2, pp. 180-189

Mansour, K.A., Bryan, F.C. & Carlson, G.W. (1997). Bowel interposition for esophageal replacement: twenty-five-year experience. *The Annals of Thoracic Surgery*, Vol.64, No.3, pp. 752-756

Marchena, G.J., Ruiz, C.E., Gomez, G.G., Vallejo, G.I., Garcia-Anguiano, F., Hernandez, R. J.M. (1997). Anastomotic stricture with the EEA-Stapler after colorectal anastomosis. *Revista Espanola de Enfermedades*, Vol.89, No.11, pp. 835-842

Marshall, J.B., Afridi, S.A., King, P.D., Barthel, J.S. & Butt, J.H. (1996). Esophageal dilation with polyvinyl (American) dilators over a marked guidewire: practice and safety at one center over a 5-yr period. *The American Journal of Gastroenterology*, Vol.91, No.8, pp. 1503-1506

Miller, K. & Moritz E. (1996). Circular stapling techniques for low anterior resection of rectal carcinoma. *Hepato-gastroenterology*, Vol.43, No.10, pp. 823-831

Moran, B.J., Blenkinsop, J. & Finnis, D. (1992). Local recurrence after anterior resection for rectal cancer using a double stapling technique. *The British Journal of Surgery*, Vol.79, No.8, pp. 836-838

Ohman, U. & Svenberg, T. (1983). EEA stapler for mid-rectum carcinoma. Review of recent literature and own initial experience. *Diseases of the Colon and Rectum*, Vol.26, No.12, pp. 775-784

Orsay, C.P., Bass, E.M., Firfer, B., Ramakrishnan, V. & Abcarian, H. (1995). Blood flow in colon anastomotic stricture formation. *Diseases of the Colon and Rectum*, Vol.38, No.2, pp. 202-206

Oz, M.C. & Forde, K.A. (1990). Endoscopic alternatives in the management of colonic strictures. *Surgery*, Vol.108, No.3, pp. 513-519

Polglase, A.L., Hughes, E.S., McDermott, F.T., Pihl, E. & Burke, F.R. (1981). A comparison of end-to-end staple and suture colorectal anastomosis in the do. *Surgery, Gynecolpgy & Obstetrics*, Vol.152, No.6, pp. 792-796

Ravitch, M.M. & Steinchen, F.M. (1979). A stapling instrument for end-to-end inverting anastomoses in the gastrointestinal tract. *Annals of Surgery*, Vol.189, No.6, pp. 791-797

Sato, H., Maeda, K., Hanai, T. & Aoyama, H. (2007). Colorectal anastomosis using a novel double-stapling technique for lower rectal carcinoma. *International Journal of Colorectal Disease*, Vol.22, No.10, pp. 1249-1253

Schlegel, R.D., Dehni, N., Parc, R., Caplin, S. & Tiret, E. (2001). Results of reoperations in colorectal anastomotic strictures. *Diseases of the Colon and Rectum*, Vol.44, No.10, pp. 1464-1468

Shikata, J. & Shida, T. (1986). Effects of tension on local blood flow in experimental intestinal anastomoses. *The Journal of Surgical Research*, Vol.40, No.2, pp. 105-111

Shimada, S., Matsuda, M., Uno, K., Matsuzaki, H., Murakami, S. & Ogawa, M. (1996). A new device for the treatment of coloproctostomic stricture after double stapling anastomoses. *Annals of Surgery*, Vol.224, No.5, pp. 603-608

Shimada, S., Honmyo, U., Hayashi, N., Matsuda, M. & Ogawa, M. (2002). Successful new treatment for intractable cervical esophageal stenosis of a jejunal segment transpositioned with a vascular anastomosis: report of a case. *Surgery Today*, Vol.32, No.11, pp. 996-999

Shimada, S., Yagi, Y., Yamamoto, K., Matsuda, M. & Baba, H. (2007). Novel treatment of intractable rectal strictures associated with anastomotic leakage using a stenosis-cutting device. *International Surgery*, Vol.92, No.2, pp. 82-88

Shirikhande, S.V., Saoji, R.R., Barreto, S.G., Kakade, A.C., Waterford, S.D., Ahire, S.B., Golowale, F.M. & Shukla, P.J. (2007). Outcomes of resection for rectal cancer in India: the impact of the double stapling technique. *World Journal of Surgical Oncology*, Vol.21, No.5, pp. 35

Smith, L.E. (1981). Anastomosis with EEA stapler after anterior colonic resection. *Diseases of the Colon and Rectum*, Vol.24, No.4, pp. 236-242

Thrsen, G. & Rosseland, A.R. (1983). Endoscopic incision of postoperative stenoses in the upper gastrointestinal tract. *Gastrointestinal Endoscopy*, Vol.29, No.1, pp. 26-29

Urayama, H., Ohtake, H., Ohmura, K. & Watanabe, Y. (1997). Pharyngoesophageal reconstruction with the use of vascular anastomoses: operative modifications and long-term prognosis. *The Journal of Thoracic and Cardiovascular Surgery*, Vol.113, No.6, pp. 975-981

Verma, J.S., Chan, A.C., Li, M.K. & Li, A.K. (1990). Low anterior resection of the rectum using a double stapling technique. *The British Journal of Surgery*, Vol.77, No.8, pp. 888-890

Vezeridis, M., Evans, J.T., Mittelman, A. & Ledesma, E.J. (1982). EEA stapler in low anterior anastomosis. *Diseases of the Colon and Rectum*, Vol.25, No.4, pp. 364-367

Vignali, A., Fazio, V.W., Lavery, I.C., Milsom, J.W., Church, J.M., Hull, T.L., Strong, S.A. & Oakley, J.R. (1997). Factors associated with the occurrence of leaks in stapled rectal anastomoses: a review of 1,014 patients. *Jounal of the American College of Surgeons*, Vol.185, No.2, pp. 105-113

Waxman, B.P. (1983). Large bowel anastomoses. II. The circular staplers. *The British Journal of Surgery*, Vol.70, No.2, pp. 64-67

Werre, A., Mulder, C., van Heteren, C. & Bilgen, E.S. (2000). Dilation of benign strictures following low anterior resection using Savary-Gilliard bougies. *Endoscopy*, Vol.32, No.5, pp. 385-388

Whitworth, P.W., Richardson, R.L. & Larson, G.M. (1988). Balloon dilation of anastomotic strictures. *Archives of Surgery*, Vol.123, No.6, pp. 759-762

12

Postoperative Ileus: Pathophysiology and Treatment

N.S. Tropskaya and T.S. Popova
The Sklifosovsky Research Institute for Emergency Medicine, Moscow, Russia

1. Introduction

Postoperative ileus (POI) is a temporary impairment of gastrointestinal (GI) motility occurring universally after major abdominal surgery (Holte & Kehlet, 2002).

For the majority of affected surgical patients, POI is transient, lasting approximately 3 to 5 days (Hotokezaka, et al., 1997). The adverse effects of POI are composed of not only physiologic effects such as reduced bowel function, exacerbation of nausea and vomiting, and increased postoperative pain, but also other clinically related effects such as delay of oral feeding, prolonged hospitalization, and increased use of human and material resources.

Determination of the end of POI is somewhat controversial. The studies in the literature have used varying end points, and each has its own weakness. Bowel sounds are sometimes used as an end point, but they require frequent auscultation, their presence does not necessarily indicate propulsive activity, and they can be the result of small-bowel activity and not colonic function (Holte & Kehlet, 2000). Flatus also is not the ideal end point. It requires a conscious patient who is comfortable reporting its occurrence to the investigator. Also, there is some question as to the correlation between flatus and bowel movements (Waldhausen, et al., 1990). Bowel movements are seemingly the most reliable end point.

The migrating myoelectric complex (MMC) is the basal level of activity in the bowel in the fasting state, serving a "housekeeping" function (Szurszewksi, 1969). The resumption of this myoelectric complex after surgery is responsible for recovery from POI.

In humans the MMC can be recognized from the lower oesophagus to the distal small intestine, but it is most prominent in proximal jejunum. This enteric rhythm usually exhibits three phases: Phase I when only slow waves are observed without spike bursts (without actual muscle contractions); phase II when spike bursts are observed on slow waves irregularly (the occurrence of intermittent muscle contractions); and phase III with spike bursts on every slow wave for a few minutes (the contractions with the maximal contractile frequency). Rats are particularly suited for studying the MMC as the cycling period is only about 15 min in the conventional state.

Motility of the GI tract is temporarily impaired after surgery and is characterized by disorganized electrical activity and lack of coordinated propulsion (Behm & Stollman, 2003). In the stomach, studies have consistently demonstrated a postoperative period of gastric hypomotility associated with irregular and disorganized electrical activity (Clevers et al., 1991). Gastric propulsion may be orad, and there may also be increased pyloric tone that contributes to abnormal gastric emptying (Dauchel et al., 1976). Motor activity is similarly disorganized in the small bowel. Morris et al. (1983) observed the disappearance of phase III contractions 2 days after the operation. Miedema et al. (2002) also detected retrograde contractions, leading to significant delays in small bowel transit. Normal colonic motility is typically the last to return after surgery. Studies evaluating postoperative colonic motility frequently have found a period of relative hypomotility that is generally associated with random, disorganized bursts of electrical activity (Wilson, 1975; Condon et al., 1986).

The type of surgical procedure performed can have significant effects on postoperative GI motility. Skin incision has no effect on the MMC activity of the bowel, whereas opening the peritoneum will completely inhibit the MMC (Livingston & Passaro, 1990).

Some controversies exist over the timing of the MMC return after abdominal surgery. Benson et al. (1994) have shown that MMCs are present in the small bowel within a few hours after surgery. On the contrary, others investigators found that MMCs were abolished for 1 or 2 days after surgery, taking from 3 to 7 days for normal pattern to reestablish (Smith et al., 1977; Morris et al., 1983; Schippers et al., 1991).

Several mechanisms are thought to play a role in POI, including sympathetic neural reflexes, local and systemic inflammatory mediators, and changes in various neural and hormonal transmitters. An imbalance between sympathetic and parasympathetic nervous-system input to the intestine has been postulated as an underlying cause. Sympathetic (adrenergic) hyperactivity results in reduction of propulsive motility, and an increase in sphincter tone. Parasympathetic (cholinergic) hypoactivity results in a decrease in gastrointestinal motility. There is finding supported the involvement nitrergic neurons in the pathogenesis of POI.

Many potential etiologic agents have been investigated to determine a cause for the development of POI. Pharmacological modulation aimed at increasing excitatory activity has principally involved the administration of para-sympathomimetic agents which increase cholinergic transmission, such as bethanecol or neostigmine (Gerring & Hunt, 1986). Similarly, cisapride works as an indirect parasympathomimetic by stimulating serotonin receptors and so enhancing acetylcholine release (Reynolds & Putman, 1992; Wiseman & Faulds, 1994). Attempts to block inhibitory components of contractility have focused on the sympathetic system. Sympathetic hyperactivity should respond to β-adrenergic blocker such as propranolol. Metaclopramide, which among other activities has antidopaminegic properties and domperidone (selective peripheral dopamine (DA_2 receptor) antagonist) have also been used to intervene in ileus cases (Reynolds & Putman, 1992). Investigations evaluating inhibitors of nitric oxide synthesis, have shown improved postoperative bowel motility in animal studies. Local anaesthetics has been most effective in the prevention of POI. Trimebutine maleate helped in improving the postoperative conditions of patients as their abdominal and colonic discomfort, abdominal pain and nausea decreased.

Although some of the mechanisms underlying the abnormal intestinal motility found after surgery have been elucidated, an integrated understanding of the pathophysiology of POI remains elusive.

2. Experimental study of postoperative ileus

We investigated the possible role of cholinergic, adrenergic, dopaminergic, serotonergic, nitrergic mechanisms, and also local anaesthetics in POI.

Objective: To investigate altered gastrointestinal motility in POI and effects of potential etiological agents on the GI electrical activity to determine a cause for the development of

POI and treatment. We were solving the following questions: 1) Whether the administration of different pharmacological agents stimulate the MMC or its separate phases; 2) Which pharmacological agents will induce early recovery of the MMC from POI?

2.1 Materials and methods

2.1.1 Experimental animals and grouping

Fifty four male Wistar rats weighing 300-350 g were used. Animals were divided into nine groups.

Control group (n = 6) which included the rats with implanted three bipolar electrodes and an infusion cannula in that the electrical activity was measured on the 10th day post surgery (after recovery).

LAP group (n = 6) in which an exploratoty laparotomy, implantation of three bipolar electrodes and an infusion cannula were considered as trauma and the study measurements were conducted on the 1st - 6th days postoperative.

Other seven LAP groups in which an exploratoty laparotomy, implantation of three bipolar electrodes and an infusion cannula were considered as trauma and the study measurements were conducted on the 1st - 6th days postoperative. These rats received from the 1st trough 3rd postoperative days neostigmine 0,2 mg/kg (n = 6), or propranolol 0,15 mg/kg (n = 6), or metaclopramide 0,5 mg/kg (n = 6), or cisapride 0,2 mg/kg (n = 6), or domperidone 0,5 mg/kg (n = 6), or L-NAME 0,1 mg/kg (n = 6), or trimebutine 2,86 mg/kg (n = 6).

2.1.2 Laparotomy

The rats were anesthetized with 5% ketamine solution i.p. in the dose of 0.3 ml/100 g body weight, and the operation was performed aseptically.

After shaving the hair on rat abdomen, an incision (about 4 cm in length) was made.

One of the three bipolar stainless steel electrodes were implanted into the muscular wall of the antrum, and the other two were implanted into the muscular wall of the small intestine at 3 cm (duodenum) and 30 cm distally to the pylorus (jejunum). An infusion cannula for drug administration was inserted into the jejunum (5cm proximal to the jejunal electrode). The wires of the electrodes and the infusion cannula were tunneled subcutaneously in the rat's tail and drawn outside at 5-6 cm of the tail tip. The incision was sutured with silk in double layers. Approximately 2 h was required from start to end of the operation.

Post-operatively, the rats are kept in individual cages with a special tether allowing the animal to move freely within the cage. This cage design enabled to manipulate with the infusion cannula for drug administration during experiment and to connect the electrodes for recording the electrical activity.

The animals were housed in an air-conditioned room at 22°C with a 12-h light cycle, fed standard laboratory diet and given water ad libitum. The animals were fasted for 24 h before surgery (ad libitum intake of water was permitted).

2.1.3 Gastrointestinal motility recordings

The rats were given no food or water during the recording of gastrointestinal motility.

In the control group, a 10-day recovery period was provided post surgery. The recording of antroduodenojejunal electromyograms was performed after the animals had been fasted for 24 h with free access to water. Fasting gastrointestinal motility was recorded for 1 h.

In the other groups gastrointestinal motility was recorded for 6 days after the operation. Fasting gastrointestinal motility was recorded for 1 h before- and for 2 h after administration of the drugs.
The electrodes were connected to the amplifier with the sensitivity of 0.1 mV and the frequency band of 0,03 - 100 Hz. The signals are entered in the computer IBM PC for the review, analysis and storage.
The evaluation of the GI electrical activity is performed using the spectral analysis (the assessment of slow waves) and non-linear filtration algorithm (assessment of spike potentials). Percentage of slow waves on which spike bursts were superimposed at the levels of stomach, duodenum and jejunum was calculated. In addition, a visual analysis of electromyograms is performed, i.e. the calculation of time parameters of electrical activity that characterize the MMC. The main feature of the MMC, the activity front or phase III, was identified as a period of clearly distinguishable intense spiking activity. The amplitude should be at least twice that of preceding baseline, and propagating aborally through the whole recording segment and followed by a period of quiescence, phase I of the MMC. Phase II was characterised as a period of irregular spiking activity preceding the activity front. Periods with no detectable spike potentials were considered as quiescence. Characteristics of the MMC, such as period of the MMC, percentage of duration of the MMC phases, duration and propagation time of phase III of the MMC were evaluated.
Period of the MMC was defined as the time lapse between the end of two consecutive phases III (for the duodenum and the jejunum).
Percentage of duration of the MMC phases was defined as the ratio between phase duration, in seconds, and period of the MMC, in seconds, and then multiplied on 100.
In case of the MMC absence than percentage of duration of the MMC phases was defined as the ratio between phase duration, in seconds, and duration of recording (3600 s), and then multiplied on 100.
Phase III duration was defined as the time lapse between beginning and end of a propagated activity front with spikes on top of every slow wave.
Phase III propagation time was defined as the time lapse between the end of a phase III at the duodenum and the jejunum.

2.1.4 Statistical analysis

Results were expressed as the Me (25; 75)% . The parameters of GI electrical activity were evaluated with the Mann-Whitney *U*-test and Friedman -ANOVA.
P values less than 0.05 were considered significant.

2.1.5 Drugs and other chemicals

L-NAME were purchased from ICN Biomedicals Inc. Propranolol (Anaprilin) was obtained from ICN Medicinal (Moscow, Russia), cisapride (Coordinax) and domperidone (Motilium) from Janssen Pharmaceutica (Beerse, Belgium), neostigmine (Proserini) from Pharmstandard-October (Moscow, Russia), metoclopramide (Cerucal) from AWD pharma (Germany), trimebutine (Tambutin) from Dae Han New Pharm. Co. (Corea). All compounds were dissolved in saline. All drugs were administered intraintestinally in volumes of 0.2 ml.
All the protocols and procedures were approved by the Institutional Review Board for Experimental Studies.

2.2 Results

2.2.1 Normal GI electrical activity

The interdigestive motility pattern, the MMC, recorded in the duodenum and proximal jejunum, was observed in all animals (control group). Approximately 5 MMC was noted during 1 h. Period of the MMC in the duodenum and in the jejunum were 700 (620; 810)s and 710 (680;770)s, respectively. Percentage of slow waves on which spike bursts were superimposed for 1 h recording at the levels of stomach, duodenum and jejunum was 12,0 (9,8; 12,2)%; 40,5 (38,9; 42,4)% and 44,0 (42,1; 46,4)%, respectively.

The MMC consisted of three distinct phases: phase I is period quiescence (only slow waves are observed without spike bursts); phase II is period of irregular activity (when spike bursts are observed on slow waves irregularly); and phase III is period of regular activity (spike bursts on every slow wave). Characteristics of the MMC are presented in Table 1.

	Duodenum	Jejunum
percentage of duration of phase I, %	37,3 (35; 41,5)	35,6 (31,5; 40,1)
percentage of duration of phase II, %	37,4 (36,8; 45)	43 (35; 44,1)
percentage of duration of phase III, %	22,9 (20; 25,2)	23,1 (21,1; 24,9)
phase III duration, s	175 (150; 180)	170 (160; 180)
phase III migration time from duodenum to jejunum, s	410 (320; 490)	

Table 1. Characteristics of the MMC

2.2.2 The effect of laparotomy on GI electrical activity

Percentage of slow waves on which spike bursts were superimposed at the levels of stomach, duodenum and jejunum was decreased on the 1st postoperative day after laparotomy in rats (Table 2). Also gastric dysrhythmias were noticed. Suppression of the MMC and weak irregular contractions were observed in all segments of the gastrointestinal tract (Figure 1). Phase III activity was absent in the duodenum and jejunum. The duration of phase II for these segments was longer than that of the normal animals (Figure 2).

Post-operative time, day	Stomach	Duodenum	Jejunum
1	4,0 (3,5; 4,5)*	22,8 (19,3; 23,4)*	24,5 (22,0; 29,8)*
2	7,0 (5,2; 7,8)*	35,2 (32,7; 35,8)*	40,4 (40,0; 42,6)
3	7,5 (6,0; 7,9)*	38,9 (36,0; 39,8)	45,6 (42,3; 46,0)
4	8,0 (6,5; 8,5)*	36,8 (36,2; 39,6)	43,8 (42,9; 44,5)
5	10,1 (9,4; 10,3)	38,8 (37,5; 39,3)	43,7 (42,5; 44,9)
6	12,0 (9,8; 12,2)	40,5 (38,9; 42,4)	44,0 (42,1; 46,4)

* - $p<0,05$ vs. control group

Table 2. Percentage of slow waves on which spike bursts were superimposed at the levels of stomach, duodenum and jejunum in each stage of the study (Me (25; 75)%).

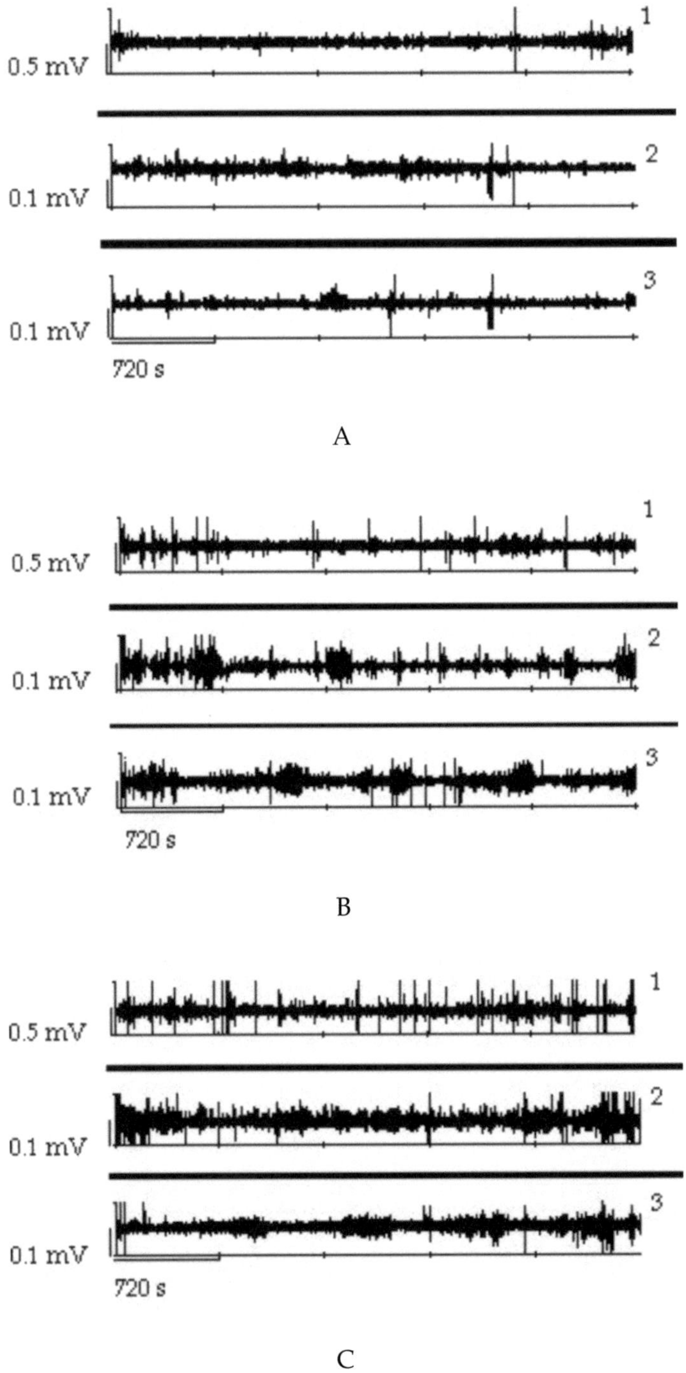

1 – stomach; 2- duodenum; 3- jejunum.
A – postoperative day 1; B – postoperative day 3; C – postoperative day 5.

Fig. 1. The effect of laparotomy on GI electrical activity.

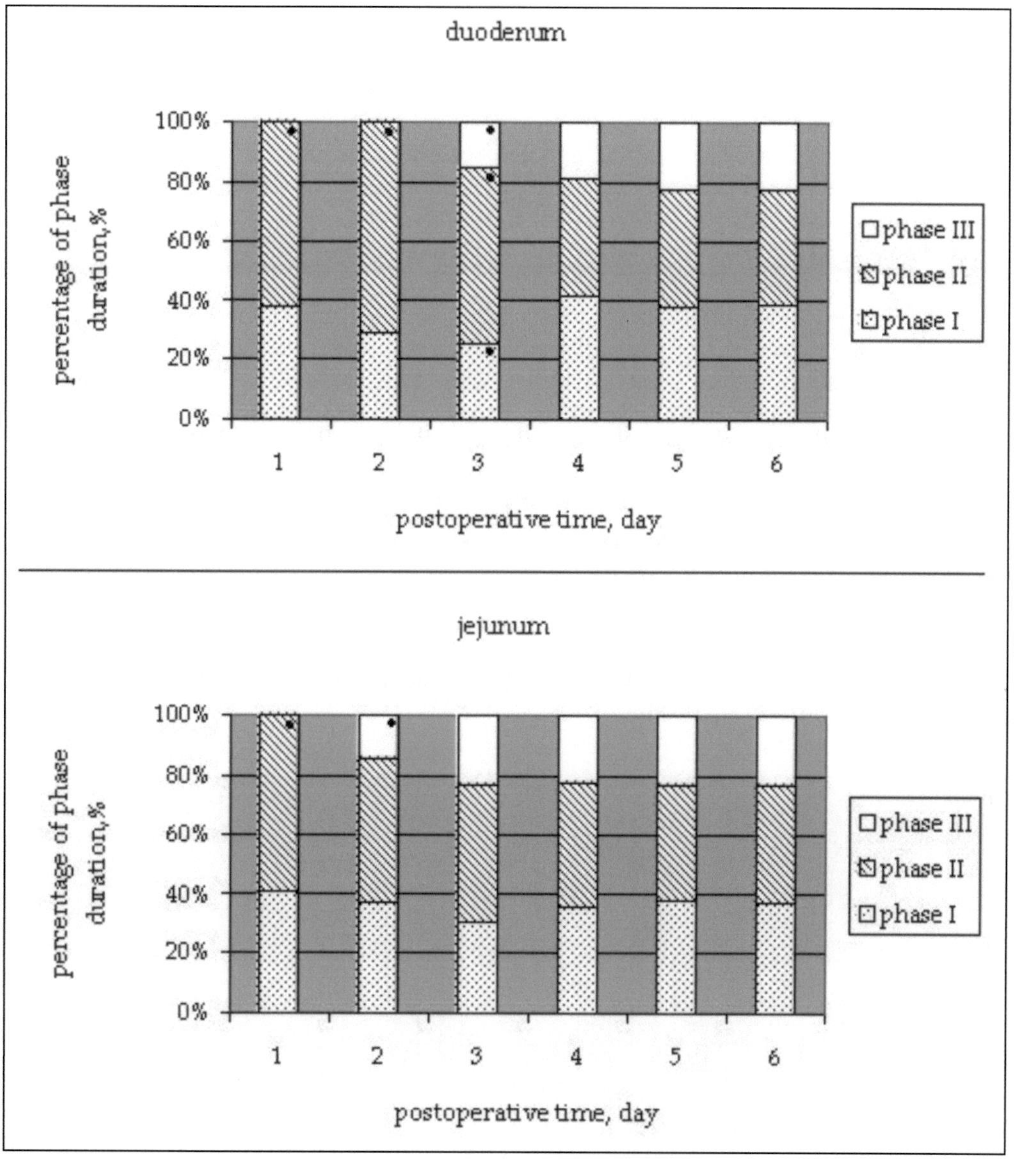

Fig. 2. Postoperative change of percentage of duration of the MMC phases (dark circle - p<0,05 vs. control group).

Percentage of slow waves on which spike bursts were superimposed at the levels of stomach and duodenum was decreased on the 2nd postoperative day. The spike activity in the jejunum returned to normal. Gastric dysrhythmias were absent. The duration of phase II for the duodenum was longer than that of normal animals, phase III was not observed. We observed appearance of phase III in the jejunum. However, the duration of phase III was shorter than that of normal animals (140 (120; 150) s, $p<0,05$).

Percentage of slow waves on which spike bursts were superimposed at the levels of stomach was decreased on the 3rd postoperative day. The spike activity in the duodenum returned to

normal. We observed all phases of the MMC in the duodenum and jejunum. However, the duration of phases for duodenum was significantly different from normal. Not all phases III migrated from the duodenum to the jejunum. Normalization of the MMC phase ratio in jejunum was noticed.
Percentage of slow waves on which spike bursts were superimposed at the levels of stomach was decreased on the 4th postoperative day. Normalization of the MMC phase ratio in duodenum was observed.
Full recovery of GI electrical activity and the MMC of small intestine we obtained on the 5th postoperative day after laparotomy.
Thus, the recovery of spike electrical activity occurs in the jejunum, then in the duodenum, and at last in the stomach. Also phase III contractions are observed at first only in the lower part of the gastrointestinal tract (jejunum) and then, gradually, in the upper part (duodenum). Normalization of spike electrical activity in the stomach occurs at the same time when the MMC from duodenum to the jejunum is observed.

2.2.3 The effects of drugs on GI electrical activity on postoperative period

Different drugs were administrated from the 1st through the 3rd postoperative days.
All drugs induced differently the increase of spike electrical activity in the stomach, duodenum and jejunum mostly significant on the 1st postoperative day (Figure 3).
The stimulating effect of cisapride on the spike electrical activity in the stomach, duodenum and jejunum was weak as compared with the other drugs while the administration of domperidone resulted in significant increase.

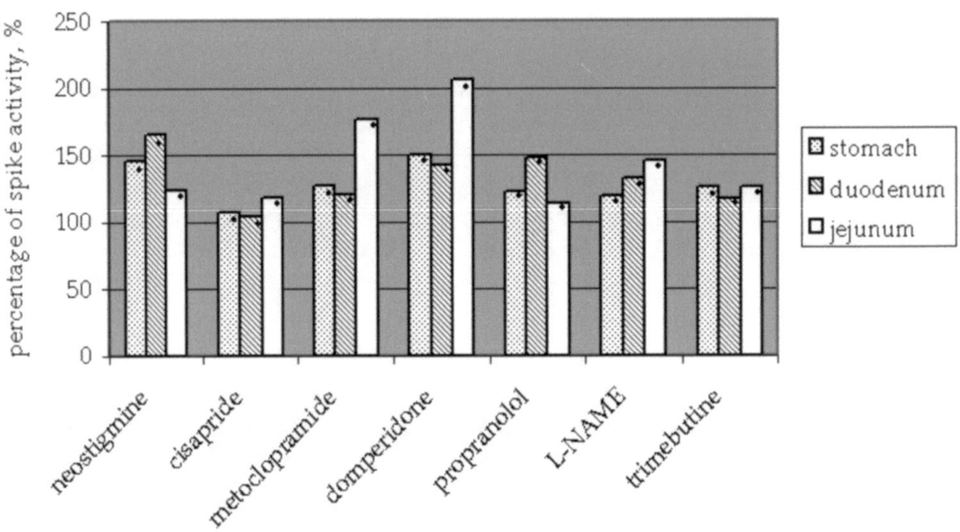

Baseline of spike activity is equal 100% (dark circle - $p<0,05$ vs. baseline).

Fig. 3. The effect of drugs on spike electrical activity on the 1st postoperative day.

As it was mentioned above, phase III was absent on the 1st postoperative day 1 in the LAP group. In connection with the fact that in the LAP group phase III appeared already on the 2nd postoperative day, in order to reveal the mechanisms which are responsible for the MMC inhibition, the effects of different etiological drugs on the 1st postoperative day were analyzed.

The different drugs stimulated different phases of the MMC in the duodenum and jejunum (Figure 4).

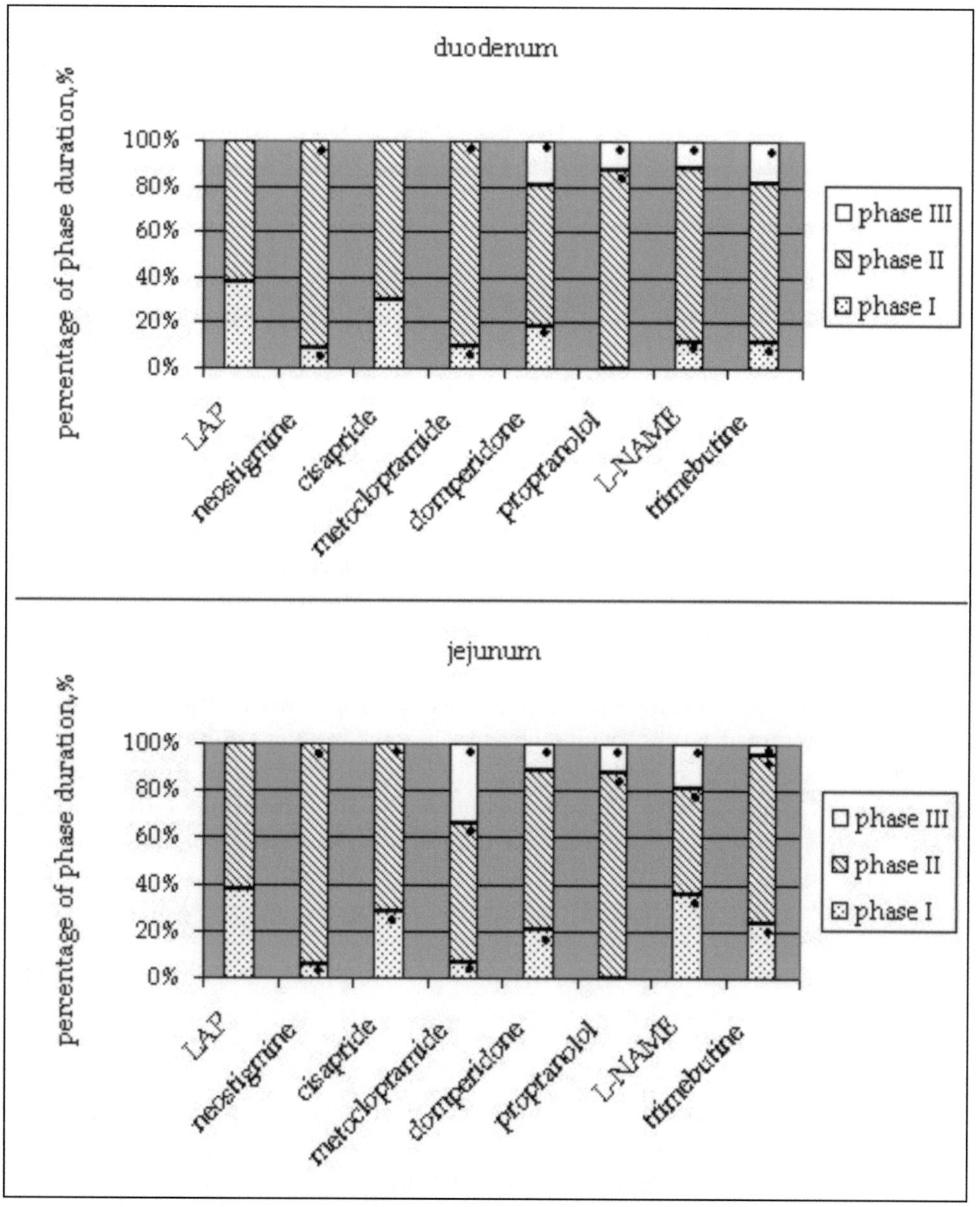

Fig. 4. The effect of drugs on percentage of phases duration of the MMC on the 1st postoperative day (dark circle - $p<0,05$ vs. LAP group).

The administration of neostigmine stimulated phase II in the duodenum and jejunum. The duration of phase II was increased. Irregular activity was represented by the groups of spike bursts (duration 20-60 s) with periods of quiescence (duration 10-20 s). The duration of phase I was decreased. We didn't observe phase III. Spastic activity was noted in the duodenum and jejunum. This type of activity consisted of the groups of spike bursts occupating 2-3 slow wave. Moreover, we observed the migrating action potential complexes (MAPCs). These complexes rapidly propagated from the duodenum to the jejunum (Fig.5).

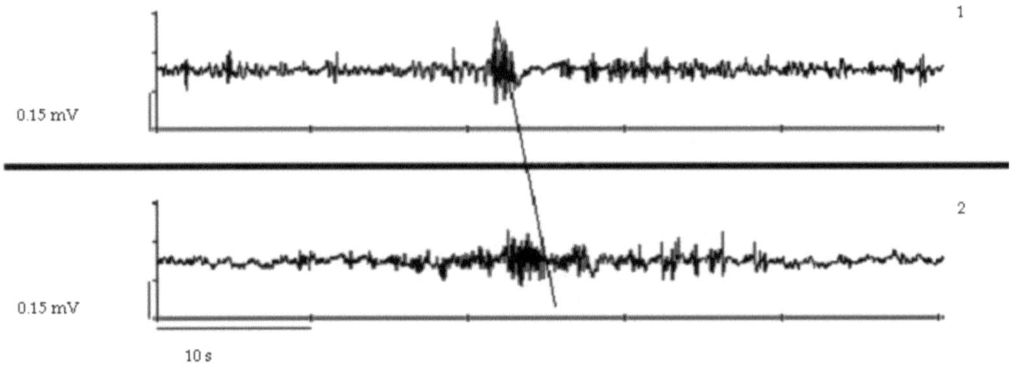

Fig. 5. Migrating action potential complex on the 1st postoperative day after administration of neostigmine
1 – duodenum; 2 - jejunum

The administration of cisapride stimulated phase II in the duodenum and jejunum. Irregular activity was represented by the groups of spike bursts (duration 20-30 s) with periods of quiescence (duration 30-60 s). The incidence of distally propagated clustered activity was observed. We didn't detect phase III.

The administration of metoclopramide stimulated phase II in the duodenum. Irregular activity was represented by the groups of spike bursts (duration 15-20 s or 30-40 s) with periods of quiescence (duration 30-40 s). We didn't observe phase III in the duodenum. Metocloptamide induced phases III in the jejunum. The duration of phase III was 100 (80; 130) s, it was less than that of the normal animals (Fig.6). The duration of phase I decreased in the duodenum and jejunum. We also observed spastic activity.

The administration of domperidone stimulated appearance of phase III both on the duodenum and jejunum.

After the administration of propranolol disappearance of phase I and appearance of phase III both on the duodenum and jejunum was observed.

After the administration of L-NAME the MMC propagating from duodenum to the jejunum was registrated (Fig. 7).

After the administration of trimebutine decrease of phase I duration and appearance of phase III in the duodenum and jejunum were observed.

So, we investigated the possible role of cholinergic, adrenergic, dopaminergic, serotonergic, nitrergic mechanisms, and also local anaesthetics in POI. We found that the administration of different pharmacological agents stimulated the MMC and its separate phases in the rat small intestine on the 1st postoperative day after laparotomy.

Neostigmine and cisapride induced phase II, but not phase III of MMC in the duodenum and jejunum. The phase II after cisapride differed from the phase II after neostigmine. The contractile pattern induced by neostigmine was spastic. We also observed occurrence the MAPCs in the duodenum and jejunum. Cisapride induced a prolonged and highly propagative phase II in the duodenum and jejunum. Metoclopramide administration resulted in occurrence of phase III only in the jejunum but not the duodenum.

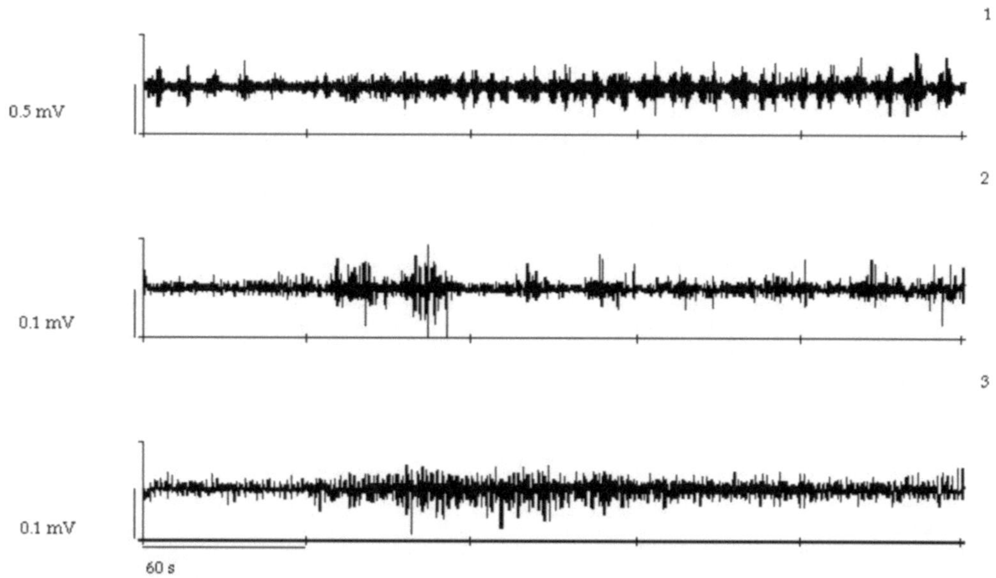

Phase II in the duodenum and phase III in the jejunum.
1 - stomach; 2- duodenum; 3 - jejunum

Fig. 6. The electrical activity of stomach, duodenum and jejunum on the 1st postoperative day after administration of metoclopramide.

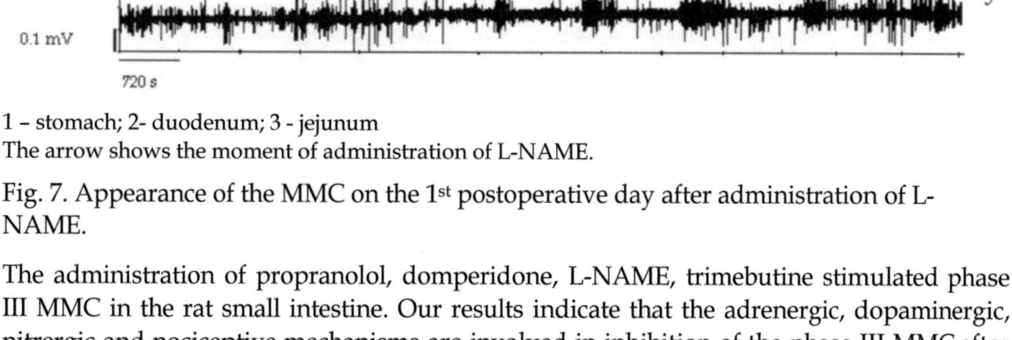

1 - stomach; 2- duodenum; 3 - jejunum
The arrow shows the moment of administration of L-NAME.

Fig. 7. Appearance of the MMC on the 1st postoperative day after administration of L-NAME.

The administration of propranolol, domperidone, L-NAME, trimebutine stimulated phase III MMC in the rat small intestine. Our results indicate that the adrenergic, dopaminergic, nitrergic and nociceptive mechanisms are involved in inhibition of the phase III MMC after surgery. Moreover, only the administration of L-NAME stimulate occurrence of the MMC propagating from the duodenum to the jejunum. Therefore, the main role in disappearance the MMC after surgery belongs to the activation of nonadrenergic noncholinergic mechanisms. In the early postoperative period, endogenous NO is a major inhibitory component that seems to constitute the common final pathway of mediators and the neural pathways inhibiting the MMC in rats.

On the 2nd postoperative day in baseline recordings in the duodenum phase III was absent in the LAP group, neostigmine and metoclopramide groups. Phase III in baseline recordings in the jejunum was observed in all groups including the LAP group, however it was absent in the group with the administration of neostigmine (Table 3).

On the 3rd postoperative day in baseline recordings in the jejunum phase III was observed in all groups, at the same time phase III in duodenum was absent only in the group with the administration of neostigmine.

Drugs	2nd postoperative day		3rd postoperative day	
	duodenum	jejunum	duodenum	jejunum
LAP	-	+	+	+
neostigmine	-	-	-	+
cisapride	+	+	+	+
metoclopramide	-	+	+	+
domperidone	+	+	+	+
propranolol	+	+	+	+
L-NAME	+	+	+	+
trimebutine	+	+	+	+

+ presence of phase III; - absence of phase III

Table 3. Phase III of the MMC on the 2nd and the 3rd postoperative days in baseline recordings in each of the groups

The administration of almost all drugs on the 1st through the 3rd postoperative day reversed recovery of GI electrical activity. All drugs, except for neostigmine induced the MMC recovery 3-4 days later after laparotomy (Figure 8).

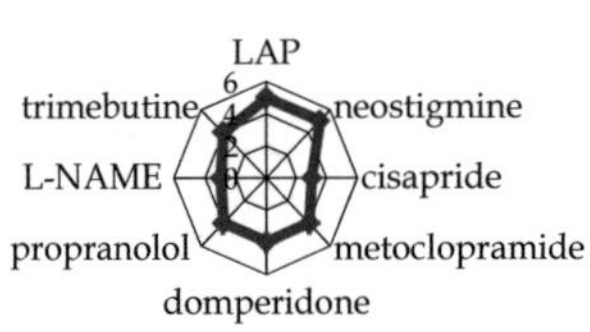

The figures show postoperative days.

Fig. 8. Time of the MMC recovery on the postoperative period.

Our finding demonstrated that cisapride, domperidone, metaclopramide, propranolol, L-NAME, trimebutine may be useful as prokinetic agents to induce early recovery of the MMC from postoperative ileus.

3. Disscusion

To observe the gastrointestinal motility under awake conditions of the rats, we implanted the infusion cannula and three electrodes at various points in the gastrointestinal tracts. Therefore, it took about 2 h from start to end of the operation and physical damage to gastrointestinal tract from the operation was greater than after laparotomy alone.

In a our study, we found that suppression of the MMC and weak irregular contractions were observed in all segments of the small intestine on the 1st postoperative day after laparotomy in rats. The time of first occurrence of phase III in the jejunum and the duodenum without drug administration was, respectively, on the 2nd and the 3rd day after laparotomy. Full recovery of GI electrical activity and the MMC of small intestine we obtained on the 5th postoperative day after laparotomy.

Clinically, the disorders of gastrointestinal motility referred to as ileus are generally present after laparotomy and require several days for recovery. During the period of post-operative ileus after laparotomy, problems arise with feeding, control of body fluids and wound healing because patients cannot eat. Early recovery from post-operative ileus would thus be beneficial. In addition, ileus after laparotomy is a major impediment to patient recovery, since it necessitates the use of a nasal tube for drainage of retained intragastric fluid and for parenteral feeding. Attempts have, therefore, been made to reduce the duration of post-operative ileus in order to permit removal of the nasal gastric tube as early as possible and to enable oral nutritional eating. It is thought that food residues and secretions remaining in the gastrointestinal tract during ileus cause abdominal distention and disorders (Tsukamoto et al., 2000).

The primary objective of pharmaceutic intervention is to augment the pathways that stimulate motility or attenuate the inhibitory neurons that predominantly suppress activity.

Studies evaluating cholinergic agonists in the setting of POI have often produced conflicting results. Acetylcholine is released from the enteric nervous system and causes increased gut wall contractility. Acetylcholine is degraded in the synaptic cleft by acetylcholinesterase. Neostigmine is a reversible inhibitor of acetylcholinesterase and as such has been investigated as a potential treatment for postoperative ileus (Luckey et al., 2003). Neostigmine is the first-line treatment for colonic ileus (De Giorgio & Knowles, 2009). Kreis et al. (2001) found that neostigmine therapy significantly increased colonic motility in the early postoperative period in patients undergoing colorectal surgery. In three randomized, placebo-controlled trials, the success rates were 85% to 94% after the first dose (Ponec et al., 1999; Amaro & Rogers, 2000; van der Spoel et al., 2001). However, it's use for impacting or in cases with excess GI distention has not been recommended due to the apparent force of drug induced contractions (Lester et al., 1998). The most common side effect is abdominal pain. In our study we found that neostigmine stimulated phase II of the MMC in the duodenum and jejunum, spastic activity and MAPC. This drug not induced early recovery of the MMC from POI. Our results no conflicted with Sarna (2006). In his opinion exogenous cholinergic agonists act concurrently and directly on circular muscle cells everywhere, resulting in stimulation of simultaneous or nonpropagating contractions. Furthermore, strong stimulation of muscarinic receptors on smooth muscle cells may uncouple slow waves at adjacent sites and suppress propagation of contractions that would further retard transit. Cholinesterase inhibitors that accumulate acetylcholine at the neuromuscular junction also stimulate nonpropagating contractions for the same reason. However, the accumulation of acetylcholine at the neuroeffector junction may also stimulate giant migrating contractions - GMCs (analog MAPCs).

Cisapride is an orally administered prokinetic agent which facilitates or restores motility throughout the length of the gastrointestinal tract. It is a substituted piperidinyl benzamide, chemically related to metoclopramide, but unlike metoclopramide, cisapride is largely devoid of central depressant or antidopaminergic effects (Wiseman & Faulds, 1994). Cisapride is a 5-HT-4 agonist that facilitates acetylcholine release from the intrinsic plexus (Tonini, 1999). Several trials have shown that cisapride actually has a beneficial effect in shortening POI (Tollesson et al., 1991; Brown et al., 1999). In our study we found that cisapride stimulated phase II of the MMC in the duodenum and jejunum. Cisapride significantly increased the incidence of distally propagated clustered activity and induced a prolonged and highly propagative phase II jejunal electrical activity. Moreover, cisapride reduced the duration of POI.

Metoclopramide, a derivative of para-aminobenzoic acid, is a dopamine antagonist with central and peripheral effects. It possesses both anti-emetic and prokinetic effects; the anti-emetic effects relate to dopamine (D_2) antagonism and serotonin (5-HT_3) receptor antagonism on vagal and brainstem pathways; the prokinetic effects result from acetylcholine release from enteric cholinergic neurons (via 5-HT_4 receptors), D_2 receptor antagonism in the myenteric plexus, and muscarinic receptor sensitization (Rabine, 2001). Metoclopramide treatment may be beneficial in the treatment of canine postoperative ileus by increasing myoelectric and contractile activity of the proximal gastrointestinal tract. Graves et al. (1989) reported that treatment with metoclopramide partially reversed the MMC phase III inhibition at the duodenum and jejunum. Motility index values were restored to preoperative baseline values with metoclopramide treatment. Other trials that assessed efficacy of metoclopramide for POI failed to show any beneficial effect (Cheape et al., 1991; Seta & Kale-Pradhan, 2001). We established that metoclopramide induced phase III in the jejunum, but not in the duodenum on the 1st and the 2nd postoperative days. However, administration of metoclopramide induced early recovery of the MMC from POI.

An important mechanism for the inhibition of motility is dopamine acting at neural D2 receptors. Previous studies have shown that stimulation of D2 receptors decreases acetylcholine release from cholinergic motoneurons innervating the gastrointestinal tract (Kurosawa, 1991). Domperidone is a dopamine antagonist that acts primarily through peripheral D_2 receptors and does not cross the blood-brain barrier; thus, its use is not associated with the majority of the central nervous system side effects of metoclopramide.

We found that administration of domperidone stimulate phase III MMC in the rat small intestine and induced early recovery of the MMC from POI.

Smith and co-workers (1977) reported a transient increase in plasma epinephrine simultaneously with a sustained increase of norepinephrine after laparotomy in the dog. In their study, ileus persisted for a long time after plasma concentrations of epinephrine returned to basal values. In addition, chemical destruction of sympathetic nerves by pretreatment with 6-hydroxydopamine prevents inhibition of gastric emptying and intestinal transit after abdominal surgery in the rat (Dubois, 1973). Increased synthesis and release of norepinephrine from the intestinal wall in the rat have been reported (Dubois et al., 1973, 1974). In our study we found that propranolol (β -adrenergic blocker) prevented inhibition of motility after laparotomy and reduce the duration of postoperative ileus.

Meile et al. (2006) investigated the effects of NO synthase inhibition on gastric, small intestinal and colonic motility in awake rats under baseline conditions and in a postoperative ileus model. L-NMMA (NO synthase inhibitior) injection prior to surgery did not prohibit intraoperative inhibition of gastrointestinal motility, but did result in immediate recovery of gastric, small intestinal and colonic motility postoperatively.
The major observation in our study is that inhibition of endogenous NO synthase by L-NAME results in early recovery of the MMC in the small intestine. In the early postoperative period, endogenous NO is a major inhibitory component that seems to constitute the common final pathway of mediators and the neural pathways inhibiting gastrointestinal motility in rats.
Trimebutine, a weak non selective opioid agonist unable to cross blood-brain barrier, has long been used in the treatment of functional bowel disease (Delvaux & Wingate, 1997). Peripheral κ-opioid agonists are not associated with GI dysmotility but they do have anti-nociceptive effects in the GI tract. For example, preclinical studies suggest that peritoneal irritation induced pain is reversed with κ-agonist. Likewise, κ - opioid agonists inhibit the response of peripheral primary afferents to colorectal distention (Corazziari, 1999; Junien & Riviere, 1995). De Winter (2003) also demonstrated that blockade of the afferent limb of the reflex pathway by peripheral κ -opioid agonists ameliorated postoperative ileus. In animal studies, bowel motility was normalized with use of fedotozine (selective κ - opioid receptor agonist) (De Winter et al., 1997; Friese et al., 1997; Riviere et al., 1994). These results support a role for peripheral κ -opioid receptors in the pathogenesis of postoperative ileus induced by abdominal surgery. N. Friese and co-workers (1997) believe that peripheral κ -opioid receptors could modulate the transmission of visceral nociceptive stimuli in the periphery and might represent an alternative to μ-agonists in the treatment of abdominal pain associated with motility and transit impairments, such as after abdominal surgery.
Moreover, a non-opioid mechanism via sodium channel blocking properties has been proposed for κ-opioid agonists suggesting that these agents may also act as a local anesthetic (Junien & Riviere, 1995; Barber & Gottschlich, 1997). Fedotozine was the first κ - agonist studied in humans. In clinical trials it proved to be better than placebo in relieving bloating, abdominal pain, postprandial fullness and nausea in patients with functional dyspepsia while it was slightly superior to placebo in getting symptom relief in patients with irritable bowel syndrome (Corazziari, 1999; Delvaux, 2001). The sodium channel-blocking activity was confirmed by the potent local anesthetic effect of trimebutine, which was 17-fold more active than lidocaine in terms of both potency and duration of action. (Roman et al., 1999). The blocking effect of trimebutine on sodium channel currents may account for this antinociceptive effect. (Roman et al., 1999). In our study we found that trimebutine stimulated phase III of the MMC in the duodenum and jejunum on the 1st postoperative day. Also administration of this drug induced early recovery of the MMC from POI. Thus, inhibition of nociceptive pathways after laparotomy is significant for occurrence of phase III and recovery of the MMC from POI.

4. Conclusion

We investigated altered gastrointestinal motility in POI and effects of potential etiological agents on gastrointestinal electrical activity to determine a cause for the development of POI and treatment. Our results are consistent with the hypothesis that small intestinal motility is under tonic inhibition by adrenergic, dopaminenergic, nitrergic and nociceptive mechanisms, and release from this inhibition results in phase III activity. The main role in disappearance the MMC after surgery belongs to the activation of nonadrenergic noncholinergic mechanisms. In the early postoperative period, endogenous NO is a major inhibitory component that seems to constitute the common final pathway of mediators and the neural pathways inhibiting the MMC in rats. The administration of almost all drugs on the 1st through the 3rd postoperative day reversed recovery of GI electrical activity. All drugs, except for neostigmine induced early recovery of the MMC from POI. Our finding demonstrated that cisapride, domperidone, metaclopramide, propranolol, L-NAME, trimebutine may be useful as prokinetic agents to induce early recovery of the MMC from POI.

5. References

Amaro, R. & Rogers, A.I. (2000) Neostigmine Infusions: New Standard of Care for Acute Colonic Pseudo-obstruction? *Am J Gastroenterol*; Vol.95, pp. 304–305.

Barber, A. & Gottschlich, R. (1997) Novel Developments with Selective, Non- peptidic Kappa-opioid Receptor Agonists, *Expert Opin Investig Drugs*, Vol.6, pp. 1351-1368.

Behm, B. & Stollman, N. (2003) Postoperative Ileus: Etiologies and Interventions, *Clinical Gastroenterology and Hepatology*, Vol.1, №2, pp. 71-80.

Benson, M. J., Roberts, J. P., Wingate, D.L. et al. (1994) Small Bowel Motility following Major Intra-Abdominal Surgery: the Effects of Opiate and Rectal Cisapride, *Gastroenterology*,Vol.106, pp. 924-936.

Brown, T.A., McDonald, J. & Williard, W. (1999) A Prospective, Randomized, Double-blinded, Placebo-controlled Trial of Cisapride After Colorectal Surgery, *Am J Surg.*,Vol.177, pp. 399-401.

Cheape, J.D., Wexner, S.D., James, K. et al. (1994) Does Metoclopramide Reduce the Length of Ileus after Colorectal Surgery? A Prospective Randomized Trial, *Dis Colon Rectum*, Vol.34, pp. 437-441.

Clevers, G.J., Smout, A.J., Van der Schee, E.J. & Akkermans, L.M. (1991) Myoelectrical and Motor Activity of the Stomach in the First Few Days after Abdominal Surgery: Evaluation by Electrogastrography and Impedance Gastrography, *J Gastroenterol Hepatol*, Vol.6, pp. 253–259.

Condon, R.E., Frantzides, C.T., Cowles, V.E. et al. (1986) Resolution of Postoperative Ileus in Humans, *Ann Surg.*, Vol.203, pp. 574–581.

Corazziari, E. (1999) Role of Opioid Ligands in the Irritable Bowel Syndrome, *Can J Gastroenterol*, Vol.13, Suppl. A, pp. 71A-75A.

Dauchel, J., Schang, J.C., Kachelhoffer, J. et al. (1976) Gastrointestinal Myoelectrical Activity During the Postoperative Period in Man, *Digestion*, Vol.14, pp. 293–303.

De Giorgio, R. & Knowles, C.H. (2009) Acute Colonic Pseudo-obstruction, *Br J Surg.*, Vol. 96, pp. 229–239.

Delvaux, M. & Wingate, D. (1997) Trimebutine: Mechanism of Action, Effects on Gastrointestinal Function and Clinical Results, *J Int Med Res.*, Vol. 25, pp. 225-246.

Delvaux, M. (2001) Pharmacology and Clinical Experience with Fedotozine, *Expert Opin Investig Drugs*, Vol.10, pp. 97-110.

De Winter, B.Y., Boeckxstaens, G.E., De Man, J.G. et al. (1997) Effects of Mu- and Kappa-opioid Receptors on Postoperative Ileus in Rats, *Eur J Pharmacol*, Vol. 339, pp. 63–67.

De Winter, B.Y. (2003) Study of the Pathogenesis of Paralytic Ileus in Animal Models of Experimentally Induced Postoperative and Septic Ileus, *Verh K Acad Geneeskd Belg.*, Vol.65, №5, pp. 293-324.

Dubois, A., Weise, V. K. & Kopin, I. J. (1973) Postoperative Ileus in the Rat: Physiopathology, Etiology and Treatment, *Ann. Surg.*, Vol.178, pp.781-786.

Dubois, A., Kopin I. J., Pettigrew, K. D. & Jacobowitz, D. M. (1974) Chemical and Histochemical Studies of Post-operative Sympathetic Nerve Activity in the Digestive Tract in Rats, *Gastroenterology*, Vol.66, pp.403-407.

Friese, N., Chevalier, E., Angel, F. et al. (1997) Reversal by Kappa-agonists of Peritoneal Irritation-induced Ileus and Visceral Pain in Rats, *Life Sci*, Vol. 60, pp. 625–634.

Gerring, E.E.L. & Hunt, J.M. (1986) Pathophysiology of Equine Ileus:Effect of Adrenergic Blockade, Parasympathetic Stimulation and Metaclopramide in an Experimental Model, *Equine Vet J.*, Vol.18, pp.249-255.

Graves, G.M., Becht, J.L. & Rawlings, C.A. (1989) Metoclopramide Reversal of Decreased Gastrointestinal Myoelectric and Contractile Activity in a Model of Canine Postoperative Ileus, *Veterinary Surgery*, Vol.18, №1, pp. 27–33.

Holte, K. & Kehlet, H. (2000) Postoperative Ileus: a Preventable Event, *Br J Surg*, Vol.87, pp.1480-1493.

Holte, K. & Kehlet, H. (2002) Postoperative Ileus: Progress Towards Effective Management, *Drugs*, Vol.62, №18, pp.2603-2615.

Hotokezaka, M., Mentis, E.P., Patel, S.P. et al. (1997) Recovery of Gastrointestinal Tract Motility and Myoelectric Activity Change After Abdominal Surgery, *Arch Surg.*,Vol.132, pp.410-417.

Junien, J.L. & Riviere, P. (1995) Review Article: the Hypersensitive Gut - Peripheral Kappa Agonists as a New Pharmacological Approach, *Aliment Pharmacol Ther*, Vol.9, pp.117-126.

Kreis, M.E., Kasparek, M., Zittel, T.T. et al. (2001) Neostigmine Increases Postoperative Colonic Motility in Patients Undergoing Colorectal Surgery, *Surgery*, Vol.130, pp.449-456.

Kurosawa, S., Hasler, W. L. & Owyang, C. (1991) Characterization of Dopamine Receptors in the Guinea Pig Stomach: Dopaminergic vs Adrenergic Receptors, *Gastroenterology*, Vol.100, pp.1224-1231, 1991.

Lester, G.D., Merritt, A.M., Neuwirth, L. et al. (1998) Effect of α2-adrenergic, Cholinergic, and Nonsteroidal Anti-inflammatory Drugs on Myoelectrical Activity of Ileum, Cecum and Right Ventral Colon and Cecal Emptying of Radiolabeled Markers in Clinically Normal Ponies, *Am J Vet Res.*, Vol.59, pp.320-327.

Livingston, E.H. & Passaro, E.P. (1990) Postoperative Ileus, *Dig Dis Sci.*, Vol.35, pp.121-132.

Luckey, A., Livingston, E.H. & Tache, Y. (2003) Mechanisms and Treatment of Postoperative Ileus, *Archives of Surgery*,Vol.138, №2, pp.206–214.

Meile, T., Glatzle, J., Habermann, F.M. et al. (2006) Nitric Oxide Synthase Inhibition Results in Immediate Postoperative Recovery of Gastric, Small Intestinal and Colonic Motility in Awake Rats, *Int J Colorectal Dis*, Vol.21, №2, pp.121-129.

Miedema, B.W., Schillie, S., Simmons, J.W. et al. (2002) Small Bowel Motility and Transit After Aortic Surgery, *J Vasc Surg.*, Vol.36, pp.19–24.

Morris, I.R., Darby, C.F., Hammond, P. & Taylor, I. (1983) Changes in Small Bowel Myoelectrical Activity following Laparotomy, *Br. J. Surg*, Vol.70,pp.547–548.

Ponec, R.J., Saunders, M.D. & Kimmey, M.B. (1999) Neostigmine for the Treatment of Acute Colonic Pseudo-obstruction, *N Engl J Med.*, Vol.341, pp.137–141.

Rabine, J.C: (2001) Management of the Patient with Gastroparesis, *J Clin Gastroenterol*, Vol. 32, pp.11-18.

Reynolds, J.C. & Putman, P.E. (1992) Prokinetic Agents, *Gastroenterol Clin of North Am*, Vol.21, pp.567-596.

Riviere, P.J., Rascaud, X., Chevalier, E. & Junien, J.L. (1994) Fedotozine Reversal of Peritoneal-irritation-induced Ileus in Rats: Possible Peripheral Action on Sensory Afferents, *J Pharmacol Exp Ther*, Vol. 270, pp.846–850.

Roman, F.J., Lanet, S., Hamon, J. et al. (1999) Pharmacological Properties of Trimebutine and N-monodesmethyltrimebutine, *J Pharmacol Exp Ther.*, Vol.289, pp.1391–1397.

Sarna, S.K. (2006) Molecular, Functional, and Pharmacological Targets for the Development of Gut Promotility Drugs, *Am.J. Physiol.(Gastrointest. Liver Physiol.)*, Vol.291, №4, pp. G545-555.

Schippers, E., Holscher, A.H., Bollschweiter, E. & Siewert, J.R. (1991) Return of Interdigestive Motor Complex after Abdominal Surgery: End of Postoperative Ileus? *Dig. Dis. Sci.*, Vol.36, pp. 621-626.

Seta, M.L. & Kale-Pradhan, P.B. (2001) Efficacy of Metoclopramide in Postoperative Ileus After Exploratory Laparotomy, *Pharmacotherapy*, Vol.21, pp. 1181-1186.

Smith, J., Kelly, K.A. & Weinshilboum, R.M. (1977) Pathophysiology of Postoperative Ileus, *Arch. Surg.*, Vol.112, pp.203–209.

Szurszewksi, J.H. (1969) A Migrating Electrical Complex of the Canine Small Intestine, *Am J Physiol*, Vol.217, pp.1757–1763.

Tollesson, P.O, Cassuto. J., Rimback, G. et al. (1991) Treatment of Postoperative Paralytic Ileus with Cisapride, *Scand J Gastroenterol*, Vol.26, pp.477-482.

Tonini, M., De Ponti, F., Di Nucci, A. & Crema, F. (1999) Review Article: Cardiac Adverse Effects of Gastrointestinal Prokinetics, *Alimentary Pharmacology & Therapeutics*, Vol.13, pp. 1585–1591.

Tsukamoto, K., Mizutani, M., Yamano, M. et al. (2000) The Effect of SK-896 on Post-operative Ileus in Dogs: Gastrointestinal Motility Pattern and Transit, *European Journal of Pharmacology*, Vol.401, pp.97–107.

van der Spoel, J.I., Oudemans-van Straaten, H.M., Stroutenbeek, C.P. et al. (2001) Neostigmine Resolves Critical Illness-related Colonic Ileus in Intensive Care Patients with Multiple Organ Failure: a Prospective, Double-blind, Placebo-controlled Trial, *Intensive Care Med.*, Vol.27, pp.822–827.

Waldhausen, J.H., Shaffrey, M.E., Skenderis, B.S. et al (1990) Gastrointestinal Myoelectric and Clinical Patterns of Recovery After Laparotomy, *Ann Surg.*, Vol.211, pp.777-784.

Wilson, J.P. (1975) Postoperative Motility of the Large Intestine in Man, *Gut*, Vol.16, pp.689–692.

Wiseman, L. & Faulds, D. (1994) Cisapride: an Updated Review of its Pharmacology and Therapeutic Efficacy as a Prokinetic in Gastrointestinal Motility Disorders, *Drugs*, Vol. 47, pp.116-152.

Part 5

Inflammatory Bowel Syndrome

13

Prospective Uses of Genetically Engineered Lactic Acid Bacteria for the Prevention of Inflammatory Bowel Diseases

Jean Guy LeBlanc[1], Silvina del Carmen[1], Fernanda Alvarenga Lima[2], Meritxell Zurita Turk[2], Anderson Miyoshi[2], Vasco Azevedo[2] and Alejandra de Moreno de LeBlanc[1]
[1]*Centro de Referencia para Lactobacilos (CERELA-CONICET), San Miguel de Tucumán, Tucumán,*
[2]*Institute of Biological Sciences, Federal University of Minas Gerais (UFMG-ICB), Belo Horizonte, MG,*
[1]*Argentina*
[2]*Brazil*

1. Introduction

Inflammatory bowel disease (IBD) is a term used to describe a group of intestinal disorders in which inflammation is a major feature. Although rare forms of IBD exist, these diseases normally pertain to ulcerative colitis (UC) (Head & Jurenka, 2003) and Crohn's disease (CD) (Baumgart & Sandborn, 2007). There is evidence that these do not represent distinct conditions but rather are the same disease with shared etiological factors (Price, 1992); however, clinical manifestations (such as the exact location of the pathology or the affected individual's immunological and constitutional endowment) are distinctive between both.

Despite many years of study, the exact etiology and pathogenesis of these disorders remain unclear but great advances have been made using experimental animal models and have provided insights into the complex, multi-factorial processes and mechanisms that can result in chronic intestinal inflammation (Elson & Weaver, 2003).

The aim of this chapter is to present an overview of the current expanding knowledge of the mechanisms by which lactic acid bacteria and other probiotic microorganisms participate in the prevention and treatment of IBD and how genetic engineering techniques can be used to improve their effectiveness or create novel therapeutic strains. In the following sections, the mechanisms by which these beneficial microorganisms exert their therapeutic effects, which include changes in the gut microbiota, stimulation of the host immune responses, enhancement of intestinal barrier function and reduction of the oxidative stress due to their antioxidant properties will be discussed.

2. Lactic acid bacteria and inflammatory bowel diseases

Lactic acid bacteria (LAB) constitute a phylogenetically heterogeneous group of ubiquitous microorganisms that are naturally present in high nutrient containing organic products such as foods and occupy a wide range of ecological niches ranging from the surface of plants to the gastro-urogenital tract of animals. Currently, the LAB group includes a large number of cocci and bacilli, such as species of the genera *Carnobacterium, Enterococcus, Lactobacillus, Lactococcus, Leuconostoc, Oenococcus, Pediococcus, Streptococcus, Tetragenococcus, Vagococcus* and *Weissella,* that normally contain a G+C content inferior to 55% in their chromosomal DNA. Although quite diverse, the members of this group have various characteristics in common, that include being: (i) Gram-positive; (ii) facultative anaerobes; (iii) non-sporulating; (iv) non-motile and (v) possess the capacity to convert sugars into lactic acid (Nouaille et al., 2003). LAB are one of the most important industrial groups of bacteria that are widely used in food production, health improvement and production of macromolecules, enzymes and metabolites.

From a historical point of view, LAB have been used since ancient times in food fermentation processes and preservation. Since the 1980's, many efforts have been made to better understand the molecular basis of LAB's technological properties in order to control the industrial processes involving these important microorganisms. Due to their lack of pathogenicity, most LAB species have received the GRAS (Generally Recognized As Safe) status by the U.S. Food and Drug Administration. In addition to their important technological properties in food production (production of lactic acid, decrease of lactose, improvement of organoleptic and physical characteristics), various species of LAB, such as *Lactobacillus casei, Lactobacillus delbrueckii, Lactobacillus acidophilus, Lactobacillus plantarum, Lactobacillus fermentum* and *Lactobacillus reuteri,* have been shown to possess therapeutic properties since they are able to prevent the development of some diseases as shown mostly using animal models and have the capacity to promote beneficial effects in human and animal health (LeBlanc et al., 2008). Because of all of their documented beneficial effects, certain strains of LAB have been designated as being *probiotic* that have been defined by the FAO/WHO as *"live microorganisms which when administered in adequate amounts confer a health benefit on the host"* (FAO/WHO, 2001). Some of the health benefits which have been claimed for probiotics include: improvement of the normal microbiota, prevention of infectious diseases and food allergies, reduction of serum cholesterol, anticarcinogenic activity, stabilization of the gut mucosal barrier, immune adjuvant properties, alleviation of intestinal bowel disease symptoms, and improvement of the digestion of lactose in intolerant hosts (Galdeano et al., 2007). The most commonly used strains as probiotics are members of lactobacilli, enterococci and bifidobacteria groups (Ouwehand et al., 2002). Currently, many products containing probiotics are available on retail shelves throughout the world because of the increase consumer demand for healthier natural foods that can increase their overall well-being (Galdeano et al., 2007). The specific health effects of selected probiotic strains have been confirmed by well documented double blind controlled human clinical trials and are becoming increasingly accepted. However, many proposed beneficial effects of probiotics still need further research and more information about their mechanisms of action is needed in order to confirm that they can be useful in the prevention and treatment of other specific diseases (Ouwehand et al., 2002).

2.1 Mechanisms of action of LAB against IBD

It has been shown that LAB and other probiotic microorganims can counteract inflammatory processes in the gut by stabilizing the microbial environment and the permeability of the intestinal barrier, and by enhancing the degradation of enteral antigens and altering their immunogenicity (Isolauri et al., 2004). Some of these disease preventing effects have been recently reviewed (del Carmen et al., 2011); however, a few examples of each of the mechanisms by which LAB exert anti-IBD effects will be given to demonstrate their potential uses.

2.1.1 Modulation of the gut microbiota

The first mechanism that LAB use to prevent IBD is the modulation of the gastrointestinal microbiota of animals. It was reported that *Lactobacillus* (*L.*) *reuteri* could be used to prevent colitis in IL-10 knock-out (KO) mice by increasing the number of LAB in the gastrointestinal tract (Madsen et al., 1999). Neonatal mice presented a decreased concentration of colonic *Lactobacillus* species and an increased concentration of mucosal adherent bacteria. Oral administration of the prebiotic lactulose increased the levels of *Lactobacillus* species and rectal swabbing with *L. reuteri* restored *Lactobacillus* levels to normal and reduced the number of adherent bacteria within the colon. These effects were associated with the attenuation of UC (Madsen et al., 1999). In a placebo-controlled trial, orally administered *L. salivarius* UCC118 reduced prevalence of colon cancer and mucosal inflammatory activity in IL-10 KO mice by modifying the intestinal microbiota in these animals: *Clostridim* (*C.*) *perfringens*, coliforms, and enterococcus levels were significantly reduced in the probiotic fed group (O'Mahony et al., 2001).

Gut microbiota can antagonize pathogenic bacteria by conferring a physiologically restrictive environment inhibiting bacterial adherence and translocation. Probiotic bacteria also decrease luminal pH, as has been demonstrated in patients with UC following ingestion of the probiotic preparation VSL#3, a mixture of 4 lactobacilli strains (*L. plantarum, L. casei, L. acidophilus,* and *L. delbrueckii ssp. bulgaricus*), 3 bifidobacteria strains (*Bifidobacterium* (*B.*) *infantis, B. breve,* and *B. longum*), and 1 strain of *Streptococcus (S.) salivarius ssp. thermophilus* (Venturi et al., 1999).

Another mechanism by which probiotics can exert a positive effect by inhibiting pathogenic microorganisms is by producing antimicrobial substances such as bacteriocins. Several bacteriocins produced by different *Lactobacillus* species have been described (Klaenhammer, 1988). The inhibitory activity of these bacteriocins varies; for example, the probiotic *L. salivarius* UCC118 produces a peptide that inhibits a broad range of pathogens such as *Bacillus, Staphylococcus, Enterococcus, Listeria,* and *Salmonella* species (Flynn et al., 2002). Lacticin 3147, a broad-spectrum bacteriocin produced by a *Lactococcus* (*Lc.*) *lactis* strain, inhibits a range of genetically distinct *C. difficile* isolated from healthy subjects, patients with IBD and from different origins (Rea et al., 2007).

The Symbiotic Instant Mixture (SIM) containing a prebiotic compound inulin, and a combination of probiotic microorganisms (*L. acidophilus* La-5 and *B. lactis* Bb-12) significantly reduced inflammation in transgenic rats that produce human HLA-B27–β2-microglobulin. The effect was enhanced by combination with metronidazole, suggesting a synergistic effect of the combination of antibiotics and probiotics in the treatment of experimental colitis (Schultz et al., 2004). In a double-blind randomized study, the efficacy of VSL#3 combined with antibiotic treatment on the post-operative recurrence of CD was compared with treatment with mesalazine alone. Combination of antibiotic and probiotic treatment was more efficient in prophylaxis of post-operative recurrence of Crohn's disease (Campieri et al., 2000).

2.1.2 Modulation of the host immune responses and enhancement of intestinal barrier function

The intestinal mucosa is the body's first line of defense against pathogenic and toxic invasions from food. After ingestion, orally administered antigens encounter the GALT (Gut Associated Lymphoid Tissue), which is a well-organized immune network that protects the host from pathogens and prevents ingested proteins from hyperstimulating the immune response through a mechanism called oral tolerance (Weiner et al., 1997).

The main mechanism of protection given by the GALT is humoral immune response mediated by secretory IgA (s-IgA) which prevents the entry of potentially harmful antigens, while also interacting with mucosal pathogens without potentiating damage. The stimulation of this immune response could thus be used to prevent certain infectious diseases that enter the host through the oral route. An increasing number of probiotic strains have shown to highly increase s-IgA, therefore the stimulation of IgA-producing cells is often considered a must in probiotic screening trials (O'Sullivan, 2001).

Numerous studies have shown that certain strains of lactobacilli and bifidobacteria can modulate the production of cytokines (mediators produced by immune cells) that are involved in the regulation, activation, growth, and differentiation of immune cells and have been recently reviewed (de Moreno de LeBlanc et al., 2011). These probiotic microorganisms are able to prevent and treat certain inflammatory diseases in the gastrointestinal tract through the repression of pro-inflammatory cytokines. In this sense, the anti-inflammatory effect of yoghurt administration to mice was studied using a TNBS induced acute intestinal inflammation model. The animals that received yoghurt continuously (before and after TNBS) had lower intestinal damages and improved anti-inflammatory response in the gut (de Moreno de LeBlanc et al., 2009). This improvement of the immune response was related with beneficial changes in the intestinal microbiota and differences in the cytokine production and secretion with increases of IL-10 and decreases of IL-17 in the mice given yoghurt. The same yoghurt was analyzed in a mouse model of recurrent inflammation where the administration of the fermented product after the acute episode, when the animals were recovered, prevented the recurrence of the inflammation (Chaves et al., 2011).

One of the central transcription factors mediating inflammatory responses is the nuclear factor κB (NF-κB). NF-κB is required for the transcriptional activation of a number of inflammatory effectors, including IL-8, TNF-α, IL-6, Cox2, iNOS and many others and, its deregulation has been detected in many inflammatory conditions. It was shown that a number of LABs can suppress inflammatory signals mediated by NF-κB. These include strains of the phylogenetically closely related species *L. acidophilus* and *L. johnsonii*, which have been isolated from the human GI tract and form part of the acidophilus complex.

One of the ways by which probiotics can exert immunomodulatory activities is by increasing IL-10 production that can in turn help in preventing certain IBD that are caused by abnormal inflammatory responses (de Moreno de LeBlanc et al., 2011). However, not all probiotic strains act in the same manner. Anti-inflammatory effects, such as stimulation of IL-10 producing cells, are strain dependent traits, and their effectiveness also depends on the concentrations used and the method of administration. By increasing IL-10 levels and in consequence decreasing inflammatory cytokines such as TNF-α, IFN-γ, and IL-17 some LAB can prevent the appearance of local inflammatory diseases and could be used as an adjunct therapy with conventional treatments (de Moreno de LeBlanc et al., 2011).

Enhancement of intestinal barrier function is another mechanism by which probiotic bacteria may benefit the host. The exact mechanisms by which probiotic bacteria enhance gut mucosal barrier function are unclear, but may relate to alterations in mucus or chloride secretion or changes in mucosal cell-cell interactions and celular stability through modulation of cytoeskeletal and tight junction protein phosphorilation (Hilsden et al., 1996, Madsen et al., 2001, Meddings, 2008, Ng et al., 2009, Schmitz et al., 1999).

Oral treatment with VSL#3 normalized colonic physiologic function and barrier integrity in IL-10 KO mice as assessed by short circuit currents, transepithelial potential differences, and mannitol fluxes in excised tissues from mice (Madsen et al., 2001).

L. plantarum and *L. reuteri* enhanced barrier function on a methotrexate-induced enterocolitis rat model (Mao et al., 1996); and colonization of healthy mice intestinal loops with *L. brevis* reduced intestinal permeability (Garcia-Lafuente et al., 2001).

Some probiotic bacteria modify MUC gene expression and mucus secretion. For example, *L. plantarum* 299v induced intestinal mucin gene (MUC2 and MUC3) expression in vitro (Mack et al., 1999). VSL#3 also induced expression of mucins in vitro and increased transepithelial resistance (TER), prevented pathogen-induced decrease in TER, and stabilized tight junctions. In this way, probiotics and protein(s) released by these organisms may functionally modulate the intestinal epithelium of the host by different mechanisms, including the competition of whole organisms for contact with the epithelial surface as well as stabilization of the cytoskeleton and barrier function and the induction of mucin expression (Otte & Podolsky, 2004).

2.1.3 Reduction of the oxidative stress

As a result of recurrent and abnormal inflammation, IBD appears to be associated with oxidative stress, which is characterized by an uncontrolled increase in reactive oxygen species (ROS) concentrations in the gastrointestinal tract. Several studies have established a correlation between the increase in ROS production and disease activity in inflamed biopsies of IBD patients. Therefore, a suggested mechanism by which LAB could prevent inflammation is through the expression of antioxidant enzymes that are able to decrease ROS levels or at least impair their formation.

ROS are normal byproducts of oxygen metabolism (such as superoxide ions, free radicals and peroxides). These small molecules can be generated in aerobiosis by flavoproteins and by phagocytes during inflammatory reactions. At low concentrations, ROS participate in cell signaling and regulatory pathways. However, when present in large amounts, they act to eliminate infectious agents by causing significant damages to cell structures and macromolecular constituents such as DNA, RNA, proteins and lipids. When ROS concentration exceeds the capacity of cell defense systems, toxicity is triggered. It is well known that oxidative damage occurs during the pathogenesis of cancer, cirrhosis, atherosclerosis and other chronic diseases. It has been shown for example that human tumor cells produce and excrete large amounts of H_2O_2 that might participate in tumor invasion and proliferation (Szatrowski & Nathan, 1991). Thus, oxidative stress plays an important role in pathologies of the gastrointestinal tract of humans such as IBD as well as in certain types of cancers.

In order to offset oxidative stress, aerobic cells like those of the normal intestinal mucosa are equipped with a complex antioxidant defense system which includes enzymatic and non-enzymatic components having synergistic and interdependent effects on each other. The normal intestinal mucosa is equipped with a network of antioxidant enzymes such as catalase (Cat), glutathione peroxidase (GSH-Px), glutathione reductase (GR), glutathione-s-transferase (GST), and superoxide dismutase (SOD) that are able to neutralize ROS. The activities of these enzymes are usually balanced to maintain a low and continual steady-state level of ROS; however, the levels of these enzymes are frequently depleted in IBD patients (Kruidenier et al., 2003). Probiotic LAB strains expressing high levels of antioxidant enzymes could increase these enzymatic activities in specific locations of the gastrointestinal tract and could thus contribute to prevent oxidative epithelial damages, giving rise to potential applications for IBD treatment or post-cancer drug treatments. Since few microorganisms produce antioxidant enzymes at the required concentrations to exert biological effects, genetic engineering strategies have been employed to produce antioxidant producing LAB, these will be discussed in another section of this chapter.

Superoxide dismutase (SOD) is considered as the first line of defense against ROS and is a member of the family of metalloenzymes that catalyze the oxido-reduction of superoxide anion to H_2O_2. There are three different forms of this enzyme according to their metal center: manganese, copper-zinc, or iron. These enzymes are found across a broad range of organisms, which can use one, two, or all three enzymes to meet their antioxidant needs. In most *Streptococcus* and *Lactococcus* spp., elimination of ROS is accomplished through the action of Mn-SOD (Sanders et al., 1995). It has also been reported that two strains of *L. fermentum*, named E-3 and E-18, and a strain of *S. thermophilus* showed significant antioxidative activity due to production of Mn-SOD (Kullisaar et al., 2002). Furthermore, recent experimental data indicate that subcutaneous treatment with SOD significantly reduces peroxidation reactions in the inflamed colon and confers significant amelioration of colonic inflammatory changes in a rat model of TNBS colitis (Segui et al., 2004). In addition, treatment with SOD decreases oxidative stress and adhesion molecule upregulation in response to abdominal irradiation in mice.

Catalase is another major antioxidant enzyme that catalyzes the decomposition of hydrogen peroxide into water and oxygen. Catalases are widespread in aerobic (facultative or not) bacteria such as *E. coli* and *Bacillus (B.) subtilis* (Rochat et al., 2005). There are two different classes of catalases according to their active-site composition: one is heme-dependent and the other, also named pseudocatalase is manganese-dependent. By definition, LAB are catalase negative microorganisms, thus genetic modifications are necessary in order for them to produce this important antioxidant enzyme.

3. Genetics of LAB and recombinant protein production strategies

Comparative genomics has facilitated our understanding of LAB evolution and has indicated that a combination of gene gain and loss occurred during the evolution of these bacteria in various environmental habitats (Makarova et al., 2006). Beginning with the genome sequencing of *Lc. lactis* IL-1403 in 1999 (Bolotin et al., 1999), by July 2011 there were 314 LAB genomes (98 complete and 216 in progress) publicly available at the National Center for Biotechnology Information (NCBI, 2011).

Lc. lactis is widely used in the dairy industry and is normally used as the model for other LAB, not only because of its economic importance, but also because of the following features: (1) it has a completely sequenced genome; (2) it is genetically easy to manipulate; and (3) many genetic tools have already been developed for this species.

Studies based on the identification and isolation of wild-type plasmids from *L. lactis* and other LAB have made it possible to develop various cloning vectors. Using molecular biology techniques, these plasmids have been manipulated so that they have become important tools for cloning and studying genes of interest, both those of prokaryotes and eukaryotes. They basically consist of (1) origin of replication (*ori*), (2) selection marker (gene) for antibiotic resistance, and (3) multiple-cloning site.

The expression of heterologous proteins in *Lc. lactis* has been favored both by advances in genetic knowledge and by new developments in molecular biology techniques. Using this duet of tools to obtain increased levels of these proteins and control their production, various vectors containing constitutive or inductive promoters were developed and currently constitute the basis of all expression systems in *Lc. lactis* and other LAB.

3.1 LAB expression systems

LAB are potential candidates to be used as vehicles for the production and delivery of heterologous proteins of vaccinal, medical, or technological interest and various delivery systems are now available for these probiotic microorganisms (Miyoshi et al., 2010). Different genetic engineering strategies in LAB have been used to: improve their carbohydrate fermenting properties (lactose, galactose), increase specific metabolite production (diaceyl, acetoin), produce or increase enzymatic activities (proteolytic enzymes, α- and β-galactosidase, α-amylase), or conferring them the capacity to produce beneficial compounds such as bacteriocins, exopolysaccharide (EPS) and other sugars, vitamins, antioxidant enzymes and anti-inflammatory cytokines (Sybesma et al., 2006).

A series of studies to develop new strains and efficient expression systems has been conducted to use LAB as "cell factories" for the production of proteins (Djordjevic & Klaenhammer, 1998). However, in order for some of these proteins (enzymes and antigens) produced by bacteria to attain the desired biological activity levels, it is necessary that they correctly target specific cellular locations: (1) cytoplasm, (2) membrane, or (3) extracellular environment.

3.1.1 Nisin-Controlled Expression (NICE) system

A versatile and tightly controlled gene expression system was first described in 1995, based on the auto-regulation mechanism of the bacteriocin nisin, denominated the Nisin-Controlled Expression (NICE) system (Kuipers et al., 1995). This system has become one of the most successful and widely used tools for regulated gene expression in Gram-positive bacteria. An extensive overview of the different applications in lactococci and other Gram-positive bacteria has been published 10 years after the NICE system was first published (Mierau & Kleerebezem, 2005) showing its potential use in: (1) over-expression of homologous and heterologous genes for functional studies and to obtain large quantities of specific gene products, (2) metabolic engineering, (3) expression of prokaryotic and eukaryotic membrane proteins, (4) protein secretion and anchoring in the cell envelope, (5) expression of genes with toxic products and analysis of essential genes and (6) large scale applications.

3.1.2 Xylose-Inducible Expression System (XIES)

Another controlled production system to target heterologous proteins to cytoplasm or extracellular medium was described for *Lc. lactis* NCDO2118 based on the use of a xylose-inducible lactococcal promoter, PxylT (Miyoshi et al., 2004). The capacities of the Xylose-Inducible Expression System (XIES) to produce cytoplasmic and secreted proteins were tested using the *Staphylococcus aureus* nuclease gene (*nuc)* fused or not to the lactococcal Usp45 signal peptide. Xylose-inducible gene expression is tightly controlled and resulted in high-level and long-term protein production, and correct targeting either to the cytoplasm or to the extracellular medium. Furthermore, this expression system is versatile and can be switched on or off easily by adding either xylose or glucose, respectively, and has potential as an alternative and useful tool for the production of proteins of interest in *Lc. lactis*.

3.1.3 pValac

A new plasmid vector for DNA delivery using lactococci, the pValac plasmid was constructed by the fusion of: i) an eukaryotic region, allowing the cloning of an antigen of interest under the control of the pCMV eukaryotic promoter to be expressed by a host cell and ii) a prokaryotic region allowing replication and selection of bacteria (Guimaraes et al., 2009). In order to evaluate pValac functionality, the *gfp* ORF was cloned into pValac (pValac:*gfp*) and was analyzed by transfection in PK15 cells. Invasiveness assays of *Lc. lactis inlA*+ strains harbouring pValac:*gfp* into Caco-2 cells demonstrated the potential of pValac to deliver DNA and trigger DNA expression by epithelial cells.

4. Prevention of IBD using genetically modified LAB

As described above, LAB are potential candidates to be used as vehicles for the production and delivery of heterologous proteins of vaccinal, medical, or technological interest and various delivery systems are now available for these probiotic microorganisms (Miyoshi et al., 2010). The use of LAB that produce anti-inflammatory compounds (such as IL-10 and antioxidant enzymes) in the treatment of colitis and IBD will be discussed in the following sections.

4.1 Antioxidant enzyme producing strains

As stated earlier, in IBD patients, oxidative stress occurs as a result of recurrent and abnormal inflammation with an associated increase in ROS concentrations.

Since few microorganisms produce antioxidant enzymes at concentrations required to exert biological effects, genetic engineering strategies have been employed to produce antioxidant producing LAB. Recent reviews have shown the potential uses of such strains in the treatment of IBD using a variety of animal models (Spyropoulos et al., 2010). LAB have been used to locally deliver antioxidant enzymes (such as SOD) directly to the intestines, an important breakthrough since oral administration of SOD is greatly limited by its short lifespan (5-10 min) in the hostile conditions of the gastrointestinal tract. It has been shown that genetically engineered *L. plantarum* and *Lc. lactis* capable of producing and releasing SOD exhibit anti-inflammatory effects in a TNBS colitis model (Han et al., 2006). Another experimental study demonstrated that *L. gasseri* producing manganese SOD had significant anti-inflammatory activity reducing the severity of colitis in IL-10-deficient mice (Carroll et al., 2007). Recent data has shown that SOD producing *L. casei* BL23 was able to significantly attenuate the TNBS-induced damages as shown by higher survival rates, decreased animal weight loss, lower bacterial translocation to the liver and the prevention of damage to the large intestines (LeBlanc et al., 2011). This is in agreement with previous results that have shown that the same SOD-expressing strain of *L. casei* was able to slightly attenuate the colonic histological damage score of a DSS-induced colitis model (Watterlot et al., 2010).

Since *Lc. lactis* has no catalase (as is also the case for the majority of LAB), the *B. subtilis* heme catalase Kat E gene was introduced into this industrially important microorganism giving rise to a strain capable of producing active catalase that can provide efficient antioxidant activity (Rochat et al., 2005). Recently, the heterologous expression of non-heme catalase in bacteria relevant to dairy industries (*L. casei*) has also been reported (Rochat et al., 2006). This latter strain offers the advantage that no exogenous heme has to be added to the culture medium in order to exert an efficient catalase activity. We have previously shown that the catalase-producing *Lc. lactis* strain was able to prevent tumor appearance in the colon (de Moreno de LeBlanc et al., 2008). In another study, we have shown that a catalase producing strain of *L. casei* BL23 significantly decreased the physiological damages caused by the TNBS administration (LeBlanc et al., 2011). This result is similar to those obtained previously where it was shown that both the native strain of *L. casei* BL23 and its catalase producing derivative presented a significant reduction of caecal and colonic inflammatory scores (Rochat et al., 2007).

4.2 IL-10 producing strains

Genetically modified *Lc. lactis* secreting IL-10 provides a novel therapeutic approach for IBD. The first description of *Lc. lactis* that can secrete biologically active IL-10 was published in 2000 (Schotte et al., 2000). In this pioneer study, murine- IL-10 was synthesized as a fusion protein, consisting of the mature part of the eukaryotic protein fused to the secretion signal of the lactococcal Usp45 protein. Intragastric administration of this recombinant *Lc. lactis* strain prevented the onset of colitis in IL-10 KO mice and caused a 50% reduction of the inflammation in DSS -induced chronic colitis (Steidler et al., 2000).

The application of IL-10 producing LAB is not only limited to the treatment of IBD. It was recently shown that treatment of asthma with a *Lc. lactis* expressing murine IL-10 was efficient since this LAB modulated experimental airway inflammation in the mouse model (Marinho et al., 2010). *Lc. lactis* producing recombinant IL-10 used in this study was efficient in suppressing lung inflammation, independently of Treg cells, since this cytokine plays a central role in the regulation of inflammatory cascades, allergen-induced airway inflammation and non-specific airway responsiveness (Tournoy et al., 2000). In another study, it was shown that oral administration of an IL-10-secreting *Lc. lactis* strain could prevent food-induced IgE sensitization in a mouse model of food allergy (Frossard et al., 2007). These studies confirm that IL-10 secreting LAB hold potential for the treatment of many inflammatory diseases where this cytokine acts as a modulating compound.

Although a clear positive effect of these recombinant strains has been demonstrated, the exact mechanism by which the beneficial effect of the IL-10-producing *Lc. lactis* on the mucosa is produced remains unclear. A recent study has demonstrated the uptake of IL-10-secreting *Lc. lactis* by the paracellular route in inflamed mucosal tissue in mouse models of chronic colitis, suggesting that IL-10 production by these LAB residing inside the mucosa in the vicinity of responsive cells can improve the local action of IL-10 in inflamed tissue and the efficiency of the treatment (Waeytens et al., 2008). In another study, it was shown that genetically engineered *Lc. lactis* secreting murine IL-10 could modulate the functions of bone marrow-derived DC in the presence of LPS (Loos et al., 2009). This data suggest that the beneficial effects of IL-10 secreting LAB during chronic colitis might involve inhibition of CD4+ Th17 cells and a reduced accumulation of these cells as well as other immune cells at the site of inflammation.

In another study, we have evaluate the anti-inflammatory effect of the administration of milks fermented by *Lc. lactis* strains that produce IL-10 under the control of the XIES, using a Trinitrobenzenesulfonic acid induced colitis murine model. Mice that received milks fermented by *Lc. lactis* strains producing IL-10 in the cytoplasm (Cyt strain) or secreted to the product (Sec strain) showed lower damage scores in their large intestines, decreased IFN-γ levels in their intestinal fluids and lower microbial translocation to liver, compared to mice receiving milk fermented by the wild-type (Wt) strain or those not receiving any treatment (unpublished data). The results obtained in this study show that the employment of fermented milks as a new form of administration of IL-10 producing *L. lactis* is effective in the prevention of IBD in a murine model. This new approach could lead to the development of novel fermented products with therapeutical purposes; suitable for specific populations suffering from gastrointestinal disorders or prone to acquiring them. Similar strains could also be included in probiotic mixtures together with other strains that are able to prevent inflammation by other mechanisms such as immune stimulation or that possess antioxidant properties.

5. Prospective uses of GM-LAB

Although there is no scientific evidence that supports the notion that genetically modified (GM) foods or microorganisms are dangerous for human consumption, it is necessary to demonstrate that these are innocuous in order to alleviate the fears held by the general public associated with the use of genetically modified organisms, if we want to use designer probiotics to extend the range of applications covered by natural probiotics. Also, the proper design of GM-LAB is essential in order to eliminate the risks of dissipation in the environment and prevent the transfer of certain genes (such as antibiotic resistance genes) to other microorganisms.

The construction of a biological containment system for a genetically modified *Lc. lactis* for intestinal delivery of human IL-10 is an important step forward for the safe use of GM-LAB for human therapeutic purposes (Steidler et al., 2003). In this study, the thymidylate synthase gene of *Lc. lactis* was replaced by the human IL-10 gene, making this strain incapable of growing when deprived of thymidine or thymine. This strain does not contain any antibiotic resistance markers and because of its thymidine auxotrophy, it cannot disseminate in the environment making it one of the safest GM strains ever engineered. This containment system was recently evaluated in CD patients and it was shown that no adverse effects were produced after consuming this GM-LAB and that it could only be recovered in feces when thymidine was added (Braat et al., 2006). Although only preliminary results from this phase 1 trial were obtained, the use of genetically modified bacteria for mucosal delivery of proteins is a feasible strategy in human with chronic intestinal inflammation (Braat et al., 2006).

Intragastric administration of *Lc. lactis* genetically modified to secrete IL-10 *in situ* in the intestine was shown to be effective in healing and preventing chronic colitis in mice. However, its use in humans is hindered by the sensitivity of *Lc. lactis* to freeze-drying and its poor survival in the gastrointestinal tract, reasons for which novel means for more effective mucosal delivery of therapeutic LAB are currently being developed (Huyghebaert et al., 2005a, b, Termont et al., 2006).

6. Conclusion

This review has shown that probiotics have been extensively used in order to prevent and treat inflammatory bowel diseases. The mechanism of action of these beneficial microorganisms, which includes changes in the gut microbiota, stimulation of the host immune responses, enhancement of intestinal barrier function and reduction of the oxidative stress due to their antioxidant properties and antioxidant enzyme production has been demonstrated principally using animal models and in specific human trials. It has recently been suggested that there is a lack of well-designed, large, randomized, placebo-controlled trials that can certify that probiotics are effective in the prevention and treatment of IBD (Mallon et al., 2007). Additional studies such as the double-blind, randomized, placebo-controlled clinical trial of the treatment of relapsing mild-to-moderate ulcerative colitis with the probiotic VSL#3 as adjunctive to a standard pharmaceutical treatment (Tursi et al., 2010) are required to confirm animal data and are necessary to convince the medical and general community of the benefits and potential application of probiotics in the prevention and treatment of IBD.

Although probiotic effects are a strain dependent trait, using modern genetic engineering techniques it is theoretically possible to obtain strains that can exert a variety of beneficial properties. For example, the introduction of antioxidant enzyme genes or cytokine producing capabilities in current probiotic strains that have natural anti-inflammatory properties, such as the ability to modulate the immune dependant anti-inflammatory processes, could generate very useful strains that could be applied in the treatment of a variety of inflammatory diseases. These strains could also be included in treatment protocols since it has been shown that probiotics can enhance the effectiveness of traditional IBD treatments. However, before proposing the genetic modification of anti-inflammatory strains, the innate mechanisms of the potential host strains should be demonstrated in properly designed large scale human clinical trials. These trials are essential in future studies using the engineered strains to demonstrate the differences between the native and modified microorganisms.

The consumption of engineered strains by humans is still highly controversial due to the public perception that genetic manipulation is not "natural". Scientists must perform well-designed studies where the results are divulged to the general populations in order to inform consumers of the obvious beneficial effects these novel techniques can confer with the minimum of risk to their health and to the environment. Throughout the course of history, most novel treatments have met resistance from potential benefactors, it is thus important to show that the potential benefits are highly superior than the risks for novel treatments to be completely accepted by the population as a whole.

7. Acknowledgment

The authors would like to thank the Consejo Nacional de Investigaciones Científicas y Técnicas (CONICET), Agencia Nacional de Promoción Científica y Tecnológica (ANPCyT), Consejo de Investigaciones de la Universidad Nacional de Tucumán (CIUNT), the Centro Argentino Brasileño de Biotecnología (CABBIO), the Coordenação de Aperfeiçoamento de Pessoal de Nível Superior (CAPES), Fundação de Amparo à Pesquisa do Estado de Minas Gerais (FAPEMIG) and the Conselho Nacional de Desenvolvimento Científico e Tecnológico (CNPq) for their financial support.

8. References

Baumgart, D. C., & Sandborn, W. J. (2007). Inflammatory bowel disease: clinical aspects and established and evolving therapies. *The Lancet* 369, pp.1641-1657.

Bolotin, A., Mauger, S., Malarme, K., Ehrlich, S. D., & Sorokin, A. (1999). Low-redundancy sequencing of the entire Lactococcus lactis IL1403 genome. *A Van Leeuw J Microb* 76(1-4), pp.27-76.

Braat, H., Rottiers, P., Hommes, D. W., Huyghebaert, N., Remaut, E., Remon, J. P., van Deventer, S. J., Neirynck, S., Peppelenbosch, M. P., & Steidler, L. (2006). A phase I trial with transgenic bacteria expressing interleukin-10 in Crohn's disease. *Clin Gastroenterol Hepatol* 4(6), pp.754-759.

Campieri, M., Rizzello, F., Venturi, A., Poggioli, G., Ugolini, F., Helwig, U., Amasini, C., Romboli, E., & Gionchetti, P. (2000). Combination of antibiotic and probiotic treatment is efficacious in prophylaxis of post-operative recurrence of Crohn's disease: a randomised controlled study v. mesalazine. *Gastroenterology* 118, pp.A4179.

Carroll, I. M., Andrus, J. M., Bruno-Barcena, J. M., Klaenhammer, T. R., Hassan, H. M., & Threadgill, D. S. (2007). Anti-inflammatory properties of Lactobacillus gasseri expressing manganese superoxide dismutase using the interleukin 10-deficient mouse model of colitis. *Am J Physiol Gastrointest Liver Physiol* 293(4), pp.G729-738.

Chaves, S., Perdigon, G., & de Moreno de LeBlanc, A. (2011). Yoghurt consumption regulates the immune cells implicated in acute intestinal inflammation and prevents the recurrence of the inflammatory process in a mouse model. *J Food Prot* 74(5), pp.801-811.

de Moreno de LeBlanc, A., Chaves, S., & Perdigon, G. (2009). Effect of yoghhurt on the cytokine profile using a murine model of intestinal inflammation. *Eur J Inflam* 7 (2), pp.97-109.

de Moreno de LeBlanc, A., del Carmen, S., Zurita-Turk, M., Santos Rochat, C., van de Guchte, M., Azevedo, V., Miyoshi, A., & LeBlanc, J. G. (2011). Importance of IL-10 modulation by probiotic microorganisms in gastrointestinal inflammatory diseases. *ISRN Gastroenterology* 1(1), pp.1-10 doi:10.5402/2011/892971.

de Moreno de LeBlanc, A., LeBlanc, J. G., Perdigon, G., Miyoshi, A., Langella, P., Azevedo, V., & Sesma, F. (2008). Oral administration of a catalase-producing Lactococcus lactis can prevent a chemically induced colon cancer in mice. *J Med Microbiol* 57(Pt 1), pp.100-105.

del Carmen, S., de Moreno de LeBlanc, A., Miyoshi, A., Santos Rochat, C., Azevedo, V., & LeBlanc, J. G. (2011). Application of probiotics in the prevention and treatment of ulcerative colitis and other inflammatory bowel diseases. *Ulcers* 1(1), pp.1-13. doi:10.1155/2011/841651

Djordjevic, G. M., & Klaenhammer, T. R. (1998). Inducible gene expression systems in Lactococcus lactis. *Mol Biotechnol* 9(2), pp.127-139.

Elson, C. O., & Weaver, C. T. (2003) Experimental mouse models of inflammatory bowel disease: new insights into pathogenic mechanisms in: *Inflammatory bowel disease. From bench to bedside,* S. R. Targan, F. Shanahan, and L. C. Karp, 2nd Edition ed, pp.67-95. Springer Science+Business Media, Inc., New York.

FAO/WHO (2001). Report of a Joint FAO/WHO Expert Consultation on Evaluation of Health and Nutritional Properties of Probiotics in Food Including Powder Milk with Live Lactic Acid Bacteria.

Flynn, S., van Sinderen, D., & Thornton, G. (2002). Characterization of the genetic locus responsible for the production of ABP-118, a novel bacteriocin produced by the probiotic bacterium Lactobacillus salivarius subsp. salivarius UCC118. *Microbiology* 148, pp.973-984.

Frossard, C. P., Steidler, L., & Eigenmann, P. A. (2007). Oral administration of an IL-10-secreting Lactococcus lactis strain prevents food-induced IgE sensitization. *J Allergy Clin Immunol* 119(4), pp.952-959.

Galdeano, C. M., de Moreno de LeBlanc, A., Vinderola, G., Bonet, M. E., & Perdigon, G. (2007). Proposed model: mechanisms of immunomodulation induced by probiotic bacteria. *Clin Vaccine Immunol* 14(5), pp.485-492.

Garcia-Lafuente, A., Antolin, M., Guarner, F., Crespo, E., & Malagelada, J. R. (2001). Modulation of colonic barrier function by the composition of the commensal flora in the rat. *Gut* 48(4), pp.503.

Guimaraes, V., Innocentin, S., Chatel, J. M., Lefevre, F., Langella, P., Azevedo, V., & Miyoshi, A. (2009). A new plasmid vector for DNA delivery using lactococci. *Genet Vaccines Ther* 7, pp.4.

Han, W., Mercenier, A., Ait-Belgnaoui, A., Pavan, S., Lamine, F., van, S., II, Kleerebezem, M., Salvador-Cartier, C., Hisbergues, M., Bueno, L., Theodorou, V., & Fioramonti, J. (2006). Improvement of an experimental colitis in rats by lactic acid bacteria producing superoxide dismutase. *Inflamm Bowel Dis* 12(11), pp.1044-1052.

Head, K. A., & Jurenka, J. S. (2003). Inflammatory bowel disease Part 1: ulcerative colitis--pathophysiology and conventional and alternative treatment options. *Altern Med Rev* 8(3), pp.247-283.

Hilsden, R. J., Meddings, J. B., & Sutherland, L. R. (1996). Intestinal permeability changes in response to acetylsalicylic acid in relatives of patients with Crohn's disease. *Gastroenterology* 110(5), pp.1395-1403.

Huyghebaert, N., Vermeire, A., Neirynck, S., Steidler, L., Remaut, E., & Remon, J. P. (2005a). Development of an enteric-coated formulation containing freeze-dried, viable recombinant Lactococcus lactis for the ileal mucosal delivery of human interleukin-10. *Eur J Pharm Biopharm* 60(3), pp.349-359.

Huyghebaert, N., Vermeire, A., Neirynck, S., Steidler, L., Remaut, E., & Remon, J. P. (2005b). Evaluation of extrusion/spheronisation, layering and compaction for the preparation of an oral, multi-particulate formulation of viable, hIL-10 producing Lactococcus lactis. *Eur J Pharm Biopharm* 59(1), pp.9-15.

Isolauri, E., Salminen, S., & Ouwehand, A. C. (2004). Microbial-gut interactions in health and disease. Probiotics. *Best Pract Res Clin Gastroenterol* 18(2), pp.299-313.

Klaenhammer, T. (1988). Bacteriocins of lactic acid bacteria. *Biochimie* 70, pp.337-349.

Kruidenier, L., van Meeteren, M. E., Kuiper, I., Jaarsma, D., Lamers, C. B., Zijlstra, F. J., & Verspaget, H. W. (2003). Attenuated mild colonic inflammation and improved survival from severe DSS-colitis of transgenic Cu/Zn-SOD mice. *Free Radic Biol Med* 34(6), pp.753-765.

Kuipers, O. P., Beerthuyzen, M. M., de Ruyter, P. G., Luesink, E. J., & de Vos, W. M. (1995). Autoregulation of nisin biosynthesis in Lactococcus lactis by signal transduction. *J Biol Chem* 270(45), pp.27299-27304.

Kullisaar, T., Zilmer, M., & Mikelsaar, M. (2002). Two antioxidative lactobacilli strains as promising probiotics. *Int J Food Microbiol* 72, pp.215-224.

LeBlanc, J. G., de Moreno de LeBlanc, A., Perdigón, G., Miyoshi, A., Rochat, T., Bermudez-Humaran, L., Langella, P., Sesma, F., & Azevedo, V. (2008). Anti-inflammatory properties of Lactic Acid Bacteria: Current knowledge, applications and prospects. *Anti-Infective Agents in Medicinal Chemistry* 7 (3), pp.148-154.

LeBlanc, J. G., del Carmen, S., Miyoshi, A., Azevedo, V., Sesma, F., Langella, P., Bermudez-Humaran, L., Watterlot, L., Perdigon, G., & de Moreno de LeBlanc, A. (2011). Use of superoxide dismutase and catalase expressing lactic acid bacteria to attenuate TNBS induced Crohn's disease in mice. *Journal of Biotechnology*. 151(3), pp.287-293.

Loos, M., Remaut, E., Rottiers, P., & De Creus, A. (2009). Genetically engineered Lactococcus lactis secreting murine IL-10 modulates the functions of bone marrow-derived dendritic cells in the presence of LPS. *Scand J Immunol* 69(2), pp.130-139.

Mack, D. R., Michail, S., Wei, S., McDougall, L., & Hollingsworth, M. A. (1999). Probiotics inhibit enteropathogenic E. coliadherence in vitro by inducing intestinal mucin gene expression. *American Journal of Physiology-Gastrointestinal and Liver Physiology* 276(4), pp.G941.

Madsen, K., Cornish, A., Soper, P., McKaigney, C., Jijon, H., Yachimec, C., Doyle, J., Jewell, L., & De Simone, C. (2001). Probiotic bacteria enhance murine and human intestinal epithelial barrier function. *Gastroenterology* 121(3), pp.580-591.

Madsen, K. L., Doyle, J. S., Jewell, L. D., Tavernini, M. M., & Fedorak, R. N. (1999). Lactobacillus species prevents colitis in interleukin 10 gene-deficient mice. *Gastroenterology* 116, pp.1107-1114.

Makarova, K., Slesarev, A., Wolf, Y., Sorokin, A., Mirkin, B., Koonin, E., Pavlov, A., Pavlova, N., Karamychev, V., Polouchine, N., Shakhova, V., Grigoriev, I., Lou, Y., Rohksar, D., Lucas, S., Huang, K., Goodstein, D. M., Hawkins, T., Plengvidhya, V., Welker, D., Hughes, J., Goh, Y., Benson, A., Baldwin, K., Lee, J. H., Diaz-Muniz, I., Dosti, B., Smeianov, V., Wechter, W., Barabote, R., Lorca, G., Altermann, E., Barrangou, R., Ganesan, B., Xie, Y., Rawsthorne, H., Tamir, D., Parker, C., Breidt, F., Broadbent, J., Hutkins, R., O'Sullivan, D., Steele, J., Unlu, G., Saier, M., Klaenhammer, T., Richardson, P., Kozyavkin, S., Weimer, B., & Mills, D. (2006). Comparative genomics of the lactic acid bacteria. *Proc Natl Acad Sci U S A* 103(42), pp.15611-15616.

Mallon, P., McKay, D., Kirk, S., & Gardiner, K. (2007). Probiotics for induction of remission in ulcerative colitis. *Cochrane Database Syst Rev* (4), pp.CD005573.

Mao, Y., Nobaek, S., Kasravi, B., Adawi, D., Stenram, U., Molin, G., & Jeppsson, B. (1996). The effects of Lactobacillus strains and oat fiber on methotrexate-induced enterocolitis in rats. *Gastroenterology* 111(2), pp.334-344.

Marinho, F. A., Pacifico, L. G., Miyoshi, A., Azevedo, V., Le Loir, Y., Guimaraes, V. D., Langella, P., Cassali, G. D., Fonseca, C. T., & Oliveira, S. C. (2010). An intranasal administration of Lactococcus lactis strains expressing recombinant interleukin-10 modulates acute allergic airway inflammation in a murine model. *Clin Exp Allergy* 40(10), pp.1541-1551.

Meddings, J. (2008). The significance of the gut barrier in disease. *Gut* 57(4), pp.438.

Mierau, I., & Kleerebezem, M. (2005). 10 years of the nisin-controlled gene expression system (NICE) in *Lactococcus lactis*. *Appl. Microbiol. Biotechnol.* 68(6), pp.705-717.

Miyoshi, A., Bermudez-Humaran, L., Pacheco de Azevedo, M., Langella, P., & Azevedo, V. (2010) Lactic Acid Bacteria as Live Vectors: Heterologous Protein Production and Delivery Systems in: *Biotechnology of Lactic Acid Bacteria Novel Applications,* F. Mozzi, R. Raya, and G. Vignolo, pp.161-176. Blackwell Publishing, Ames, Iowa, USA.

Miyoshi, A., Jamet, E., Commissaire, J., Renault, P., Langella, P., & Azevedo, V. (2004). A xylose-inducible expression system for Lactococcus lactis. *FEMS Microbiol Lett* 239(2), pp.205-212.

NCBI. 2011. Microbial genomes (http://www.ncbi.nlm.nih.gov/genomes/MICROBES/microbial_taxtree.html).

Ng, S. C., Hart, A. L., Kamm, M. A., Stagg, A. J., & Knight, S. C. (2009). Mechanisms of action of probiotics: recent advances. *Inflammatory bowel diseases* 15(2), pp.300-310.

Nouaille, S., Ribeiro, L. A., Miyoshi, A., Pontes, D., Le Loir, Y., Oliveira, S. C., Langella, P., & Azevedo, V. (2003). Heterologous protein production and delivery systems for Lactococcus lactis. *Genet Mol Res* 2(1), pp.102-111.

O'Sullivan, D. J. (2001). Screening of intestinal microflora for effective probiotic bacteria. *J Agric Food Chem* 49(4), pp.1751-1760.

O'Mahony, L., Feeney, M., O'Halloran, S., Murphy, L., Kiely, B., Fitzgibbon, J., Lee, G., O'Sullivan, G., Shanahan, F., & Collins, J. K. (2001). Probiotic impact on microbial flora, inflammation and tumour development in IL-10 knockout mice. *Aliment Pharmacol Ther* 15, pp.1219-1225.

Otte, J., & Podolsky, D. (2004). Functional modulation of enterocytes by Gram-positive and Gram-negative microorganisms. *Am J Physiol Gastrointest Liver Physiol* 286, pp.G613-G626.

Ouwehand, A. C., Salminen, S., & Isolauri, E. (2002). Probiotics: an overview of beneficial effects. *Antonie Van Leeuwenhoek* 82(1-4), pp.279-289.

Price, A. B. (1992) Inflammatory Bowel Disease in: *Oxford Textbook of Pathology,* J. O. D. McGee, P. G. Isaacson, and N. A. Wright, pp.1234-1254. Oxford University Press, Oxford. UK.

Rea, M., Clayton, E., & O'Connor, P. (2007). Antimicrobial activity of lacticin 3,147 against clinical Clostridium difficile strains. *J Med Microbiol* 56, pp.940 -946.

Rochat, T., Bermudez-Humaran, L., Gratadoux, J. J., Fourage, C., Hoebler, C., Corthier, G., & Langella, P. (2007). Anti-inflammatory effects of Lactobacillus casei BL23 producing or not a manganese-dependant catalase on DSS-induced colitis in mice. *Microb Cell Fact* 6(22), pp.1-10.

Rochat, T., Gratadoux, J. J., Gruss, A., Corthier, G., Maguin, E., Langella, P., & van de Guchte, M. (2006). Production of a heterologous nonheme catalase by Lactobacillus casei: an efficient tool for removal of H2O2 and protection of Lactobacillus bulgaricus from oxidative stress in milk. *Appl Environ Microbiol* 72(8), pp.5143-5149.

Rochat, T., Miyoshi, A., Gratadoux, J. J., Duwat, P., Sourice, S., Azevedo, V., & Langella, P. (2005). High-level resistance to oxidative stress in Lactococcus lactis conferred by Bacillus subtilis catalase KatE. *Microbiology* 151(Pt 9), pp.3011-3018.

Sanders, J. W., Leenhouts, K. J., Haandrikman, A. J., Venema, G., & Kok, J. (1995). Stress response in Lactococcus lactis: cloning, expression analysis, and mutation of the lactococcal superoxide dismutase gene. *J Bacteriol* 177(18), pp.5254-5260.

Schmitz, H., Barmeyer, C., Fromm, M. L., Runkel, N., Foss, H. D., Bentzel, C. J., Riecken, E. O., & Schulzke, J. D. (1999). Altered tight junction structure contributes to the impaired epithelial barrier function in ulcerative colitis. *Gastroenterology* 116(2), pp.301-309.

Schotte, L., Steidler, L., Vandekerckhove, J., & Remaut, E. (2000). Secretion of biologically active murine interleukin-10 by Lactococcus lactis. *Enzyme and Microbial Technology* 27, pp.761–765.

Schultz, M., Munro, K., Tannock, G. W., Melchner, I., Göttl, C., Schwietz, H., Schölmerich, J., & Rath, H. C. (2004). Effects of feeding a probiotic preparation (SIM) containing inulin on the severity of colitis and on the composition of the intestinal microflora in HLA-B27 transgenic rats. *Clin Diagn Lab Immunol* 11, pp.581-587.

Segui, J., Gironella, M., Sans, M., Granell, S., Gil, F., Gimeno, M., Coronel, P., Pique, J. M., & Panes, J. (2004). Superoxide dismutase ameliorates TNBS-induced colitis by reducing oxidative stress, adhesion molecule expression, and leukocyte recruitment into the inflamed intestine. *J Leukoc Biol* 76(3), pp.537-544.

Spyropoulos, B., Misiakos, E., Fotiadis, C., & Stoidis, C. (2010). Antioxidant Properties of Probiotics and Their Protective Effects in the Pathogenesis of Radiation-Induced Enteritis and Colitis. *Digestive Diseases and Sciences*, pp.1-10.

Steidler, L., Hans, W., Schotte, L., Neirynck, S., Obermeier, F., Falk, W., Fiers, W., & Remaut, E. (2000). Treatment of murine colitis by Lactococcus lactis secreting interleukin-10. *Science* 289(5483), pp.1352-1355.

Steidler, L., Neirynck, S., Huyghebaert, N., Snoeck, V., Vermeire, A., Goddeeris, B., Cox, E., Remon, J. P., & Remaut, E. (2003). Biological containment of genetically modified Lactococcus lactis for intestinal delivery of human interleukin 10. *Nat Biotechnol* 21(7), pp.785-789.

Sybesma, W., Hugenholtz, J., de Vos, W. M., & Smid, E. J. (2006). Safe use of genetically modified lactic acid bacteria in food. Bridging the gap between consumers, green groups, and industry. *Elect. J. Biotechnol.* 9(4), pp.424-448.

Szatrowski, T. P., & Nathan, C. F. (1991). Production of large amounts of hydrogen peroxide by human tumor cells. *Cancer Res* 51(3), pp.794-798.

Termont, S., Vandenbroucke, K., Iserentant, D., Neirynck, S., Steidler, L., Remaut, E., & Rottiers, P. (2006). Intracellular accumulation of trehalose protects Lactococcus lactis from freeze-drying damage and bile toxicity and increases gastric acid resistance. *Appl Environ Microbiol* 72(12), pp.7694-7700.

Tournoy, K. G., Kips, J. C., & Pauwels, R. A. (2000). Endogenous interleukin-10 suppresses allergen-induced airway inflammation and nonspecific airway responsiveness. *Clin Exp Allergy* 30(6), pp.775-783.

Tursi, A., Brandimarte, G., Papa, A., Giglio, A., Elisei, W., Giorgetti, G. M., Forti, G., Morini, S., Hassan, C., Pistoia, M. A., Modeo, M. E., Rodino, S., D'Amico, T., Sebkova, L., Sacca, N., Di Giulio, E., Luzza, F., Imeneo, M., Larussa, T., Di Rosa, S., Annese, V., Danese, S., & Gasbarrini, A. (2010). Treatment of relapsing mild-to-moderate ulcerative colitis with the probiotic VSL#3 as adjunctive to a standard pharmaceutical treatment: a double-blind, randomized, placebo-controlled study. *Am J Gastroenterol* 105(10), pp.2218-2227.

Venturi, A., Gionchetti, P., Rizzello, F., Johansson, R., Zucconi, E., Brigidi, P., Matteuzzi, D., & Campieri, M. (1999). Impact on the composition of the faecal flora by a new probiotic preparation: preliminary data on maintenance treatment of patients with ulcerative colitis. *Aliment Pharmacol Ther* 13(8), pp.1103-1108.

Waeytens, A., Ferdinande, L., Neirynck, S., Rottiers, P., De Vos, M., Steidler, L., & Cuvelier, C. A. (2008). Paracellular entry of interleukin-10 producing Lactococcus lactis in inflamed intestinal mucosa in mice. *Inflamm Bowel Dis* 14(4), pp.471-479.

Watterlot, L., Rochat, T., Sokol, H., Cherbuy, C., Bouloufa, I., Lefevre, F., Gratadoux, J. J., Honvo-Hueto, E., Chilmonczyk, S., Blugeon, S., Corthier, G., Langella, P., & Bermudez-Humaran, L. G. (2010). Intragastric administration of a superoxide dismutase-producing recombinant Lactobacillus casei BL23 strain attenuates DSS colitis in mice. *Int J Food Microbiol* 144(1), pp.35-41.

Weiner, H. L., Gonnella, P. A., Slavin, A., & Maron, R. (1997). Oral tolerance: cytokine milieu in the gut and modulation of tolerance by cytokines. *Res Immunol* 148(8-9), pp.528-533.

14

Prognostic Relevance of Subjective Theories of Illness on the Clinical and Psychological Parameters in Irritable Bowel Syndrome Patients – A Longitudinal Study

A. Riedl[1], J. Maass[1], A. Ahnis[1], A. Stengel[1],
H. Mönnikes[2], B.F. Klapp[1] and H. Fliege[1]
[1]*Division of Psychosomatic Medicine and Psychotherapy, Department of Medicine, Charité-Universitätsmedizin Berlin, Campus Mitte*
[2]*Department of Medicine and Institute of Neurogastroenterology, Martin-Luther-Hospital*
Germany

1. Introduction

Irritable bowel syndrome (IBS) is a highly prevalent functional gastrointestinal disorder that is characterised by abdominal pain associated with altered stool frequency and/or consistency. The criteria for IBS were last specified by the Rome Committee in 2006 (Drossmann et al., 2006):

Chronic or recurrent abdominal pain or symptoms of not less than three months duration during the last 6 months and associated with not less than 2 of the following 3 criteria: • improvement in the symptoms following defecation • alteration in stool frequency and/or • alteration in stool consistency

Table 1. Rome III criteria for the diagnosis of IBS, adapted from Drossman et al., 2006

While the exact cause of IBS is still not known, multiple factors, such as visceral hypersensitivity (alterations in gastrointestinal sensitivity), motility disturbances, psychosocial factors and immune-mediated factors, are thought to contribute to the symptom complex of IBS (Mathew & Bhatia, 2009). These changes seem to be triggered by stress (Mayer et al., 2001). However, there is no uniform, scientifically-based model of the etiology of IBS that patients could use for orientation.

Patients with IBS have been repeatedly described as lacking health-related quality of life compared to healthy controls (Dancey et al., 2002). The majority of patients with IBS symptoms do not consult a healthcare professional. One of the main reasons that patients decline to consult a doctor is not the severity of symptoms but rather the fear of a serious illness (Whitehead et al., 2002) or other psychological or somatic comorbidities (Riedl et al., 2008).

The course of chronic diseases puts high demands on the coping behaviours of patients. To cope with a chronic disease, patients develop explanations, convictions and expectations concerning the origin of the disease that can be subsumed as subjective theories of illness (Faller, 1993). Based on their research into subjective causes, patients retrospectively ascribe a meaning to their illnesses by attempting to understand why they occurred in the first place, whether they could be influenced in the future and how relapses could be prevented. This subjective theorisation contributes to patients' coping mechanisms (Hampson et al., 1990). Because of these subjective theories of illness, the patient is enabled to make predictions and decisions concerning therapeutic options or the handling of their medical conditions (Faller, 1993). Furthermore, there is evidence that subjective theories of illness affect compliance and cooperation in the relationship between the doctor and the patient (Leventhal et al., 1980) and the restoration of fitness for work (Lacroix et al., 1991, Schiaffino et al., 1998). Subjective causal assumptions are especially important for the sufferers of diseases for which a uniform, evidence-based etiological model providing patients with orientation has not been developed, as is the case for IBS. Subjective causal assumptions and their effects on clinical parameters in IBS and on disease perception are poorly understood and have been insufficiently evaluated.

This study is based on an adaptation (Figure 1) of the Common Sense Model of Illness Representation by Leventhal et al. (1980).

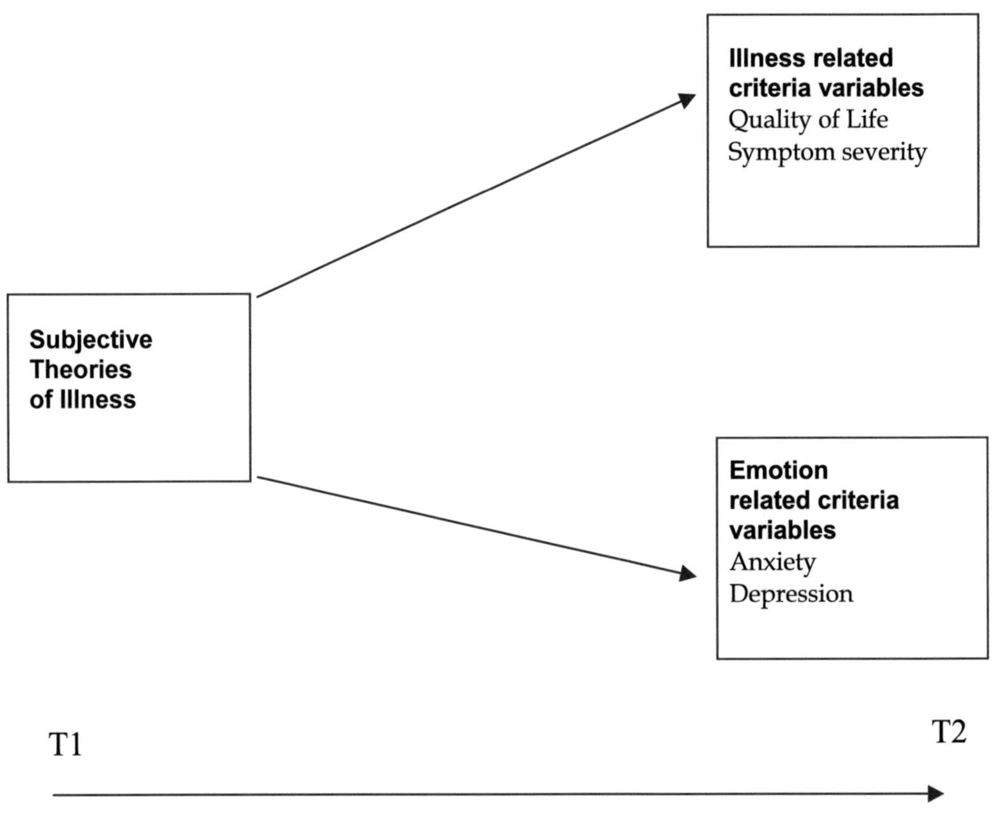

Fig. 1. Adaptation of the Common Sense Model of Illness Representation by Leventhal et al. (1980); Hagger & Orbell (2003)

This model describes the link between subjective theories of illness, coping behaviour and quality of life and is considered the most influential theoretical model regarding the regulatory processes of patients dealing with diseases (Leventhal et al., 1980) . Leventhal et al. stated that patients develop ideas about their illnesses within five representational dimensions: identity; causal attributions; expectations of duration; expectations of consequences; and perceived control and curability. The identity of an illness is characterised by its symptoms and the diagnosis itself. The search for the causes of a disease (causal attributions) represents a fundamental part of subjective theories of illness. In addition to this retrospective cognition, these subjective theories of illness also contain prospective assumptions, including expectations of disease duration and its consequences. Leventhal et al. (1980) also described anticipated control as a dimension of subjective theories of illness. In the present study, we focused on the investigation of causal attributions.

Evidence for the validity of the Common Sense Model of Illness Representation (Leventhal et al., 1980) has been found in various cross-sectional studies (Hagger & Orbell, 2003; Rutter & Rutter, 2002). However, few studies have validated this model on the longitudinal axis (Hagger & Orbell, 2003; Kaptein et al., 2003), and the only longitudinal study investigating the influence of subjective theories of illness in IBS patients showed that theories remained stable over one year (Rutter & Rutter, 2007). "Psychological causal assumptions" and "severity of expected consequences" proved to be predictors for anxiety and depression. However, subjective theories of illness were not significantly predictive for the "quality of life"parameter (Rutter & Rutter, 2007). Because they did not examine the possible consequences of subjective theories on clinical symptoms in this study, no conclusion can be drawn concerning somatic outcome.

We recently reported a correlation between subjective theories of illness, symptom severity and quality of life. Due to this study' s cross-sectional study design, we were not able to test for causality at this time (Riedl et al., 2009).

Therefore, we designed the following study to examine whether patients' causal attributions would have prognostic relevance with regard to symptoms and patient quality of life over the course of an illness.

Based on the Common Sense Model, this study evaluated whether subjective theories of illness in IBS patients could affect clinical outcome parameters, such as symptom severity, quality of life, anxiety and depression, after one year. Furthermore, we evaluated whether subjective theories of illness change over time in IBS patients.

2. Methods

2.1 Measurements

2.1.1 Subjective theories of illness

To encompass a wide range of causal assumptions in addition to the causal assumptions questionnaire (SKT) by Faller (Faller & Walitzer, 2001), we included a second Cause Questionnaire that was developed by Fliege (Fliege et al., 2003) and was originally intended for chronic inflammatory bowel disease (IBD) patients; it was subsequently modified for IBS (Riedl et al., 2009). This latter questionnaire includes the items "dysfunctional stress regulation" and "fatalism", which are two elements that are not covered by the SKT.

2.1.2 Causal assumptions questionnaire (SKT)

The SKT (Faller & Walitzer, 2001) includes 16 items that are rated on a 5-point response scale. Validated in 197 patients attending a psychotherapist clinic, this questionnaire displays good psychometric characteristics. The items are assigned to four scales by factor analysis. These scales are as follows:

Scale I, Intrapsychic causes, with four items (Could your disorder result from (1) internal conflicts, (2) internal anxiety, (3) poor coping with problems and/or (4) lack of self-confidence?);

Scale II, Social causes, with three items (stress through worries about family and partnership setting, lack of understanding through other people and conflicts with other people);

Scale III, Interpersonal causes, with six items (unhealthy lifestyle, difficulties in professional life, common life stress, environmental stress, financial problems and social circumstances); and

Scale IV, Somatic causes, with three items (somatic disease, poor circulation and weather).

The parameters for internal consistency, expressed as Cronbach' s α, are good for scales I and III (scale I: T1 = 0.84, T2 = 0.93; scale III: T1 = 0.7, T2 = 0.68) and satisfactory for scales II and IV (scale II: T1 = 0.76, T2 = 0.57; scale IV: T1 = 0.56, T2 = 0.57).

2.1.3 Cause questionnaire for chronic IBD patients

For our purposes, the original questionnaire developed by Fliege et al. (2003) to assess causal assumptions in IBS patients required a change of instructions. The term chronic IBD was replaced with IBS, but the original wording of the items was retained. The questionnaire includes 16 items that are assigned to five scales (dysfunctional stress regulation, interactionality, lifestyle, physiology and fatalism) with 5-point response formats. For the present study, only two scales were included ("dysfunctional stress regulation" and "fatalism") to enrich the SKT, which lacks these items.

The scale "fatalism" only comprises two items: higher power and destiny/fate (Spearman' s r: T1 = 0.56, T2 = 0.55).

The scale "dysfunctional stress regulation" is based on four items: wrong stress coping, high workload, inability to relax and disposition to be overly sensitive to negative situations (Cronbach' s α: T1 = 0.76, T2 = 0.78).

2.1.4 Outcome

2.1.5 Beck Depression Inventory (BDI)

The BDI (Hautzinger, 1991) is a self-rating scale for the assessment of depressive symptoms; it contains 21 items (Cronbach' s α T1 = 0.86, T2 = 0.72).

2.1.6 Hospital Anxiety and Depression Scale (HADS)

The HADS (Herrmann, 1997), which is a 14-item scale, was specifically developed for use by individuals with somatic diseases. It measures patients degrees of anxiety and depression based on their self-ratings. For the present study, only the anxiety scale was used (Cronbach' s α: T1 = 0.76, T2 = 0.78).

2.1.7 Health-related quality of life (SF-12)

The SF-12 (Bullinger, 1996) is a brief version of the SF-36, which measures two components of quality of life: mental well being and physical condition (Cronbach' s α: T1 = 0.67 and 0.64, T2 = 0.66 and 0.71).

2.1.8 Questionnaire for gastrointestinal symptoms

The somatic parameters were assessed with the aid of a questionnaire that was specifically developed for and routinely employed by the Outpatient Clinic for Gastrointestinal Motility Disorders and Functional Gastrointestinal Diseases at Charité University Medical Center. Subjects were asked to check the frequency and severity of 13 symptoms that are typical of irritable bowel syndrome (pain, pressure, cramps in the upper and lower abdomen, the feeling of being bloated, the unpleasant passing of gas, diarrhoea, constipation, alternating diarrhoea and constipation, the feeling that the bowels have not been completely evacuated and loud or bothersome bowel sounds [borborygmi]).

The total scores were calculated as the sum of the products of frequencies ("How frequently have you suffered from your symptoms", rated on a scale from 0 = never to 4 = constantly) and severities ("How bad were your symptoms", rated on a scale from 0 = no symptoms to 5 = very severe) of the monitored symptoms (Cronbach's α: T1 = 0.88, T2 = 0.75).

3. Participants and study design

Patients received questionnaires on hand-held computers during their waits at the Outpatient Clinic for Gastrointestinal Motility Disorders and Functional Gastrointestinal Diseases at Charité-University Medical Center, Campus Virchow (Berlin, Germany). Patients were included in the study based on the Rome III criteria following a medical examination (all subtypes were included using the Bristol stool scale). The criteria for exclusion were as follows: age <18 years, lack of cooperation and the indication of another disease explaining the symptoms (such as chronic inflammatory bowel disease (IBD), lactose or fructose intolerance, malignant disease or the abuse of alcohol other drugs).

After the criteria for inclusion or exclusion had been checked, 88 patients were able to be included in the study at T1. Patient recruitment at T1 took place from November 2006 to March 2007. Questionnaires were mailed to these 88 patients after one year for follow-up evaluations (T2, November 2007 to March 2008). Of these patients, 49 subjects returned the questionnaire, and 3 had moved to unknown addresses. Of the 49 data sets received, 44 were completed and included in the follow-up study.

The sample comprised 30 females (68%) and 14 males (32%). The mean age was 46 years (SD = 15.23 years, range = 19-72 years).

4. Statistical analysis

All analyses were carried out with the statistics program SPSS, version 14.0. The descriptive parameters were calculated for each scale, and the normal distribution was assessed by the Kolmogorov- Smirnov test.

Intercorrelation was calculated by the Pearson correlation coefficient, and predictors for clinical and psychological outcome criteria of causal assumptions were tested by multiple stepwise linear regression analyses. All scales covering the subjective theories of illness at T1 that significantly correlated with the criteria variables at T2 (see Table 2) were included in the regression analyses. Furthermore, the base level (T1) of criteria variables was enclosed as an autoregressor in all regression analyses. Other predicting effects that exceeded the autoregressor can be considered to be robust.

5. Results

5.1 Characteristics of causal assumptions at T1 and T2

The SKT was dominated by the "intrapsychic causes scale" (M = 2.50, SD = 0.18 at T1 and M = 2.55, SD = 0.17 at T2) and the "social causes scale" (M = 1.89, SD = 0.11 at T1 and M = 2.02, SD = 0.97 at T2), followed by "somatic causal attributions" (M = 1.78, SD = 0.11 at T1 and M = 2.08, SD = 0.12 at T2) and "interpersonal causal attributions" (M = 1.80, SD = 0.13 at T1 and M = 2.02, SD = 0.13 at T2).

In the causal assumptions questionnaire (SKT), the highest mean corresponded to the scale "dysfunctional stress regulation" (M = 1.97, SD = 0.15 at T1 and M = 2.07, SD = 0.13 at T2). The "fatalism scale" produced the lowest meanof all scales (M = 0.51, SD = 0.13 at T1 and M = 0.55, SD = 0.12 at T2).

5.2 Stability of causal assumptions over the course of one year

To assess the stability of causal assumptions over the course of one year, mean comparisons were performed using a t-test.

Except for the scale "somatic causes" (p = 0.01), there were no significant changes supporting consistency in the attribution of causal assumptions. The score of "somatic causes" increased after one year.

5.3 Correlations and regression analyses

Table 2 depicts the correlations of causal assumptions at T1 and outcome at T2.

	Physical QoL[1] at T2	*Mental QoL [1] at T2*	*Anxiety at T2*	*Depression at T2*	*Symptom severity at T2*
Causal assumptions at T1					
Dysfunctional Stressregulation	.31*	-.41**	.65**	.26	.36*
Fatalism	-.23	-.36*	.44*	.53*	.25
Intrapsychic causes	.21	-.39**	.61**	.44**	.34*
Interpersonal causes	.07	-.44**	.58**	.51	.27
Social causes	.03	-.29	.44**	.19	.47**
Somatic causes	-.37*	.02	.12	.01	.21

[1]QoL = Quality of life
Note * $p < 0.05$, ** $p < 0.01$

Table 2. Correlations between causal assumptions at T1 and outcome variables at T2.

No differences between causal assumptions with regard to age, gender or IBS-subgroups were found. Thus, these socio-demographic variables were not considered for later analysis. To examine the overall relationship between the predictor variables and the outcome variables, all correlating predictors were entered stepwise in a linear regression analysis.

Table 3 shows the last step of each regression. β (beta coefficient) is the standardised regression coefficient of the last step of each regression. It shows, which regressor (in this

Outcome Symptom Severity					
Predictors	*β*	*R^2 Step 1*	*ΔR^2 Step 2*		
Social causes	0.33*	0.22 ($p < 0.01$)			
Symptom intensity at T1	0.43**		0.17 ($p < 0.01$)		
Outcome Depression					
Predictors	*β*	*R^2 Step 1*	*ΔR^2 Step 2*	*ΔR^2 Step 3*	
Fatalism	0.05	0.31 ($p < 0.001$)			
Interpersonal causes	0.15		0.08 ($p < 0.05$)		
Value depression at T1	0.74***			0.35 ($p < 0.001$)	
Outcome Anxiety					
Predictors	*β*	*R^2 Step 1*	*ΔR^2 Step 2*	*ΔR^2 Step 3*	
Dysfunctional stress regulation	0.25*	0.42 ($p < 0.001$)			
Interpersonal causes	0.25*		0.12 ($p < 0.001$)		
Anxiety at T1	0.46**			0.11 ($p < 0.001$)	
Outcome Mental Quality of Life					
Predictors	*β*	*R^2 Step 1*	*ΔR^2 Step 2*	*ΔR^2 Step 3*	
Interpersonal causes	0.25	0.21 ($p < 0.01$)			
Dysfunctional stress regulation	-0.09		0.08 ($p < 0.05$)		
Psychological quality of life at T1	0.71***			0.27 ($p < 0.001$)	
Outcome Physical Quality of Life					
Predictors	*β*	*R^2 Step 1*	*ΔR^2 Step 2*	*ΔR^2 Step 3*	*ΔR^2Step4*
Somatic causes	-0.13	0.13 ($p < 0.05$)			
Dysfunctional stress regulation	0.28*		0.11 ($p < 0.05$)		
Fatalism	-0.35*			0.08 ($p < 0.05$)	
Physical quality of life at T1	0.49**				0.18 ($p < 0.001$)

β = standardised coefficient; Regression value of the last step

*** < 0.001, **p = 0.01; * p < 0.05.

Table 3. Regressions of causal assumptions and autoregressor (T1) of all outcome variables (T2).

case subjective causal assumptions) makes the maximum contribution to the prognosis of the dependent variable (in this case outcome variables).
R^2, the coefficient of determination, is a measure of the portion of the variance explained, ΔR^2 stands for the changes in the amount of the variance explained effected by the subjective causal assumptions entered in the last step.

5.3.1 Causal assumptions and IBS symptom severity

In addition to the autoregressor, symptom severity was only predicated by the scale "social causes" (ß = 0.33, $p < 0.05$). Social causal assumptions accounted for 22% of the variance in symptom severity at T2.

5.3.2 Causal assumptions and depression

The first step showed the scale "fatalism" to be a significant predictor for depression. It explained 31% of the recorded variance (step 1: *ß* = 0.55; $p < 0.001$). Another 8% of this variance was explained in the second step by the scale "interpersonal reasons" (step 2: *ß* = 0.34; $p < 0.05$). In tests, the influence of causal assumptions was not significant beyond the influence of the base level of depression at T1. Thus, the base level for depression proved to be the only significant predictor of depression at T2 (*ß* = 0.74; $p < 0.001$) (35% of variance explained).

5.3.3 Causal assumptions and anxiety

Causal assumptions explained 54% of the variance of "anxiety" at T2 (Table 3). Furthermore, the scales "dysfunctional stress regulation" and "interpersonal causes" were equally prognostic for "anxiety".

5.3.4 Causal assumptions and mental quality of life

Causal assumptions explained 29% of the variance, and the base level explained another 27% of the variance. No significant effects of the causal assumptions "interpersonal cause" (step 1: ß = -0.46, $p < 0.01$; step 2: ß = -0.35, $p < 0.05$) and "dysfunctional stress regulation" (step 2: ß = -0.30, $p < 0.05$) were found after checking for the base level of mental quality of life at T1. Thus, no significant effect of causal assumptions on mental quality of life was found after considering the autoregressor.

5.3.5 Causal assumptions and physical quality of life

The scales "dysfunctional stress regulation" and "fatalism" significantly predicted patients' physical quality of life at T2 (19% of variance explained).

6. Discussion

In this study, we longitudinally assessed subjective theories of illness in IBS and their prognostic relevance based on the Common Sense Model of Illness. Two questions were asked: 1.) do subjective theories of illness in IBS change over time, and 2.) can they predict clinical and psychological outcomes?
All causal items had relatively small means and standard deviations, indicating that patients likely give little significance to single causes. This finding may represent a study limitation. It might be possible that the questionnaires that were used did not properly reflect causal

assumptions. "Intrapsychic factors", "social factors" and "dysfunctional stress regulation" received the strongest agreement. In IBS patients, causal assumptions that were based on stress and intrapsychic factors are particularly relevant because they reflect scientific aetiology models that show connections between coping experience and symptom reinforcement.

We assessed beliefs at two time points. Except for the scale "somatic causes", the results of the comparisons of the means of causal assumptions at T1 and T2 were not significant. Therefore, our results indicate a consistency of causal assumptions over time and support known data regarding IBS (Rutter & Rutter, 2007). Leventhal et al. (1980) argued that patients' illness representations are constantly being updated as new illness experiences and knowledge are acquired. This argument cannot be supported by our findings, except for those in the "somatic causes" scale, possibly due to the fact that over time, IBS patients increase their knowledge about scientific, physical explanations for their symptoms. Similar to Rutter & Rutter (2007), we predominantly found no change in individuals' illness representations across the two measured time points. This finding supports the hypothesis that IBS is a chronic disease and distinguishes it from Leventhal' s model, which was designed largely around acute illnesses. The stability of illness cognitions in IBS patients over time is an important clinical finding that, if replicated in further, larger studies, will provide strong indicators for psychological interventions with these patients.

While Rutter and Rutter (2007) used longitudinal data but only predicted psychological outcomes, we focused this study on the prediction of variables of clinical outcomes such as symptom severity, allowing us to demonstrate for the first time that subjective theories of illness have prognostic relevance in IBS. Through these results, we show a strong predictive value of subjective theories of illness based on symptom severity and psychological factors (anxiety).

Via the direct regression path, subjective causal assumptions explained 22% of the variance in symptom severity, in which particularly social causes significantly predicted symptom severity after one year. Patients who strongly attributed their illnesses to social causes (stress through worries in family and partnership setting, lack of understanding through other people and conflicts with other people) reported elevated symptom severity after one year.

Furthermore, subjective causal assumptions explained 54% of the variance in anxiety after one year. Patients who attributed the cause of their disease to dysfunctional stress regulation (coping with stress incorrectly, high workload, inability to relax or disposition to be overly sensitive to negative situations) or interpersonal causes (unhealthy lifestyle, difficulties in professional life, common life stress, environmental stress, financial problems or social circumstances) showed higher values for anxiety after one year.

Subjective theories of illness proved to be predictive with regard to physical quality of life but not predictive of mental quality of life. Patients who attributed the cause of their illnesses to fatalism (higher power and destiny/fate) reported an impaired physical quality of life, while causal attribution to dysfunctional stress regulation resulted in an improvement of physical quality of life after one year.

Subjective theories of illness were not predictive for depression during the course of the study. This finding could be due to the fact that depression is considered to be more of a chronic comorbidity in IBS patients and is thus a stable variable that is weakly influenced by subjective theories of illness. However, in the first step of the regression analysis, 31% of the

variance for depression was explained by fatalist causal assumptions, and only after adjusting for the base level did this predictive value become insignificant, suggesting that fatalism and depression may be confounded in these responses.
Our results confirm the presumption of the Common Sense Model of Illness because they show that subjective theories of illness have direct and fundamental prognostic value for clinical and psychological factors in IBS. The longitudinal prognostic relations of subjective theories of illness to symptom severity, anxiety and physical quality of life are still preserved when the base level of criteria variables is adjusted for statistical controls. Thus, the effect of the predictors can be considered robust.
Our findings point to the relevance of subjective causal assumptions in IBS by revealing several partly differential connections between single causal dimensions and outcome variables. Some of the study weaknesses include a relatively small sample size and a significant loss to follow-up. The small sample size is limiting given the number of variables that could be included in the regressions.

7. Conclusion

This study of the treatment of IBS patients is significant with regard to the information gain that occurs in subjective theories of illness and to the relevance of these theories for symptoms of anxiety and depression and for quality of life and symptom severity.
Social causal attributions that relate to interpersonal and domestic conflicts are prognostic for perceived increased symptom severity. It should be noted that subjective theories of illness point to a worsened disease course in IBS patients, which should be sufficient to include maladaptive causal assumptions in the focus of (psycho-) therapeutic treatment.
Dysfunctional stress regulation (coping with stress incorrectly, high workload, inability to relax or disposition to be overly sensitive to negative situations) and interpersonal causes (unhealthy lifestyle, difficulties in professional life, common life stress, environmental stress, financial problems or social circumstances) have prognostic value for the increased occurrence of anxieties. This causal relation could be the product of a chronic distress burden caused by real social problems and therefore might be considered an indirect prognostic factor for the development of anxiety in IBS. IBS patients have a lifetime prevalence (up to 90%) of developing a psychiatric comorbidity such as an anxiety disorder (Lydiard et al., 1993). Thus, it becomes evident that the knowledge of prognostic factors, such as subjective theories of illness, is valuable for preventive and therapeutic care. To counteract the development of anxious or depressive symptoms in the course of IBS, adverse subjective theories of illness should be recognised as early as possible and adapted if necessary.
The medical histories of patients with IBS should include an assessment of subjective theories of illness. It seems especially important that, for the clinical course of the disease, physicians inquire about and treat adverse prognostic factors in the social environment (stress through worries in family and partnership setting, lack of understanding through other people and conflicts with other people) as early as possible. The knowledge of the content and significance of the concepts that patients develop to explain their disease will enable healthcare professionals to better understand treatment approaches and patient expectations and improve doctor-patient relationships in the treatment of irritable bowel syndrome.

8. References

Bullinger, M. (1996). Assessment of health related quality of life with the SF-36 Health Survey. *Rehabilitation*, 35(3)

Dancey, C. P., Hutton-Young S. A. , Moye S. & Devins G.M. (2002). Perceived stigma, illness intrusiveness and quality of life in men and women with irritable bowel syndrome. *Psychology, Health & Medicine* 7(4), 381-395

Drossmann, D.A, Corrazziari, E., Delvaux, M., Spiller, R., Talley, N.J. &Thompson, W.G (2006). Rome III: The functional Gastrointestinal Disorders. Degnon Associates (McLean,VA)

Faller, H. (1993). Subjective illness theories: determinants or epiphenomena of coping with illness? A comparison of methods in patients with bronchial cancer. Z Psychosom Med Psychoanal. , 39(4), 356-74

Faller, H. & Walitzer, S. (2001). Causal attribution and personality in psychotherapy patients. *Z Psychosom Med P sychother*, 47(3), 234-49

Fliege, H., Drandarevski, A., Klapp, B.F. & Rose, M. (2003). Causal attribution of patients with inflammatory bowel syndrome. *Z Klin Psychol Psychother*, 32(4), 276-285

Hagger, M. & Orbell, S. (2003). A Meta-Analytic Review of the Common-Sense Model of Illness Representation. *Psychology and Health*, 18, 141-184

Hampson, S.E., Galsgow, R.E. & Toobert, D.J. (1990). Personal models of diabetes and their relations to self-care activities. *Health Psychology,*, 9, 632-646

Hautzinger, M. (1991). The Beck Depression Inventory in clinical practice. Nervenarzt, 62(11), 689 - 96

Herrmann, C.(1997). International experiences with the Hospital Anxiety and Depression Scale - a review of validation data and clinical results. *J Psychosom Res*, 42(1), 17-41

Kaptein, A.A., Scharloo, M., Helder, D.I., Kleijn, W.C., Van Korlaar, I.M. & Woertman, M.(2003). Representation of chronic illnesses. In: LD cameron & H. Leventhal 2003. *The Self-regulation of health and illness behaviour* (pp-97-118). London: Routledge Taylor & Francis Group

Lacroix, J.M., Martin, B., Avendano, M. & Goldstein, R. (1991). Symptom schemata in chronic respiratory patients. *Health Psychology*, 10, 268-273

Leventhal, H., Meyer, D. & Nerenz, D. (1980). The common sense representation of illness danger. *Contributions to medical psychology*, 2, 7-30

Lydiard, R. B., Fossey, M.D., Marsh, W. & Ballenger, J. C. (1993). Prevalence of psychiatric disorders in patients with irritable bowel syndrome. *Psychosomatics*, 34, 229-234

Mathew, P. & Bhatia S.J. (2009). Pathogenesis and management of irritable bowel syndrome. *Trop Gastroenterol*, 30(1), 19-25

Mayer, E.A., Naliboff, B.D. & Chang, L. (2001). Basic pathophysiologic mechanisms in Irritable Bowel Syndrome. *Dig Dis*, 19, 212-218

Riedl, A., Schmidtmann, M., Stengel, A., Goebel, M., Klapp, B.F. & Mönnikes, H. (2008) Somatic Comorbidities of the Irritable Bowel Syndrome - A systematic analysis. *J Psychosom Res*, 64(6), 573-582

Riedl, A., Maass, J., Schmidtmann, M., Fliege, H., Klapp, B.F. & Mönnikes, H. (2009). Subjective Theories of Illness affects Clinical and Psychological Outcome in Patients with Irritable Bowel Syndrome. *J Psychosom Res*, 67(5), 449-55

Rutter, C.L & Rutter, D. (2002). Illness representation, coping and outcome in irritable bowel syndrome (IBS). *British Journal of Health Psychology*, 7, 377-391

Rutter, C.L. & Rutter, R. (2007). Longitudinal Analysis of the Illness Representation Model in Patients with Irritable Bowel Syndrome (IBS). Illness representation, coping and outcome in IBS. *Journal of Health Psychology*, 12(1), 141-148

Schiaffino, K.M., Shawaryn, M.A. & Blum, D. (1998). Examining the impact of illness representations on psychological adjustment to chronic illnesses. *Health Psychol* ,17, 262-268

Whitehead, W. E., Palsson, O. & Jones, K. R. (2002). Systematic review of the comorbidity of irritable bowel syndrome with other disorders: What are the causes and implications? *Gastroenterology*, 122, 1140-1156

15

Modulation of Visceral Pain by Stress: Implications in Irritable Bowel Syndrome

Agata Mulak, Muriel Larauche and Yvette Taché
University of California Los Angeles
USA

1. Introduction

Stress-related changes in visceral perception resulting in enhanced sensitivity to physiological and/or experimental visceral stimuli along with hypervigilance are considered to play a critical role in the pathophysiology of irritable bowel syndrome (IBS) (Elsenbruch et al., 2010; Mayer et al., 2008; Mulak & Bonaz, 2004; Posserud et al., 2004). Visceral hypersensitivity present in about two-thirds of IBS patients has been considered a biological marker in IBS (Bouin et al., 2002; Mertz et al., 1995). Numerous studies have also reported coexisting somatic hypersensitivity in IBS, although results are not unanimous (Chang et al., 2000; Iovino et al., 2006), most likely due to methodological issues, heterogeneity of IBS patient subgroups, or concomitant disorders (e.g., fibromyalgia) (Moshiree et al., 2007; Verne et al., 2001). The widespread character of hypersensitivity has been related to both peripheral and central mechanisms (Azpiroz et al., 2007; Piché et al., 2010). Alterations in the central nervous system (CNS) circuitries responsive to visceral input have been recently delineated in IBS patients compared with healthy subjects using functional brain imaging techniques (Song et al., 2006; Wilder-Smith et al., 2004). Evidence of spinal nociceptive facilitation in IBS has been also provided (Coffin et al., 2004).

Over the past 15 years, various animal models have been developed to gain a deeper insight into the central and peripheral mechanisms of visceral hypersensitivity (Holschneider et al., 2011; Mayer et al., 2008). However, only recently has the role of alterations in descending pain modulatory pathways in the pathophysiology of IBS and experimental models of IBS been recognized (Berman et al., 2008; Larauche et al., 2011a; Larauche et al., 2011b; Wilder-Smith et al., 2004). In this chapter, we will review the recent developments on stress-related modulation of visceral sensitivity to colorectal distension (CRD), with a special focus on alterations in stress-induced visceral analgesia and pain inhibitory mechanisms.

2. Mechanisms of widespread hypersensitivity in IBS

Several underlying mechanisms have been implicated independently or synergistically to account for the widespread hypersensitivity in IBS. Changes in excitability of central neurons and processes called 'central sensitization' contribute to the maintenance of secondary hyperalgesia (i.e. increased sensitivity to stimuli from uninjured tissues adjacent to or at some distance from the site of injury). Spinal sensitization could explain both visceral hypersensitivity and secondary hyperalgesia found in lumbosacral dermatomes, consistent with the viscerosomatic convergence on spinal neurons (Verne et al., 2001). In support of this contention, the local rectal application of lidocaine reversed visceral and cutaneous hyperalgesia in the lower limbs of IBS patients (Verne et al., 2003). Likewise, in animal models, 25% of rats receiving intracolonic administration of trinitrobenzene sulfonic acid to induce colitis displayed long-lasting hypersensitivity to both rectal distension and somatic stimuli such as heat stimulus applied to the foot or tail (Zhou et al., 2008). The hypersensitivity was the most pronounced in lumbosacral dermatomes, and intracolonic lidocaine administration normalized both rectal and somatic hypersensitivity (Zhou et al., 2008). In addition, an altered descending modulation (discussed in the next paragraph) may also play an important role. Pain facilitation processes associated with psychological factors are important components contributing to the hypersensitivity as well, along with pain inhibition deficits observed in IBS. In fact, heightened levels of anxiety and depression in IBS patients correlate with lower sensory thresholds to gut distension (Bouin et al., 2002; Posserud et al., 2004).

3. Descending pain modulatory system

The periaqueductal gray matter (PAG) and the nucleus raphe magnus, as well as nearby structures of the rostral ventromedial medulla (RVM) with their projections to the spinal dorsal horn, constitute a pain-control system that 'descends' from the brain onto the spinal cord (Vanegas & Schaible, 2004). Importantly, this endogenous descending pain modulatory system consists not only of inhibitory, but also facilitatory pathways. Persistent nociception simultaneously triggers descending facilitation and inhibition. For instance, in models of inflammation following the subcutaneous injection of irritants, descending pain inhibition predominates over facilitation in response to input from the inflamed tissue, therefore attenuating primary hyperalgesia. In the case of secondary hyperalgesia, descending facilitation predominates over inhibition in pain circuits with input from adjacent tissues (Vanegas & Schaible, 2004). The importance of facilitation of the spinal nociceptive processing has been recently recognized as a potential mechanism contributing to the pathophysiology of chronic pain conditions, including numerous functional disorders, such as IBS (Coffin et al., 2004). In these disorders characterized by persistent pain or discomfort without clearly defined tissue pathology, normally innocuous stimulation is incorrectly interpreted as noxious, which may originate from input to the RVM from sites rostral in the brain (e.g., via cortical, amygdalar or hypothalamic efferents), and be affected by a state of attention, anxiety, or cognitive perception (Urban & Gebhart, 1999).

Numerous studies using inflammatory, neurogenic, or neuropathic models of hyperalgesia have shown that the RVM plays a key role in central sensitization which underlies the pathogenesis of chronic pain disorders. For example, visceral hyperalgesia associated with colonic inflammation could be reversed by the intra-RVM administration of an *N*-methyl-D-aspartic acid receptor antagonist, suggesting tonic activity at glutamatergic synapses in the RVM (Coutinho et al., 1998). Other neuropeptide modulators present in the rodent RVM such as neurotensin or cholecystokinin have also been identified to be tonically active following peripheral tissue insult or inflammation (Friedrich & Gebhart, 2003; Gui et al., 2004; Gebhart, 2004). A noteworthy aspect - in the RVM there are different electrophysiologically defined cells, termed ON cells, which are thought to facilitate nociception, and OFF cells that inhibit nociception processing (Mason, 2005). Descending inhibitory influences from the RVM are confined to the dorsolateral funiculi whereas facilitatory influences descend the spinal cord in the ventral/ventrolateral cord (Gebhart, 2004).

4. Monitoring of visceral pain in rodents

The assessment of pseudoaffective reflex responses (and to a lesser degree, behavioral responses) to controlled isobaric distensions of the distal colon has become the primary readout and the standard assay for the measurement of visceral pain in rodents since its development in 1988 by Ness and Gebhart (Ness & Gebhart, 1988). When applied to rats, CRD produces a range of autonomic and behavioral pseudoaffective reflexes (changes in arterial pressure and heart rate, passive avoidance behaviors, and contraction of abdominal musculature). Monitoring the contraction of abdominal muscles or visceromotor response (VMR) is the most commonly used index of visceral pain response in rats and mice. In conscious animals, it can be directly assessed by electromyographic (EMG) signals monitored via surgically-implanted recording electrodes into the external or internal abdominal muscle, where the electrode device is either externalized through the skin (abdomen, neck) (Bradesi et al., 2005; Christianson & Gebhart, 2007; Larsson et al., 2003) or connected to radiotelemetric implants into the abdominal cavity (Welting et al., 2005). Although the method is of significant value in the field of visceral pain, it has experimental shortfalls such as damage to EMG electrodes, loss of signal, and electrical interferences, which is of particular concern in chronic experimental settings. Additionally, EMG implantation requires surgery that encompasses skin and/or muscle incision depending on the technique used (subcutaneous abdominal electrodes or intraperitoneal cannula) and chronic implantation of a foreign body. Even though no data are available in the literature in relation to the immune impact of chronic EMG electrodes placed into the abdominal wall, such intervention could induce a host-tissue response with local micro-inflammation (neutrophils, lymphocytes and macrophages) as it has been shown for other types of implants in the skin and peritoneum (Klueh & Kreutzer, 2005). A recent report suggests that the preconditions of animals (EMG surgery, post-surgical delivery of antibiotic and single housing) have a considerable impact on the visceral pain responses to CRD, particularly in the context of stress studies (Larauche et al., 2010). Other approaches consist of recording manometric changes in the pressure of the balloon inserted into the distal colon (Arvidsson et al., 2006) or changes in pressure inside the colonic lumen (Larauche et al., 2009; Larauche et al., 2010). These two techniques present the advantage of being minimally invasive as they do not require surgery and post-surgical treatments such as antibiotics or analgesics which can affect the visceral pain responses and still remain an objective and sensitive measure of abdominal contractions. However, they entail the partial restraint of animals in Bollman cages, a context to which they need to be habituated and which by itself may bring a component of stress. Behavioral approaches such as operant behavioral assays (Ness & Gebhart, 1988) have also been used in early studies and capitalized on the learning and fear behaviors of animals in response to painful CRD. Furthermore, visual monitoring of the abdominal withdrawal reflex (Al-Chaer et al., 2000) has been applied in a few studies, and while having the great advantage of being one of the less invasive techniques employed to date, it is a very subjective method. Indirect endpoints, such as the marker of neuronal activation, Fos protein or extracellular signal-regulated protein kinase expression induced in neurons at specific sites in the CNS (Million et al., 2006; Wu et al., 2010), as well as functional brain imaging of integrated brain responses to nociceptive stimuli (Wang et al.,

2008), have also been utilized in some animal studies. These approaches allow for direct assessment of neuronal circuitries activated by the visceral pain stimulus and, in the case of functional brain imaging, are very similar to the monitoring of CRD responses in IBS patients and healthy subjects. Unfortunately, in animals these brain mapping techniques require euthanasia and limit the assessment to specific time points. However, as more stringent brain imaging approaches are developed in rodents, they will open new venues to parallel human studies (Coello et al., 2011; Lee et al., 2010).

We recently developed an alternative non-invasive method to study visceral sensitivity to CRD in conscious mice, using a commercially-available miniaturized pressure catheter to record intraluminal colonic pressure (ICP) (Larauche et al., 2010). Briefly, a PE50 catheter was taped 2 cm below the pressure sensor of a miniaturized pressure transducer catheter (SPR-524 Mikro-Tip catheter; Millar Instruments, Houston, TX). A custom-made balloon (1-cm width x 2-cm length) (Arvidsson et al., 2006; Christianson & Gebhart, 2007; Kamp et al., 2003) prepared from a polyethylene plastic bag was tied over the catheter at 1 cm below the pressure sensor with silk 4.0. Ligature points were covered with parafilm to prevent any air from leaking. To validate the technique, we monitored the VMR to graded phasic CRD by simultaneously recording ICP and EMG signals in mice chronically implanted with electrodes. We found an excellent correlation between signals from ICP and EMG during consecutive ascending phasic distensions between 15 to 60 mmHg when recorded simultaneously in the same mice. We also showed that the colonic pain pressure threshold to CRD detected by both methods were similar (about 32 mmHg), and consistent with values previously reported using EMG and manometry (Arvidsson et al., 2006; Kamp et al., 2003). As colonic pressure could be altered following abdominal contractions and/or contractions of the colonic wall, we assessed the effects of atropine, a muscarinic blocker known to inhibit colonic motility (Gourcerol et al., 2009), on the VMR to CRD monitored by ICP in naïve mice (Larauche et al., 2010). We found that atropine did not significantly modify the phasic CRD-associated ICP changes (Larauche et al., 2010), while inhibiting distal colonic motility measured by ICP changes in conscious mice maintained under similar recording conditions (Gourcerol et al., 2009). In addition, with the use of the non-invasive method, it has been confirmed that buprenorphine, a partial agonist for mu-opioid receptors, inhibited visceral sensitivity to graded phasic ascending CRD which is consistent with opioid-induced reduction of basal visceral response to CRD in both rats and mice (Danzebrink et al., 1995; Larsson et al., 2003). Conversely, an hyperalgesic response to CRD can be induced after the intraperitoneal injection of cortagine, a selective corticotropin releasing factor receptor subtype 1 (CRF_1) agonist, known to act directly on the CRF_1 receptor expressed in the colon (Larauche et al., 2009). A similar, non-invasive method to monitor VMR has also been validated in rats (Larauche et al., 2009). Taken together, these data have established the reliability of ICP method to assess the modulation of visceral sensitivity in conscious rodents (Larauche et al., 2010).

5. Stress-induced modulation of visceral pain

By convention, stressors are categorized as exteroceptive (psychological or neurogenic) and interoceptive (physical, systemic, visceral or immune) (Herman & Cullinan, 1997; Sawchenko et al., 2000). Both have been applied to rodents to investigate the relationship between stress and visceral pain modulation (Mayer & Collins, 2002). Dual visceral pain responses - hyperalgesia and analgesia have been described in rodents. Stress-induced

hyperalgesia has been examined in detail in several recent reviews (Larauche et al., 2011a; Larauche et al., 2011b; Mayer, 2008) to which the reader is referred to. By contrast, while extensively described in the somatic pain field (Butler & Finn, 2009), to date stress-related activation of descending inhibitory pathways under conditions of visceral pain has received less attention. Opioids have been implicated in descending inhibition of visceral sensitivity to CRD following an acute stress. This is evidenced by the fact that naloxone unmasked water avoidance stress (WAS)-induced hyperalgesia to CRD in normal Long-Evans rats and exacerbated the pain response to CRD in maternally-separated rats (Coutinho et al., 2002). In another study, a non-opioid, neurotensin-dependent visceral analgesic response was induced in wild-type mice 6 h after exposure to an acute session of WAS, while neurotensin knock-out mice under the same conditions had no analgesia (Gui et al., 2004). In addition, male Sprague-Dawley rats exhibited stronger analgesia to WAS than females (Gui et al., 2004). In another experimental model, a daily short period (15 min) pup separation from the mother, occurring from postnatal days 2 to 14, decreased VMR to CRD performed immediately after WAS and prevented the development of hyperalgesia 24 h after WAS in adult male Long-Evans rats (Schwetz et al., 2005). These data suggest a potential upregulation of endogenous pain-modulatory systems by this short maternal separation stress (Schwetz et al., 2005). Similar findings have been recently reported in adult Wistar rats handled daily for 9 days which develop visceral hypoalgesia in response to CRD that becomes significant 7 days after the last handling (Winston et al., 2010). These studies point to different types of mild psychological or environmental stressors–induced naloxone dependent or independent visceral analgesia as reported for somatic pain (Butler & Finn, 2009) and indicate a potential sex difference in such a stress-related analgesic response.
However, importantly, we recently demonstrated that mice that had undergone surgery for the placement of EMG electrodes on the abdominal wall and were subsequently singly housed to avoid deterioration of the implanted electrodes by cage-mates, developed visceral hyperalgesia in response to repeated WAS (1h/day for 10 consecutive days), while mice tested for visceral pain using the non-invasive solid-state intraluminal pressure recording and kept group housed, developed a strong visceral analgesia under otherwise similar conditions of repeated intermittent WAS (Larauche et al., 2010). Collectively, these data demonstrate that the state of the tested animal (naïve vs exposed to surgery), its social environment (group housing vs single housing, cage enrichment or not), the handling performed by the investigator, the methods used to record visceromotor responses (EMG requiring surgery and antibiotic post surgery vs manometry not requiring surgery/antibiotic), as well as the animal sex can significantly affect the analgesic response to exteroceptive stressors. Therefore these preconditions should be carefully detailed in describing the experimental setting and taken into consideration in the study design and interpretations of the data when investigating the influence of stress on visceral sensitivity in experimental animals.

6. Deficit in pain inhibition in IBS

The stress-related analgesic response bears very relevant implications to the understanding of analgesic mechanisms that can be impaired in visceral pain-associated pathologies such as IBS. Deficits in stress-related descending pain inhibition may lay at the origin of both somatic and visceral hypersensitivity. Alteration in pain inhibitory modulation was observed in IBS patients under conditions of counter-irritation, a clinically well-recognized phenomenon frequently described as "pain inhibits pain" (Le Bars et al., 1979; Wilder-Smith et al., 2004). It occurs when response from a painful stimulus is inhibited by another, often spatially distant and noxious and relates to mechanisms named diffuse noxious inhibitory controls (DNICs) (Le Bars et al., 1979). Counter-irritation modulated via CNS mechanisms usually produces robust pain inhibition with residual analgesia persisting during the recovery period. Studies using the DNIC model to quantify the central pain sensitization in patients with chronic pain syndrome showed that defective DNIC is a risk factor for developing these disorders (Edwards et al., 2003; Lautenbacher & Rollman, 1997). Interestingly, many IBS patients display a reduced inhibition of evoked somatic or rectal pain that normally occur when a noxious stimulus is simultaneously applied to another body area, e.g. hot or cold water immersion tests (King et al., 2009; Wilder-Smith et al., 2004). Recent studies assessing the correlation between visceral and somatic hypersensitivity in diarrhea-predominant IBS patients have shown that patients with rectal hypersensitivity display a clear concomitant deficit in somatic pain inhibition (Piché et al., 2010). The observed somatic hypersensitivity to cutaneous heat stimulation involved different regions of the body but was more pronounced in dermatomes in which afferents converge on spinal neurons receiving bowel afferents. These data suggest that the coexisting visceral and somatic hypersensitivity may depend on both viscerosomatic convergence and generalized spinal hyperexcitability (Piché et al., 2010). A deficit in endogenous pain modulation and somatic hypersensitivity have also been demonstrated in other recent studies in IBS patients (Heymen et al., 2010; Wilder-Smith et al. 2004). Moreover, the spinal transmission of nociceptive signals in IBS patients was investigated by analyzing the effects of rectal distensions on EMG recordings of the somatic nociceptive flexion (RIII) reflex, an objective index of spinal somatic nociceptive processes (Coffin et al., 2004). The results indicated that the RIII reflex was significantly facilitated during slow ramp distension, whereas inhibitions induced by rapid distensions were significantly reduced in IBS patients compared to healthy controls (Coffin et al., 2004). Therefore both reduction in inhibition and active facilitation could contribute to central sensitization and secondary hyperalgesia in IBS (Price et al., 2009).

7. Conclusions

Based on recent clinical findings demonstrating that IBS patients have a compromised engagement of the inhibitory descending pain modulation systems (Berman et al., 2008; Coffin et al., 2004; Piché et al., 2010; Song et al., 2006; Wilder-Smith et al., 2004), gaining a deeper understanding of mechanisms involved in the expression of stress-induced visceral analgesia, or lack thereof, are promising avenues to be explored and may lead to new therapeutic targets for IBS. Therefore the use of non-invasive methods of monitoring VMR that allows the unraveling of the analgesic influence of stress on visceral pain represents a step forward to gain insight into the underlying mechanisms, in particular the neural substrates and neurochemistry of stress-related analgesia as established in the somatic pain field (Butler & Finn, 2009).

8. Acknowledgements

This review is supported by the VA Research Career Scientist Award, NIH grants R01 DK-57238 and DK 33061 and P50 DK-64539 (YT) and K01 DK088937 (ML). The authors thank Ms. Eugenia Hu for reviewing the manuscript.

9. References

Al-Chaer, E.D.; Kawasaki, M. & Pasricha, P.J. (2000). A new model of chronic visceral hypersensitivity in adult rats induced by colon irritation during postnatal development. *Gastroenterology,* 119, 5, pp. 1276-1285, ISSN 0016-5085

Arvidsson, S.; Larsson, M.; Larsson, H.; Lindström, E. & Martinez, V. (2006). Assessment of visceral pain-related pseudo-affective responses to colorectal distension in mice by intracolonic manometric recordings. *J. Pain,* 7, 2, pp. 108-118, ISSN 1526-5900

Azpiroz, F.; Bouin, M.; Camilleri, M.; Mayer, E.A.; Poitras, P.; Serra, J. & Spiller, R.C. (2007). Mechanisms of hypersensitivity in IBS and functional disorders. *Neurogastroenterol. Motil.,* 19, 1 Suppl, pp. 62-88, ISSN 1350-1925

Berman, S.M.; Naliboff, B.D.; Suyenobu, B.; Labus, J.S.; Stains, J.; Ohning, G.; Kilpatrick, L.; Bueller, J.A.; Ruby, K.; Jarcho, J. & Mayer, E.A. (2008). Reduced brainstem inhibition during anticipated pelvic visceral pain correlates with enhanced brain response to the visceral stimulus in women with irritable bowel syndrome. *J. Neurosci.,* 28, 2, pp. 349-359, ISSN 0270-6474

Bouin, M.; Plourde, V.; Boivin, M.; Riberdy, M.; Lupien, F.; Laganière, M.; Verrier, P. & Poitras, P. (2002). Rectal distention testing in patients with irritable bowel syndrome: sensitivity, specificity, and predictive values of pain sensory thresholds. *Gastroenterology,* 122, 7, pp. 1771-1777, ISSN 0016-5085

Bradesi, S.; Schwetz, I.; Ennes, H.S.; Lamy, C.M.; Ohning, G.; Fanselow, M.; Pothoulakis, C.; McRoberts, J.A. & Mayer, E.A. (2005). Repeated exposure to water avoidance stress in rats: a new model for sustained visceral hyperalgesia. *Am. J. Physiol. Gastrointest. Liver Physiol.,* 289, 1, pp. G42-G53, ISSN 0193-1857

Butler, R.K. & Finn, D.P. (2009). Stress-induced analgesia. *Prog. Neurobiol.,* 88, 3, pp. 184-202, ISSN 0301-0082

Chang, L.; Mayer, E.A.; Johnson, T.; FitzGerald, L.Z. & Naliboff, B. (2000). Differences in somatic perception in female patients with irritable bowel syndrome with and without fibromyalgia. *Pain,* 84, 2-3, pp. 297-307, ISSN 0304-3959

Christianson, J.A. & Gebhart, G.F. (2007). Assessment of colon sensitivity by luminal distension in mice. *Nat. Protoc.,* 2, 10, pp. 2624-2631, ISSN 1754-2189

Coello, C.; Hjornevik, T.; Courivaud, F. & Willoch, F. (2011). Anatomical standardization of small animal brain FDG-PET images using synthetic functional template: Experimental comparison with anatomical template. *J. Neurosci. Methods,* 199, 1, pp. 166-172, ISSN 0165-0270

Coffin, B.; Bouhassira, D.; Sabate, J.M.; Barbe, L. & Jian, R. (2004). Alteration of the spinal modulation of nociceptive processing in patients with irritable bowel syndrome. *Gut,* 53, 10, pp. 1465-1470, ISSN 0017-5749

Coutinho, S.V.; Plotsky, P.M.; Sablad, M.; Miller, J.C.; Zhou, H.; Bayati, A.I.; McRoberts, J.A. & Mayer, E.A. (2002). Neonatal maternal separation alters stress-induced responses to viscerosomatic nociceptive stimuli in rat. *Am. J. Physiol. Gastrointest. Liver Physiol.,* 282, 2, pp. G307-G316, ISSN 0193-1857

Coutinho, S.V.; Urban, M.O. & Gebhart, G.F. (1998). Role of glutamate receptors and nitric oxide in the rostral ventromedial medulla in visceral hyperalgesia. *Pain,* 78, 1, pp. 59-69, ISSN 0304-3959

Danzebrink, R.M.; Green, S.A. & Gebhart, G.F. (1995). Spinal mu and delta, but not kappa, opioid-receptor agonists attenuate responses to noxious colorectal distension in the rat. *Pain,* 63, 1, pp. 39-47, ISSN 0304-3959

Edwards, R.R.; Ness, T.J.; Weigent, D.A. & Fillingim, R.B. (2003). Individual differences in diffuse noxious inhibitory controls (DNIC): association with clinical variables. *Pain,* 106, 3, pp. 427-437, ISSN 0304-3959

Elsenbruch, S.; Rosenberger, C.; Bingel, U.; Forsting, M.; Schedlowski, M. & Gizewski, E.R. (2010). Patients with irritable bowel syndrome have altered emotional modulation of neural responses to visceral stimuli. *Gastroenterology,* 139, 4, pp. 1310-1319, ISSN 0016-5085

Friedrich, A.E. & Gebhart, G.F. (2003). Modulation of visceral hyperalgesia by morphine and cholecystokinin from the rat rostroventral medial medulla. *Pain,* 104, 1-2, pp. 93-101, ISSN 0304-3959

Gebhart, G.F. (2004). Descending modulation of pain. *Neurosci. Biobehav. Rev.,* 27, 8, pp. 729-737, ISSN 0149-7634

Gourcerol, G.; Wang, L.; Adelson, D.W.; Larauche, M.; Taché, Y. & Million, M. (2009). Cholinergic giant migrating contractions in conscious mice colon assessed by using a novel non-invasive solid-state manometry method: modulation by stressors. *Am. J. Physiol. Gastrointest. Liver Physiol.,* 296, 5, pp. G992-G1002, ISSN 0193-1857

Gui, X.; Carraway, R.E. & Dobner, P.R. (2004). Endogenous neurotensin facilitates visceral nociception and is required for stress-induced antinociception in mice and rats. *Neuroscience,* 126, 4, pp. 1023-1032, ISSN 0306-4522

Herman, J.P. & Cullinan, W.E. (1997). Neurocircuitry of stress: central control of the hypothalamo-pituitary-adrenocortical axis. *Trends Neurosci.,* 20, 2, pp. 78-84, ISSN 0166-2236

Heymen, S.; Maixner, W.; Whitehead, W.E.; Klatzkin, R.R.; Mechlin, B. & Light, K.C. (2010). Central processing of noxious somatic stimuli in patients with irritable bowel syndrome compared with healthy controls. *Clin. J. Pain,* 26, 2, pp. 104-109, ISSN 1536-5409

Holschneider, D.P.; Bradesi, S. & Mayer, E.A. (2011). The role of experimental models in developing new treatments for irritable bowel syndrome. *Expert. Rev. Gastroenterol. Hepatol.,* 5, 1, pp. 43-57, ISSN 1747-4124

Iovino, P.; Tremolaterra, F.; Consalvo, D.; Sabbatini, F.; Mazzacca, G. & Ciacci, C. (2006). Perception of electrocutaneous stimuli in irritable bowel syndrome. *Am. J. Gastroenterol.,* 101, 3, pp. 596-603, ISSN 0002-9270

Kamp, E.H.; Jones, R.C., III; Tillman, S.R. & Gebhart, G.F. (2003). Quantitative assessment and characterization of visceral nociception and hyperalgesia in mice. *Am. J. Physiol. Gastrointest. Liver Physiol.,* 284, 3, pp. G434-G444, ISSN 0193-1857

King, C.D.; Wong, F.; Currie, T.; Mauderli, A.P.; Fillingim, R.B. & Riley, J.L., 3rd (2009). Deficiency in endogenous modulation of prolonged heat pain in patients with Irritable Bowel Syndrome and Temporomandibular Disorder. *Pain,* 143, 3, pp. 172-178, ISSN 0304-3959

Klueh, U. & Kreutzer, D.L. (2005). Murine model of implantable glucose sensors: a novel model for glucose sensor development. *Diabetes Technol. Ther.,* 7, 5, pp. 727-737, ISSN 1520-9156

Larauche, M.; Gourcerol, G.; Million, M.; Adelson, D.W. & Taché, Y. (2010). Repeated psychological stress-induced alterations of visceral sensitivity and colonic motor functions in mice: Influence of surgery and postoperative single housing on visceromotor responses. *Stress,* 13, 4, pp. 343-354, ISSN 1025-3890

Larauche, M.; Gourcerol, G.; Wang, L.; Pambukchian, K.; Brunnhuber, S.; Adelson, D.W.; Rivier, J.; Million, M. & Taché, Y. (2009). Cortagine, a CRF1 agonist, induces stresslike alterations of colonic function and visceral hypersensitivity in rodents primarily through peripheral pathways. *Am. J. Physiol. Gastrointest. Liver Physiol.*, 297, 1, pp. G215-G227, ISSN 0193-1857

Larauche, M.; Mulak, A. & Taché, Y. (2011a). Stress and visceral pain: From animal models to clinical therapies. *Exp. Neurol.*, Published Online First *doi:10.1016/j.expneurol.2011.04.020*, ISSN 0014-4886

Larauche, M.; Mulak, A. & Taché, Y. (2011b). Stress-related alterations of visceral sensation: animal models for IBS study. *J. Neurogastroenterol. Motil.*, Published Online First *doi:10.5056/jnm.2011.17.3.212.*, ISSN 2093-0879

Larsson, M.; Arvidsson, S.; Ekman, C. & Bayati, A. (2003). A model for chronic quantitative studies of colorectal sensitivity using balloon distension in conscious mice - effects of opioid receptor agonists. *Neurogastroenterol. Motil.*, 15, 4, pp. 371-381, ISSN 1350-1925

Lautenbacher, S. & Rollman, G.B. (1997). Possible deficiencies of pain modulation in fibromyalgia. *Clin. J. Pain*, 13, 3, pp. 189-196, ISSN 1536-5409

Le Bars, B.D.; Dickenson, A.H. & Besson, J.M. (1979). Diffuse noxious inhibitory controls (DNIC). I. Effects on dorsal horn convergent neurones in the rat. *Pain*, 6, 3, pp. 283-304, ISSN 0304-3959

Lee, J.H.; Durand, R.; Gradinaru, V.; Zhang, F.; Goshen, I.; Kim, D.S.; Fenno, L.E.; Ramakrishnan, C. & Deisseroth, K. (2010). Global and local fMRI signals driven by neurons defined optogenetically by type and wiring. *Nature*, 465, 7299, pp. 788-792, ISSN 0028-0836

Mason, P. (2005). Ventromedial medulla: pain modulation and beyond. *J. Comp. Neurol.*, 493, 1, pp. 2-8, ISSN 0021-9967

Martinez, V.; Thakur, S.; Mogil, J.S.; Taché, Y. & Mayer, E.A. (1999). Differential effects of chemical and mechanical colonic irritation on behavioral pain response to intraperitoneal acetic acid in mice. *Pain*, 81, 1-2, pp. 179-186, ISSN 0304-3959

Mayer, E.A.; Bradesi, S.; Chang, L.; Spiegel, B.M.; Bueller, J.A. & Naliboff, B.D. (2008). Functional GI disorders: from animal models to drug development. *Gut*, 57, 3, pp. 384-404, ISSN 0017-5749

Mayer, E.A. & Collins, S.M. (2002). Evolving pathophysiologic models of functional gastrointestinal disorders. *Gastroenterology*, 122, 7, pp. 2032-2048, ISSN 0016-5085

Mertz, H.; Naliboff, B.; Munakata, J.; Niazi, N. & Mayer, E.A. (1995). Altered rectal perception is a biological marker of patients with irritable bowel syndrome. *Gastroenterology*, 109, 1, pp. 40-52, ISSN 0016-5085

Million, M.; Wang, L.; Wang, Y.; Adelson, D.W.; Yuan, P.Q.; Maillot, C.; Coutinho, S.V.; McRoberts, J.A.; Bayati, A.; Mattsson, H.; Wu, V.; Wei, J.Y.; Rivier, J.; Vale, W.; Mayer, E.A. & Taché, Y. (2006). CRF2 receptor activation prevents colorectal distension induced visceral pain and spinal ERK1/2 phosphorylation in rats. *Gut*, 55, 2, pp. 172-181, ISSN 0017-5749

Moshiree, B.; Price, D.D.; Robinson, M.E.; Gaible, R. & Verne, G.N. (2007). Thermal and visceral hypersensitivity in irritable bowel syndrome patients with and without fibromyalgia. *Clin. J. Pain*, 23, 4, pp. 323-330, ISSN 1536-5409

Mulak, A. & Bonaz, B. (2004). Irritable bowel syndrome: a model of the brain-gut interactions. *Med. Sci. Monit.*, 10, 4, pp. RA55-62, ISSN 1234-1010

Ness, T.J. & Gebhart, G.F. (1988). Colorectal distension as a noxious visceral stimulus: physiologic and pharmacologic characterization of pseudaffective reflexes in the rat. *Brain Res.*, 450, 1-2, pp. 153-169, ISSN 0006-8993

Piché, M.; Arsenault, M.; Poitras, P.; Rainville, P. & Bouin, M. (2010). Widespread hypersensitivity is related to altered pain inhibition processes in irritable bowel syndrome. *Pain*, 148, 1, pp. 49-58, ISSN 0304-3959

Posserud, I.; Agerforz, P.; Ekman, R.; Bjornsson, E.S.; Abrahamsson, H. & Simren, M. (2004). Altered visceral perceptual and neuroendocrine response in patients with irritable bowel syndrome during mental stress. *Gut,* 53, 8, pp. 1102-1108, ISSN 0017-5749

Price, D.D.; Craggs, J.G.; Zhou, Q.; Verne, G.N.; Perlstein, W.M. & Robinson, M.E. (2009). Widespread hyperalgesia in irritable bowel syndrome is dynamically maintained by tonic visceral impulse input and placebo/nocebo factors: evidence from human psychophysics, animal models, and neuroimaging. *Neuroimage,* 47, 3, pp. 995-1001, ISSN 1053-8119

Sawchenko, P.E.; Li, H.Y. & Ericsson, A. (2000). Circuits and mechanisms governing hypothalamic responses to stress: a tale of two paradigms. *Prog. Brain Res.,* 122, 61-78, ISSN 0079-6123

Schwetz, I.; McRoberts, J.A.; Coutinho, S.V.; Bradesi, S.; Gale, G.; Fanselow, M.; Million, M.; Ohning, G.; Taché, Y.; Plotsky, P.M. & Mayer, E.A. (2005). Corticotropin-releasing factor receptor 1 mediates acute and delayed stress-induced visceral hyperalgesia in maternally separated Long-Evans rats. *Am. J. Physiol. Gastrointest. Liver Physiol.,* 289, 4, pp. G704-G712, ISSN 0193-1857

Song, G.H.; Venkatraman, V.; Ho, K.Y.; Chee, M.W.; Yeoh, K.G. & Wilder-Smith, C.H. (2006). Cortical effects of anticipation and endogenous modulation of visceral pain assessed by functional brain MRI in irritable bowel syndrome patients and healthy controls. *Pain,* 126, 1-3, pp. 79-90, ISSN 0304-3959

Urban, M.O. & Gebhart G.F. (1999). Central mechanisms in pain. *Med. Clin. North Am.,* 83, 3, pp. 585-596, ISSN 0025-7125

Vanegas, H. & Schaible, H.G. (2004). Descending control of persistent pain: inhibitory or facilitatory? *Brain Res. Rev.,* 46, 3, pp. 295-309, ISSN 0165-0173

Verne, G.N.; Robinson, M.E. & Price, D.D. (2001). Hypersensitivity to visceral and cutaneous pain in the irritable bowel syndrome. *Pain,* 93, 1, pp. 7-14, ISSN 0304-3959

Verne, G.N.; Robinson, M.E.; Vase, L. & Price, D.D. (2003). Reversal of visceral and cutaneous hyperalgesia by local rectal anesthesia in irritable bowel syndrome (IBS) patients. *Pain,* 105, 1-2, pp. 223-230, ISSN 0304-3959

Wang, Z.; Bradesi, S.; Maarek, J.M.; Lee, K.; Winchester, W.J.; Mayer, E.A. & Holschneider, D.P. (2008). Regional brain activation in conscious, nonrestrained rats in response to noxious visceral stimulation. *Pain,* 138, 1, pp. 233-243, ISSN 0304-3959

Welting, O.; van den Wijngaard, R.M.; de Jonge, W.J.; Holman, R. & Boeckxstaens, G.E. (2005). Assessment of visceral sensitivity using radio telemetry in a rat model of maternal separation. *Neurogastroenterol. Motil.,* 17, 6, pp. 838-845, ISSN 1350-1925

Wilder-Smith, C.H.; Schindler, D.; Lovblad, K.; Redmond, S.M. & Nirkko, A. (2004). Brain functional magnetic resonance imaging of rectal pain and activation of endogenous inhibitory mechanisms in irritable bowel syndrome patient subgroups and healthy controls. *Gut,* 53, 11, pp. 1595-1601, ISSN 0017-5749

Winston, J.H.; Xu, G.Y. & Sarna, S.K. (2010). Adrenergic stimulation mediates visceral hypersensitivity to colorectal distension following heterotypic chronic stress. *Gastroenterology,* 138, 1, pp. 294-304, ISSN 0016-5085

Wu, J.C.; Ziea, E.T.; Lao, L.; Lam, E.F.; Chan, C.S.; Liang, A.Y.; Chu, S.L.; Yew, D.T.; Berman, B.M. & Sung, J.J. (2010). Effect of electroacupuncture on visceral hyperalgesia, serotonin and fos expression in an animal model of irritable bowel syndrome. *J. Neurogastroenterol. Motil.,* 16, 3, pp. 306-314, ISSN 2093-0879

Zhou, Q.; Price, D.D. & Verne, G.N. (2008). Reversal of visceral and somatic hypersensitivity in a subset of hypersensitive rats by intracolonic lidocaine. *Pain,* 139, 1, pp. 218-224, ISSN 0304-3959

16

Dysbiosis of the Intestinal Microbiota in IBS

Anna Lyra and Sampo Lahtinen
Danisco, Health & Nutrition
Finland

1. Introduction

The human gastrointestinal (GI) microbiota is a rich and dynamic community inhabited by approximately 10^{14} bacteria, most of which have not yet been cultivated in the laboratory (Zoetendal *et al*, 2006). The GI microbiota has been suggested as one of the etiological factors in irritable bowel syndrome (IBS), with a putative role in the development and maintenance of IBS symptoms (for a review, see Bolino & Bercik, 2010). The worldwide prevalence of IBS is 10-20% among adults and adolescents, depending on the diagnostic criteria applied (Longstreth *et al*, 2006). Abdominal pain or discomfort, irregular bowel movements and constipation or diarrhoea are common symptoms of IBS. Symptoms outside the GI tract, such as fatigue, anxiety and depression, are also often encountered. At its worst, IBS can cause significant effects on patients' well-being, but it is not known to predispose to any severe illnesses. Patients can be grouped into three subtypes according to bowel habits: diarrhoea-predominant (IBS-D), constipation-predominant (IBS-C) or mixed-subtype (IBS-M). However, the symptom subtype of each patient may vary over time (Longstreth *et al*, 2006).

Compared to non-IBS controls, subjects with IBS have been associated with a greater temporal instability of the GI microbiota and quantitative changes have been detected within several distinct bacterial groups or species-like phylotypes, which are defined based solely on sequence data (see Table 1 for references). In analyses covering the overall microbial community, IBS subjects have shown a tendency to cluster apart from the healthy control subjects (Ponnusamy *et al*, 2011; Rajilić-Stojanović, 2007). Moreover, the IBS symptom-subgroups IBS have been proposed to differ from each other according to the GI microbiota of subjects within these groups (Lyra *et al*, 2009; Malinen *et al*, 2005; Rajilic-Stojanovic, 2007). The most distinctive symptom sub-type is IBS-D, which could also be a result of the impact of the diarrhoea on the microbial environment in the gut. In addition, comparatively low quantities of bifidobacteria, which are generally considered beneficial to health, have been detected in several IBS studies (Balsari *et al*, 1982; Enck *et al*, 2009; Kerckhoffs *et al*, 2009; Krogius-Kurikka *et al*, 2009; Si *et al*, 2004). This finding, though still preliminary, encourages development of probiotic and prebiotic therapies for IBS. On the other hand, elevated numbers of Proteobacteria and Firmicutes, including *Ruminococcus* -like phylotypes, *Lactobacillus* sp. and *Veillonella* sp., have been reported.

Quantitative and qualitative microbial alterations in the GI tract of IBS subjects may have a functional role in the syndrome aetiology or merely reflect the status of the gut, but still have diagnostic or prognostic value in clinical practise and research (Kassinen, 2009;

Salonen *et al*, 2010). In the following chapter, these IBS-related alterations within the human GI microbiota are reviewed.

2. Intestinal microbiota

The intestinal microbiota is individual-specific and relatively stable through time (Zoetendal *et al*, 1998). From a microbial point of view, a tremendous variety of physiologically connected environments exists in the human GI tract. The mouth and stomach harbour their distinct microbiotas (Bik *et al*, 2006; Zaura *et al*, 2009). In the small intestine, the bacterial load and diversity rise from 10^4 to 10^8 cells per millilitre of intestinal content towards the distal ileum. *Veillonella, Streptococcus, Clostridium* cluster I and *Enterococcus* form the core genera of the small intestinal lumen (Booijink *et al*, 2010). Reaching the colon, the transit slows down and the bacterial density rises from 10^8 in the caecum and ascending colon to an average of 10^{11} to 10^{12} cells of bacteria per gram in faeces. The proportion of obligate anaerobic bacteria expands to 99%. The phyla Firmicutes, Bacteroidetes, Actinobacteria, Proteobacteria, Fusobacteria and Verrucomicrobia are present in the colon (Andersson *et al*, 2008; Kurokawa *et al*, 2007). In the small and large intestines, the mucosal and luminal microbiotas are distinct from each other (Booijink *et al*, 2007; Zoetendal *et al*, 2002). Recently it has been shown that the human GI microbiota roughly groups into three entorotypes, with either *Bacteroides, Prevotella* or *Ruminococcus* predominating (Arumugam *et al*, 2011).

The GI microbiota has a dynamic mutualistic relationship with its host affecting host nutrition and metabolism, immunocompetence and tolerance, GI tract surface maturation and function and even behaviour, thus possessing a potentially tremendous impact on host well-being (for review see Sekirov *et al*, 2010). Multiple theories linking IBS aetiology with the intestinal microbiota have been proposed, which, together with the discovered IBS-associated GI microbiota alterations, imply that bacteria may well play a role in IBS aetiology.

3. Gut microbiota in IBS

Alterations in the GI microbiota related to IBS have been investigated since the early 1980s' by conventional culture-based methods and an array of molecular methods (Table 1). Several of the published studies are based on the same Finnish sample panel originating from a probiotic intervention and additional healthy control subjects. For clarity, these studies are represented under a separate sub-heading in Table 1. Besides differing from control subjects, IBS also differs from IBD including Crohn's disease and ulcerative colitis (Enck *et al*, 2009; Ponnusamy *et al*, 2011).

Study	Samples	Method	Outcome for IBS[1] subjects
Balsari *et al*, 1982	20 IBS, 20 Controls	Culturing	Less coliforms, lactobacilli and bifidobacteria
Si *et al*, 2004	25 IBS, 25 Controls	Culturing	Less bifidobacteia More *Enterobacteriaceae*
Rajilić-Stojanović, 2007	20 IBS, 20 Controls	HITChip	Distinctive clustering; Subtype-specific alterations; Higher inter-individual variation

Kerckhoffs *et al*, 2009	41 IBS 26 Controls	FISH, qPCR; Fecal and mucosal brush samples	Bifidobacteria in feces and *Bifidobacterium catenulatum* on the mucosa decreased
Enck *et al*, 2009	7765 IBS, 198 CD, 515 UC, 10478 Other GI diag.	Culturing	Less bifidobacteria than in samples of subjects with other GI complaints
Malinen *et al*, 2010	44 IBS	qPCR, Questionnaires	Previously IBS associated phylotype now associated with sensation of symptoms
Codling *et al*, 2010	47 IBS, 33 Controls	DGGE; Fecal and mucosal samples	Lower inter-individual variation
Tana *et al*, 2010	26 IBS, 26 Controls	qPCR, culturing, SCFA, questionnaires, X-ray	*Veillonella* and lactobacilli elevated; Acetic, propionic and total SCFA elevated and correlated with symptoms
Noor *et al*, 2010	11 IBS, 13 UC, 22 Controls	DGGE	Less diversity among *Bacteroides*
Carroll *et al*, 2010	10 IBS-D, 10 Controls	Culturing, qPCR; Fecal and mucosal biopsy samples	Less aerobes and more lactobacilli in feces
Carroll *et al*, 2011	16 IBS-D, 21 Controls	T-RFLP; Fecal and mucosal biopsy samples	The microbial profiles grouped according to origin (mucosal or luminal) rather than health status. Microbial composition at both mucosa and lumen altered in IBS-D.
Ponnusamy *et al*, 2011	11 IBS, 8 non-IBS patients	DGGE, qPCR	Higher diversity of total bacteria, *Bacteroides* and *Lactobacillus;* Elevated amino acids and phenolic compounds
Saulnier *et al*, 2011	22 Pediatric IBS, 22 Control children	Pyrosequencing, PhyloChip	Gammaproteobacteria including *Haemophilus influenzae* elevated; *Ruminococcus* –like phylotype associated with IBS; *Allistipes* correlated with pain
Studies on a Finnish sample set[2]			
Study / Method	**Healthy controls**	**IBS subjects on placebo**	**IBS subjects on probiotic[3]**
Kajander *et al.*, 2005; Intervention	NA	Analysed as control	Total symptom score reduced (borborygmi)
Malinen *et al.*, 2005; qPCR 300 gut species	Analyzed as control	High *Lactobacillus* sp. in IBS-D Low *Veillonella* sp. in IBS-C	NA
Mättö *et al.*, 2005; Culturing, DGGE	Analysed as control	More coliforms; Higher aerobe:anaerobe ratio	NA

Maukonen *et al.*, 2006; DGGE, TRAC,	Analysed as control	Less *Clostridium coccoides-Eubacterium rectale* in IBS-C (RNA); Less stable microbiota (RNA)	NA
Kajander *et al.*, 2007; qPCR 300 gut species	NA	Analyzed as control	No alteration
Kassinen *et al.*, 2007; G+C%, sequencing, qPCR	Analyzed as control	Altered community structure; 3 altering phylotypes	NA
Lyra *et al.*, 2009; qPCR 14 phylotypes	Two associated phylotypes	IBS-D and IBS-C associated phylotypes; IBS-D distinguishable	NA
Krogius-Kurikka *et al.*, 2009; G+C%, sequencing	Actinobacteria abundant	NA	NA
Krogius-Kurikka *et al.*, 2009; G+C%, sequencing, qPCR	More Actinobacteria and Bacteroidetes	IBS-D enriched with Proteobacteria and Firmicutes, especially Lachnospiraceae	NA
Lyra *et al.*, 2010; qPCR 8 phylotypes	NA	Analyzed as control	Quantities shifted towards healthy like levels
Rinttilä *et al.*, 2011; qPCR 12 pathogens	Analyzed as control	*Staphylococcus aureus* more prevalent in IBS	NA

[1]The abbreviations in order of appearance stand for IBS, irritable bowel syndrome; HITCip, Human Intestinal Tract Chip; FISH, fluorescent *in situ* hybridization; qPCR, real-time quantitative PCR; CD, Crohn's disease; UC, ulcerative colitis; GI, gastrointestinal; DGGE, denaturing gradient gel electrophoresis; SCFA, short chain fatty acids; IBS-D, diarrhea-predominant IBS; T-RFLP, terminal-restriction fragment length polymorphism; NA, not analyzed; and IBS-C, constipation-predominant IBS.
[2]The sample set consisted of probiotic intervention samples from the intervnetion by Kajander *et al.*, (2005) and additional control samples from subjects devoid of gastrointestinal symptoms. The detected alterations are given under the sample group they apply to.
[3]The probiotic supplement was a combination of *L. rhamnosus* GG and Lc705, *B. breve* Bb99 and *P. freudenreichii* ssp. *shermanii* JS administered for 6 months at a daily dose of 8–9 x 10^9 CFU with equal amounts of each strain (Kajander *et al*, 2005).

Table 1. Studies on irritable bowel syndrome (IBS) related intestinal microbiota.

3.1 Culture-based analyses

Using culture-based techniques, the GI microbiota of IBS patients was characterized as having less coliforms, lactobacilli and bifidobacteria in a study with 20 IBS patients and 20 controls (Balsari *et al*, 1982). Likewise, in a later study (Si *et al*, 2004) with 25 IBS patients fulfilling the Rome II criteria and 25 controls, lower levels of bifidobacteria were detected in IBS patients, but the level of bacteria belonging to the family *Enterobacteriaceae* was higher in IBS patients. Contrary to Balsari *et al.* (1982), Mättö *et al.* (2005) detected more coliforms in IBS subjects' and no difference in the bifidobacterial counts using culture-based methods, whereas the number of coliforms and aerobe:anaerobe ratio were elevated (26 IBS and 25 control subjects). In 2009, Enck and colleagues conducted an impressive culturing study by analysing the intestinal microbiota of a total of 34 313 subjects of varying conditions (Enck *et al*, 2009). Routine analyses were applied to *Clostridium difficile, Bifidobacterium* spp., *Bacteroides* spp., *Escherichia coli, Enterococcus* spp. and *Lactobacillus* spp. A total of 7 765 IBS subjects were included in the final data analysis revealing a significantly lower abundance of *Bifidobaterium* spp. In the latest study based on culturing, aerobes were elevated in the faecal samples of IBS-D patients compared with control subjects, whereas anaerobes, *Clostridium* spp., *Bacteroides* spp., *Lactobacillus* spp., *Bifidobacterium* spp., and *Escherichia coli* were not altered in IBS-D (Carroll *et al*, 2010).

Taken together, evidence for increased numbers of aerobes and comparably low counts of bifidobacteria exist from culture based analyses with the latter giving good grounds for prebiotic and probiotic therapy research. The results on coliforms are contradictory between different studies.

3.2 Community structure with molecular methods

The overall microbial community from faecal samples of IBS subjects has been analysed applying denaturing gradient gel electrophoresis (DGGE), microarray (HITCip and PhyloChip), and sequencing (conventional Sanger sequencing and 2nd generation 454 pyrosequencing). All of these methods are capable of detecting the unculturable species in the microbiota, although they bear restrictions due to primer and probe dependency and technical biases. The main advantage is the possibility to gain a non-restricted overview and with sequencing, to able to design targeted primers and probes for applications based on PCR or hybridization.

Greater temporal instability of the intestinal microbiota of IBS patients compared with that of healthy controls has been detected with RNA-based DGGE (Maukonen *et al*, 2006). Applying DNA-based DGGE on the same sample set did not show IBS related temporal variation (Maukonen *et al*, 2006), but variation due to antibiotic therapy was observed (Mättö *et al*, 2005). The inter-individual variability has been assessed in two studies with contradictory results. With the HITChip microarray analysis IBS subjects showed significantly more inter-individual variation compared with the controls (Rajilić-Stojanović, 2007), whereas with DGGE more variation was seen amongst control subjects (Codling *et al*, 2010). This discrepancy is likely due to methodological differences as the probe or primer based bacterial targets differ.

Moreover, the biodiversity, an expression of species richness and abundance, is decreased in IBS (Noor *et al*, 2010). Loss of species richness was especially evident among *Bacteroides* species, which was speculated to suggest their putative protective role in the GI tract (Noor *et al*, 2010). Krogius-Kurikka *et al.* (2009) also found IBS-D related GI microbiota to lack diversity in a sequencing analysis, but the number of samples pooled prior to analysis was lower in the IBS-D sample possibly affecting the result (Krogius-Kurikka *et al*, 2009). On the other hand, Saulnier and colleagues (2011) analysed multiple samples from 22 pediatric IBS patients and 22 control subjects with 454 pyrosequencing (54 287 reads per sample) and a portion of the samples further with the PhyloChip which targets revealing no significant difference in bacterial bacterial quantities or richness, although qualitative changes were detected between the two subject groups and in relation to perception of pain (Saulnier *et al*, 2011).

Thus, at least for adult IBS subjects, the diversity and species richness in the GI microbiota are diminished, which would together with the alternating symptoms explain a higher temporal and inter-individual variation in the gut microbiota. A less stable microbiota is potentially more vulnerable to external interference (infection, antibiotics, stress), possibly leading to a recurrent aberration in gut function.

3.3 From community to phylotype level

In addition to the overall community structure and stability in the GI tract, the thousands of bacterial species therein, referred to as phylotypes when based only on molecular data, are important. Aspects such as their absolute and relative abundance, prevalence and association to symptoms sub-types and perception have been studied.

The sample set studied by Mättö *et al.* (2005) and Maukonen *et al.* (2006) was further studied using 20 quantitative real-time PCR (qPCR) assays covering approximately 300 bacterial species (27 IBS patients and 22 controls gave faecal samples at the first time-point; 21 IBS patients and 15 controls gave faecal samples at three time-points at three-month intervals) (Malinen *et al*, 2005). The first time-point was analysed with IBS subjects divided into symptom subgroups; IBS-D, IBS-C and IBS-M. Statistically significant differences were observed with real-time PCR assays targeting *Lactobacillus* spp. (less abundant in IBS-D than in IBS-C), *Veillonella* spp. (less abundant in controls than in IBS-C) and *Bifidobacterium* spp. (less abundant in IBS-D than in all other groups). The *Clostridium coccoides* and *Bifidobacterium catenulatum* group assays detected more target bacteria in controls than in IBS patients when the results from the three different time-points were averaged and the IBS subjects analysed as a single group.

Thereafter, the samples were analysed with percent guanine plus cytosine (%G+C) profiling (Kassinen *et al*, 2007): The pooled symptom subtype profiles diverged with the %G+C profiling and the three most diverging fractions were subsequently studied using 16S rDNA Sanger sequencing. Real-time PCR assays targeting specifically the alterations between the sequesnce libraries of IBS and control subjects were designed and applied in several studies highlighting a ruminococcal phylotype in relation to IBS-D and a taxonomically unclassifiable phylotype with the control subjects and IBS subjects under probiotic theraphy (Lyra *et al*, 2010; Lyra *et al*, 2009; Malinen *et al*, 2010).

Ruminococcal bacteria have also been associated with Crohn's disease and pediatric IBS (Frank *et al*, 2007; Martinez-Medina *et al*, 2006; Saulnier *et al*, 2011). Ruminococci include mucolytic bacteria with a possible competitive advantage in a disturbed gut with excessive mucus secretion. Novel uncultured bacterial phylotypes discovered in relation to IBS and health may also perform well as diagnostic microbiome signatures (Kassinen *et al*, 2007; Lyra *et al*, 2009; Saulnier *et al*, 2011) although their possible relation to the syndrome is mere speculation at this stage. The genera *Bifidobacterium, Coriobacterium* and *Collinsella* within the phylum Actinobacteria have been less abundant in IBS patients (Enck *et al*, 2009; Kassinen *et al*, 2007; Kerckhoffs *et al*, 2009; Lyra *et al*, 2009). Correspondingly, redused levels of Actinobacteria including bifidobacteria have been associated with Crohn's disease patients

(Fyderek *et al*, 2009; Manichanh *et al*, 2006; Sokol *et al*, 2009), and *Collinsella aerofaciens* has been associated with a low risk of colon cancer (Moore & Moore, 1995).

These more specific changes, once well established in relation to both healthy and non-IBS GI patient controls, have potential in diagnostics and tailor-made therapeutic approaches. The possibility of finding a causative agent for IBS, for instance among the ruminococcal phylotypes, is intriguing though still a future challenge.

3.4 Microarray analyses

Two 16S rRNA gene sequence based microarrays with a wide array of target phylotypes have been applied to IBS samples. The advantage of microarrays is their semi-quantitative nature, high-throughput capability and more straightforward applicability to diagnostic and therapeutic applications.

The first microarray analysis focusing on IBS-associated GI microbiota applying a microarray (The Human Intestinal Tract Chip, HITChip) was published in 2007 (Rajilic-Stojanovic, 2007). The HITChip is a 16S rRNA gene-based phylogenetic microarray specifically designed to target the human intestinal microbiota (Rajilic-Stojanovic *et al*, 2009). It is unable to quantify phylotypes directly, but relative changes in hybridization signals can be detected between 0.1% and 3% subpopulations in an artificial mixture of 30 phylotypes (Rajilic-Stojanovic, 2007). The HITChip study on IBS encompassed 20 IBS patients sub-grouped according to symptom subtype and 20 healthy controls. With a hierarchical cluster analysis, the phylogenetic fingerprints of the faecal microbiota of IBS patients and controls grouped into two distinctive groups, with one dominated by IBS patients' samples (14 IBS patients and 4 controls) and the other by healthy controls' samples (16 controls and 6 IBS patients). The clustering did not correlate with the IBS symptom subtype. Stronger variation in the composition of the microbiota was seen among the IBS patients' profiles.

Within the phylotypes targeted by the HITChip, the IBS-C group of IBS patients had lower levels of *Bacteroides* species (*Bacteroides ovatus, Bacteroides uniformis, Bacteroides vulgatus*) and *Clostridium stercorarium*-like bacteria and higher levels of *Bacillus* spp.; the IBS-D patients were characterized by higher levels of *Aneuribacillus* spp., *Streptococcus mitis* and *Streptococcus intermedius*-like bacterial phylotypes from the order *Bacilli*. Various IBS-subgroup dependent differences were detected within *Clostridium* cluster XIVa (*C. coccoides* group). For instance, *Roseburia intestinalis* was more abundant in IBS-D and Ruminococcus gnavus in alternating-type IBS than in healthy controls. Several phylotypes within the *Clostridium* cluster IV (the *Clostridium leptum* -group) were more prominent in IBS-C than in IBS-D. (Rajilic-Stojanovic, 2007)

The other microarray analysis was done on pediatric IBS subjects applying the PhyloChip (Saulnier *et al*, 2011). PhyloChip targets a wider array of microbes not specifically restricted to the expected human intestinal tract inhabitants (Brodie *et al*, 2006) although it is well applicable also to analysing intestinal microbiota (Nelson *et al*, 2011; Saulnier *et al*, 2011). Saulnier and colleagues (2011) discovered that Proteobacteria, especially Gammaproteobacteria, are abundant in pediatric IBS subjects. Within these Gammaproteobacteria the species *Haemophilus parainfluenzae* was commonly encountered. Similarly the pyrosequencing analysis revealed elevated numbers of Protebacteria and unclassified ruminococcal phylotypes in association to pediatric IBS and (Saulnier *et al*, 2011). In the PhyloChip analysis, several *Bacteroides* phylotypes, including a *Bacteroides vulgatus* -like phylotype, were elevated in healthy children (Saulnier *et al*, 2011), as has previously been noted in the case of adult subjects with ulcerative colitis (UC) or IBS (Noor *et al*, 2010).

These efficient high-throughput methods have potential for analyzing large enough sample sets to identify common alterations in the heterogeneous IBS subject population. So far too few studies have been published for making a consensus on the results. In addition, it would be beneficial if the sampling schema would include several samples linked to thorough symptom data from each subject as both the microbiota and the symptoms in IBS are prone to alter over time.

3.5 The mucosal microbiota

The mucosal microbiota is of special interest in health related studies as it is in an intimate contact with the host. In a healthy intestine, the mucosal microbiota resides on the mucosal lining of the epithelium, whereas in a damaged intestine straight contact with the host epithelium is plausible. Fluorescent in situ hybridization (FISH) applied on mucosal samples of patients with IBD, IBS or no GI symptoms revealed that mucosal bacteria were more abundant in IBS patients than in healthy controls, although the difference was less evident than with the IBD patients (Swidsinski *et al*, 2005). The proportional amounts of the different bacterial groups targeted in the FISH analysis (*Bacteroides-Prevotella, Bacteroides fragilis, Eubacterium rectale-Clostridium coccoides, Faecalibacterium prausnitzii* and *Enterococcus faecalis*), however, were similar between IBS patients and controls (Swidsinski *et al*, 2005). Likewise, Carroll and colleagues (2010) found no significant difference between the abundances of cultured bacteria (aerobic, anaerobes, *Clostridium* spp., *Bacteroides* spp., *Lactobacillus* spp., *Bifidobacterium* spp., and *Escherichia coli*). With qPCR, elevated levels of *Pseudomonas aeruginosa*, a gram-negative opportunistic pathogen, have been detected in duodenal brush samples of IBS patients. Nevertheless, a recent terminal-restriction fragment length polymorphism (T-RFLP) analysis was able to differentiate between the composition of IBS-D patients' and control subjects' mucosal microbiota, although the overall microbial profiles clustered according to site of sampling (mucosal or luminal) rather than health status (IBS-D or healthy control) (Carroll *et al*, 2011).

Taken together, no drastic alteration in the mucosal microbiota of IBS subjects has been defined. The mucosal and luminal microbiotas differ in IBS subjects as they do in healthy controls, underlying the importance of research on this specific niche. One reason for the small number of mucosal IBS studies is the invasive nature of mucosal sampling as colonoscopy is not a regular procedure in IBS diagnostics or treatment.

4. Microbial metabolites and enzymes

4.1 Short Chain Fatty Acids (SCFAs)

The principal products of microbial carbohydrate metabolism in the human GI tract are short-chain fatty acids (SCFAs), which can be absorbed by the human host. The SCFAs produced throughout the GI tract are mainly acetate, butyrate and propionate, but in the colon acetate predominates (Cummings *et al*, 1987). The colonic epithelial cells prefers butyrate over other SCFAs as an energy source, and butyrate has been shown to have a positive effect on health (Pryde *et al*, 2002). The most abundant intestinal butyrate-producing bacteria are Firmicutes from Clostridial clusters XIVa and IV (*Clostridium, Eubacterium, Fusobacterium*) (Pryde *et al*, 2002). Starch fermentation by starch-degrading bacteria results in comparatively high amounts of butyrate (Chassard *et al*, 2008). Starch-degrading bacteria, including *Ruminococcus bromii* (Clostridium cluster IV), *Eubacterium rectale* (Clostridium cluster XIVa) and bifidobacteria (Leitch *et al*, 2007), comprise approximately 10% of culturable bacteria in faecal samples (Chassard *et al*, 2008).

Reduced amounts of total SCFAs due to lower levels of acetate and propionate have been measured in association with IBS-D, while an elevated concentration of n-butyrate seemed to be characteristic of IBS-D (Treem *et al*, 1996). Tana and colleagues (2010) analysed the microbiota and SCFAs from faecal samples donated by 26 IBS and 26 control subjects. Contrary to Treem *et al.* (1996), the IBS subjects had elevated numbers of *Veillonella* spp. and *Lactobacillus* spp. together with higher concentrations of total organic acids and acetic and propionic acid. The increase in acidic metabolites was more pronounced in the group of IBS subjects with worse GI symptoms, quality of life and emotional status according to subjective evaluation (Tana *et al*, 2010).

Colonic gas production (H_2 and CH_4) has been shown to be greater in patients with IBS (Rome II criteria) compared with controls using a standardized diet, which might be associated with alterations in the activity of hydrogen-consuming bacteria (King *et al*, 1998). An exclusion diet, mainly devoid of dairy products and cereals other than rice, reduced IBS symptoms and lowered the maximum gas excretion (King *et al*, 1998). Furthermore, functional constipation and IBS-C have been associated with methane production according to breath testing in a recent meta-analysis (Kunkel *et al*, 2011).

Thus, although the results on microbial metabolites in the colon are still scarce and to some extent contradictory, they have been linked to symptom severity and defecation habit sub-type. The elevated amount of butyrate among IBS-D subjects in one study is surprising, as butyrate is considered to have a positive effect on health.

4.2 Luminal proteases

Certain studies have suggested an association between luminal proteases and IBS. An elevated faecal serine protease activity has been associated with IBS-D (Roka *et al*, 2007). The faecal supernatants from IBS-D patients caused increased colonic paracellular permeability when administered to the mucosal side of a mouse colon strip and increased visceral hypersensitivity in mice (Gecse *et al*, 2008). Gecse *et al.* (2008) also showed that the effect on mucosal permeability is mediated by serine protease through protease-activated receptor two (PAR-2). Pre-incubation with serine protease inhibitors decreased the effect of the faecal supernatant from the IBS-D patients on the colonic paracellular permeability of mouse colon strips. Furthermore, the use of colonic strips derived from PAR-2-deficient mice completely removed the increase in colonic paracellular permeability. The elevated serine protease activity in IBS-D patients was suggested to be of microbial origin (Gecse *et al*, 2008). The PAR-2 mediated increase in visceral hypersensitivity appears to be specifically related to IBS-D in comparison to inflammatory bowel diseases (IBD) (Annahazi *et al*, 2009).

The evidence for the role of luminal proteases in IBS symptoms is at its early stage, but intriguing. It links the GI microbiota with the host's IBS symptoms through increased gut permeability and visceral hypersensitivity.

5. Post-infectious IBS

In a large cohort study (over 500 000 patients), gastroenteritis was concluded to increase the risk of developing IBS by a factor of ten (Rodriguez & Ruigomez, 1999). Post-infectious IBS

(PI-IBS) has been reported after *Campylobacter, Shigella* and *Salmonella* infections (Ji *et al,* 2005; Mearin *et al,* 2005; Spiller *et al,* 2000) and *Staphylococcus aureus* has been detected in a comparatively high prevalence in IBS subjects (Rinttilä *et al,* 2011). Nevertheless, PI-IBS appears to be a non-specific response (Spiller, 2007). Typically PI-IBS is characterized by loose stools, less depression and anxiety and increased enterochromaffin cells in mucosal biopsies compared with non-PI-IBS (Dunlop *et al,* 2003; Neal *et al,* 2002). Detecting an infectious agent from random IBS subjects is unlikely (Rinttilä *et al,* 2011), but this still does not rule out the possibility of an earlier infectious event having etiological importance.
Since the initial gastroenteritis triggering PI-IBS is a coincidental event, and among PI-IBS patients the symptoms are relatively homogeneous and psychological abnormalities are less common than in other IBS patients, PI-IBS presents a clearer model for studying the possible mechanisms underlying IBS (Spiller, 2007). On the other hand, PI-IBS may be etiologically too distinct to represent the whole of IBS subtype variety.
In addition to acute gastroenteritis triggering IBS symptomology, low-grade inflammation with focus on mast cells and monocytes has been suggested to have a pivotal role in IBS aetiology (for review see Ohman & Simren, 2010). Low-grade mucosal inflammation (Barbara *et al,* 2007; Chadwick *et al,* 2002; Dunlop *et al,* 2003; Ohman *et al,* 2005) and stable alterations in mucosal gene expression (Aerssens *et al,* 2008) of IBS patients of all symptom subtypes have been detected. Furthermore, the basal and *E. coli* lipopolysaccharide induced release of pro-inflammatory cytokines from peripheral blood mononuclear cells has been shown to be elevated in IBS-D patients compared to healthy controls (Liebregts *et al,* 2007). Additionally, antibodies against certain bacterial flagellin have been detected in IBS patients, particularly in PI-IBS patients, with a higher frequency than in healthy controls (Schoepfer *et al,* 2008).
Taken together, PI-IBS is a widely accepted sub-type of IBS which can reside from a variety of causative agents. Minimizing risk, severity and length of acute gastroenteritis would likely lower the risk of recurrent functional GI disturbances such as IBS.

6. Probiotics for balancing the GI microbiota in IBS

Being a syndrome diagnosed based on subjective assessment of GI function, the most important outcome in IBS intervention studies is the patients' sensation of symptom relief. This is usually assessed by applying GI symptom questionnaires. According to a recent meta-analysis, the separate IBS symptoms (abdominal pain, bloating and flatulence) and their composite sum have all been significantly improved with probiotics (Hoveyda *et al.* 2009).
From the microbiological point of view, it is of interest to see whether the symptom improvement during the intervention is linked to alteration within the GI microbiota – putatively to a state that better resembles that of healthy-like control subjects. If no change in the microbiota is seen in a specific study, this doesn't necessarily mean there hasn't been one as the methodology used may have missed the targets of interest. This has been the case for a multispecies supplement intervention trial with *L. rhamnosus* GG, *L. rhamnosus* LC705, *B. breve* Bb99 and *P. freudenreichii* ssp. *shermanii* JS (Kajander *et al,* 2005), first assessed by qPCR assays targeting known GI bacteria (Kajander *et al,* 2007) and thereafter by targeting IBS associated phylotypes (Lyra *et al,* 2010). The analyses of 300 known GI bacteria showed no alterations due to the intervention (Kajander *et al,* 2007), but a vast number of phylotypes may have been missed with analyses restricted by primer target selection, whereas in the

latter study, when the same samples were screened with qPCR assays targeting specifically IBS associated phylotypes (Lyra *et al*, 2010), alterations towards levels previously measured in controls devoid of GI symptoms (Lyra *et al*, 2009) were measured.

Nobaek and co-workers (2000) have analysed abundances of *Enterobacteriacea*, sulphate-reducing bacteria and *Enterococci* in IBS subjects consuming a rose-hip drink with *Lactobacillus plantarum* (DSM 9843). No alterations were detected in the probiotic group, but the probiotic strain was detected in faecal and rectal mucosal samples (Nobaek *et al*, 2000). Here again, the analysis method covered only a minor portion of the entire microbiota.

In addition to affecting the bacterial levels and the stability of the GI microbiota, the relief of bloating and distention with probiotics may be linked to an effect on microbial metabolism (Schmulson & Chang, 2011).

7. Conclusion

Dysbiosis of the intestinal microbiota in IBS has been detected on several levels: the overall community appears to be less diverse with more variation between individuals and over time. These phenomena may reduce the resilience of the microbiota to external stressors, and both trigger and sustain functional aberrations in the gut. In addition to overall dysbiosis, specific bacterial groups are either elevated (*Lactobacillus, Veillonella, Ruminococcus, Enterobacteria,* aerobes as a group, *S. aureus*) or reduced (*Bifidobactrium, B. catenulatum, Bacteroides*) in IBS, but with the exception of bifidobacteria, the available data is not yet conclusive. Ruminococcal phylotypes have been associated specifically with IBS and also with inflammatory states in the intestinal tract in several studies and certainly deserve more attention. The analytical methodologies available for studying the GI microbiota have developed immensely in the past decade and the discovery of efficient microbial signature based diagnostic and therapeutic methods even for such a heterogeneous and subjectively defined patient group as IBS can be expected in the near future.

8. References

Aerssens J, Camilleri M, Talloen W, Thielemans L, Gohlmann HW, Van Den Wyngaert I, Thielemans T, De Hoogt R, Andrews CN, Bharucha AE, Carlson PJ, Busciglio I, Burton DD, Smyrk T, Urrutia R, Coulie B (2008) Alterations in mucosal immunity identified in the colon of patients with irritable bowel syndrome. *Clin Gastroenterol Hepatol* 6: 194-205

Andersson AF, Lindberg M, Jakobsson H, Backhed F, Nyren P, Engstrand L (2008) Comparative analysis of human gut microbiota by barcoded pyrosequencing. *PLoS One* 3: e2836

Annahazi A, Gecse K, Dabek M, Ait-Belgnaoui A, Rosztoczy A, Roka R, Molnar T, Theodorou V, Wittmann T, Bueno L, Eutamene H (2009) Fecal proteases from diarrheic-IBS and ulcerative colitis patients exert opposite effect on visceral sensitivity in mice. *Pain* 144: 209-217

Arumugam M, Raes J, Pelletier E, Le Paslier D, Yamada T, Mende DR, Fernandes GR, Tap J, Bruls T, Batto JM, Bertalan M, Borruel N, Casellas F, Fernandez L, Gautier L, Hansen T, Hattori M, Hayashi T, Kleerebezem M, Kurokawa K, Leclerc M, Levenez F, Manichanh C, Nielsen HB, Nielsen T, Pons N, Poulain J, Qin J, Sicheritz-Ponten T, Tims S, Torrents D, Ugarte E, Zoetendal EG, Wang J, Guarner F, Pedersen O, de

Vos WM, Brunak S, Dore J, Antolin M, Artiguenave F, Blottiere HM, Almeida M, Brechot C, Cara C, Chervaux C, Cultrone A, Delorme C, Denariaz G, Dervyn R, Foerstner KU, Friss C, van de Guchte M, Guedon E, Haimet F, Huber W, van Hylckama-Vlieg J, Jamet A, Juste C, Kaci G, Knol J, Lakhdari O, Layec S, Le Roux K, Maguin E, Merieux A, Melo Minardi R, M'Rini C, Muller J, Oozeer R, Parkhill J, Renault P, Rescigno M, Sanchez N, Sunagawa S, Torrejon A, Turner K, Vandemeulebrouck G, Varela E, Winogradsky Y, Zeller G, Weissenbach J, Ehrlich SD, Bork P (2011) Enterotypes of the human gut microbiome. *Nature* 473: 174-180

Balsari A, Ceccarelli A, Dubini F, Fesce E, Poli G (1982) The fecal microbial population in the irritable bowel syndrome. *Microbiologica* 5: 185-194

Barbara G, Wang B, Stanghellini V, de Giorgio R, Cremon C, Di Nardo G, Trevisani M, Campi B, Geppetti P, Tonini M, Bunnett NW, Grundy D, Corinaldesi R (2007) Mast cell-dependent excitation of visceral-nociceptive sensory neurons in irritable bowel syndrome. *Gastroenterology* 132: 26-37

Bik EM, Eckburg PB, Gill SR, Nelson KE, Purdom EA, Francois F, Perez-Perez G, Blaser MJ, Relman DA (2006) Molecular analysis of the bacterial microbiota in the human stomach. *Proc Natl Acad Sci U S A* 103: 732-737

Bolino CM, Bercik P (2010) Pathogenic factors involved in the development of irritable bowel syndrome: focus on a microbial role. *Infect Dis Clin North Am* 24: 961-975, ix

Booijink CC, El-Aidy S, Rajilic-Stojanovic M, Heilig HG, Troost FJ, Smidt H, Kleerebezem M, De Vos WM, Zoetendal EG (2010) High temporal and inter-individual variation detected in the human ileal microbiota. *Environ Microbiol* 12: 3213-3227

Booijink CC, Zoetendal EG, Kleerebezem M, de Vos WM (2007) Microbial communities in the human small intestine: coupling diversity to metagenomics. *Future Microbiol* 2: 285-295

Brodie EL, Desantis TZ, Joyner DC, Baek SM, Larsen JT, Andersen GL, Hazen TC, Richardson PM, Herman DJ, Tokunaga TK, Wan JM, Firestone MK (2006) Application of a high-density oligonucleotide microarray approach to study bacterial population dynamics during uranium reduction and reoxidation. *Appl Environ Microbiol* 72: 6288-6298

Carroll IM, Chang YH, Park J, Sartor RB, Ringel Y (2010) Luminal and mucosal-associated intestinal microbiota in patients with diarrhea-predominant irritable bowel syndrome. *Gut Pathog* 2: 19

Carroll IM, Ringel-Kulka T, Keku TO, Chang YH, Packey CD, Sartor RB, Ringel Y (2011) Molecular Analysis of the Luminal and Mucosal-Associated Intestinal Microbiota in Diarrhea-Predominant Irritable Bowel Syndrome. *Am J Physiol Gastrointest Liver Physiol*

Chadwick VS, Chen W, Shu D, Paulus B, Bethwaite P, Tie A, Wilson I (2002) Activation of the mucosal immune system in irritable bowel syndrome. *Gastroenterology* 122: 1778-1783

Chassard C, Scott KP, Marquet P, Martin JC, Del'homme C, Dapoigny M, Flint HJ, Bernalier-Donadille A (2008) Assessment of metabolic diversity within the intestinal microbiota from healthy humans using combined molecular and cultural approaches. *FEMS Microbiol Ecol* 66: 496-504

Codling C, O'Mahony L, Shanahan F, Quigley EM, Marchesi JR (2010) A molecular analysis of fecal and mucosal bacterial communities in irritable bowel syndrome. *Dig Dis Sci* 55: 392-397

Cummings JH, Pomare EW, Branch WJ, Naylor CP, Macfarlane GT (1987) Short chain fatty acids in human large intestine, portal, hepatic and venous blood. *Gut* 28: 1221-1227

Dunlop SP, Jenkins D, Spiller RC (2003) Distinctive clinical, psychological, and histological features of postinfective irritable bowel syndrome. *Am J Gastroenterol* 98: 1578-1583

Enck P, Zimmermann K, Rusch K, Schwiertz A, Klosterhalfen S, Frick JS (2009) The effects of ageing on the colonic bacterial microflora in adults. *Z Gastroenterol* 47: 653-658

Frank DN, St Amand AL, Feldman RA, Boedeker EC, Harpaz N, Pace NR (2007) Molecular-phylogenetic characterization of microbial community imbalances in human inflammatory bowel diseases. *Proc Natl Acad Sci U S A* 104: 13780-13785

Fyderek K, Strus M, Kowalska-Duplaga K, Gosiewski T, Wedrychowicz A, Jedynak-Wasowicz U, Sladek M, Pieczarkowski S, Adamski P, Kochan P, Heczko PB (2009) Mucosal bacterial microflora and mucus layer thickness in adolescents with inflammatory bowel disease. *World J Gastroenterol* 15: 5287-5294

Gecse K, Roka R, Ferrier L, Leveque M, Eutamene H, Cartier C, Ait-Belgnaoui A, Rosztoczy A, Izbeki F, Fioramonti J, Wittmann T, Bueno L (2008) Increased faecal serine protease activity in diarrhoeic IBS patients: a colonic lumenal factor impairing colonic permeability and sensitivity. *Gut* 57: 591-599

Ji S, Park H, Lee D, Song YK, Choi JP, Lee SI (2005) Post-infectious irritable bowel syndrome in patients with Shigella infection. *J Gastroenterol Hepatol* 20: 381-386

Kajander K, Hatakka K, Poussa T, Färkkilä M, Korpela R (2005) A probiotic mixture alleviates symptoms in irritable bowel syndrome patients: a controlled 6-month intervention. *Aliment Pharmacol Ther* 22: 387-394

Kajander K, Krogius-Kurikka L, Rinttilä T, Karjalainen H, Palva A, Korpela R (2007) Effects of multispecies probiotic supplementation on intestinal microbiota in irritable bowel syndrome. *Aliment Pharmacol Ther* 26: 463-473

Kassinen A, Krogius-Kurikka L, Mäkivuokko H, Rinttilä T, Paulin L, Corander J, Malinen E, Apajalahti J, Palva A (2007) The fecal microbiota of irritable bowel syndrome patients differs significantly from that of healthy subjects. *Gastroenterology* 133: 24-33

Kassinen A (née Lyra) (2009) Alterations in the intestinal microbiota of subjects diagnosed with irritable bowel syndrome. PhD Thesis, Faculty of Veterinary Medicine, University of Helsinki, Hesinki

Kerckhoffs AP, Samsom M, van der Rest ME, de Vogel J, Knol J, Ben-Amor K, Akkermans LM (2009) Lower Bifidobacteria counts in both duodenal mucosa-associated and fecal microbiota in irritable bowel syndrome patients. *World J Gastroenterol* 15: 2887-2892

King TS, Elia M, Hunter JO (1998) Abnormal colonic fermentation in irritable bowel syndrome. *Lancet* 352: 1187-1189

Krogius-Kurikka L, Lyra A, Malinen E, Aarnikunnas J, Tuimala J, Paulin L, Makivuokko H, Kajander K, Palva A (2009) Microbial community analysis reveals high level phylogenetic alterations in the overall gastrointestinal microbiota of diarrhoea-predominant irritable bowel syndrome sufferers. *BMC Gastroenterol* 9: 95

Kunkel D, Basseri RJ, Makhani MD, Chong K, Chang C, Pimentel M (2011) Methane on breath testing is associated with constipation: a systematic review and meta-analysis. *Dig Dis Sci* 56: 1612-1618

Kurokawa K, Itoh T, Kuwahara T, Oshima K, Toh H, Toyoda A, Takami H, Morita H, Sharma VK, Srivastava TP, Taylor TD, Noguchi H, Mori H, Ogura Y, Ehrlich DS, Itoh K, Takagi T, Sakaki Y, Hayashi T, Hattori M (2007) Comparative metagenomics revealed commonly enriched gene sets in human gut microbiomes. *DNA Res* 14: 169-181

Leitch EC, Walker AW, Duncan SH, Holtrop G, Flint HJ (2007) Selective colonization of insoluble substrates by human faecal bacteria. *Environ Microbiol* 9: 667-679

Liebregts T, Adam B, Bredack C, Roth A, Heinzel S, Lester S, Downie-Doyle S, Smith E, Drew P, Talley NJ, Holtmann G (2007) Immune activation in patients with irritable bowel syndrome. *Gastroenterology* 132: 913-920

Longstreth GF, Thompson WG, Chey WD, Houghton LA, Mearin F, Spiller RC (2006) Functional bowel disorders. *Gastroenterology* 130: 1480-1491

Lyra A, Krogius-Kurikka L, Nikkila J, Malinen E, Kajander K, Kurikka K, Korpela R, Palva A (2010) Effect of a multispecies probiotic supplement on quantity of irritable bowel syndrome-related intestinal microbial phylotypes. *BMC Gastroenterol* 10: 110

Lyra A, Rinttilä T, Nikkila J, Krogius-Kurikka L, Kajander K, Malinen E, Mättö J, Makela L, Palva A (2009) Diarrhoea-predominant irritable bowel syndrome distinguishable by 16S rRNA gene phylotype quantification. *World J Gastroenterol* 15: 5936-5945

Malinen E, Krogius-Kurikka L, Lyra A, Nikkilä J, Jääskeläinen A, Rinttilä T, Vilpponen-Salmela T, von Wright AJ, Palva A (2010) Association of symptoms with gastrointestinal microbiota in irritable bowel syndrome. *World J Gastroenterol* 16: 4532-4540

Malinen E, Rinttilä T, Kajander K, Mättö J, Kassinen A, Krogius L, Saarela M, Korpela R, Palva A (2005) Analysis of the fecal microbiota of irritable bowel syndrome patients and healthy controls with real-time PCR. *Am J Gastroenterol* 100: 373-382

Manichanh C, Rigottier-Gois L, Bonnaud E, Gloux K, Pelletier E, Frangeul L, Nalin R, Jarrin C, Chardon P, Marteau P, Roca J, Dore J (2006) Reduced diversity of faecal microbiota in Crohn's disease revealed by a metagenomic approach. *Gut* 55: 205-211

Martinez-Medina M, Aldeguer X, Gonzalez-Huix F, Acero D, Garcia-Gil LJ (2006) Abnormal microbiota composition in the ileocolonic mucosa of Crohn's disease patients as revealed by polymerase chain reaction-denaturing gradient gel electrophoresis. *Inflamm Bowel Dis* 12: 1136-1145

Mättö J, Maunuksela L, Kajander K, Palva A, Korpela R, Kassinen A, Saarela M (2005) Composition and temporal stability of gastrointestinal microbiota in irritable bowel syndrome--a longitudinal study in IBS and control subjects. *FEMS Immunol Med Microbiol* 43: 213-222

Maukonen J, Satokari R, Mättö J, Söderlund H, Mattila-Sandholm T, Saarela M (2006) Prevalence and temporal stability of selected clostridial groups in irritable bowel syndrome in relation to predominant faecal bacteria. *J Med Microbiol* 55: 625-633

Mearin F, Perez-Oliveras M, Perello A, Vinyet J, Ibanez A, Coderch J, Perona M (2005) Dyspepsia and irritable bowel syndrome after a Salmonella gastroenteritis outbreak: one-year follow-up cohort study. *Gastroenterology* 129: 98-104

Moore WE, Moore LH (1995) Intestinal floras of populations that have a high risk of colon cancer. *Appl Environ Microbiol* 61: 3202-3207

Neal KR, Barker L, Spiller RC (2002) Prognosis in post-infective irritable bowel syndrome: a six year follow up study. *Gut* 51: 410-413

Nelson TA, Holmes S, Alekseyenko AV, Shenoy M, Desantis T, Wu CH, Andersen GL, Winston J, Sonnenburg J, Pasricha PJ, Spormann A (2011) PhyloChip microarray analysis reveals altered gastrointestinal microbial communities in a rat model of colonic hypersensitivity. *Neurogastroenterol Motil* 23: 169-177, e141-162

Nobaek S, Johansson ML, Molin G, Ahrne S, Jeppsson B (2000) Alteration of intestinal microflora is associated with reduction in abdominal bloating and pain in patients with irritable bowel syndrome. *Am J Gastroenterol* 95: 1231-1238

Noor SO, Ridgway K, Scovell L, Kemsley EK, Lund EK, Jamieson C, Johnson IT, Narbad A (2010) Ulcerative colitis and irritable bowel patients exhibit distinct abnormalities of the gut microbiota. *BMC Gastroenterol* 10: 134

Ohman L, Isaksson S, Lundgren A, Simren M, Sjovall H (2005) A controlled study of colonic immune activity and beta7+ blood T lymphocytes in patients with irritable bowel syndrome. *Clin Gastroenterol Hepatol* 3: 980-986

Ohman L, Simren M (2010) Pathogenesis of IBS: role of inflammation, immunity and neuroimmune interactions. *Nat Rev Gastroenterol Hepatol* 7: 163-173

Ponnusamy K, Choi JN, Kim J, Lee SY, Lee CH (2011) Microbial community and metabolomic comparison of irritable bowel syndrome faeces. *J Med Microbiol* 60: 817-827

Pryde SE, Duncan SH, Hold GL, Stewart CS, Flint HJ (2002) The microbiology of butyrate formation in the human colon. *FEMS Microbiol Lett* 217: 133-139

Rajilić-Stojanović M (2007) Diveresity of the Human Gastrointestinal Microbiota - Novel Perspectives from High Throughput Analyses. PhD Thesis, Wageningen University, Wageningen

Rajilić-Stojanović M, Heilig HG, Molenaar D, Kajander K, Surakka A, Smidt H, de Vos WM (2009) Development and application of the human intestinal tract chip, a phylogenetic microarray: analysis of universally conserved phylotypes in the abundant microbiota of young and elderly adults. *Environ Microbiol* 11: 1736-1751

Rinttilä T, Lyra A, Krogius-Kurikka L, Palva A (2011) Real-time PCR analysis of enteric pathogens from fecal samples of irritable bowel syndrome subjects. *Gut Pathog* 3: 6

Rodriguez LA, Ruigomez A (1999) Increased risk of irritable bowel syndrome after bacterial gastroenteritis: cohort study. *BMJ* 318: 565-566

Roka R, Rosztoczy A, Leveque M, Izbeki F, Nagy F, Molnar T, Lonovics J, Garcia-Villar R, Fioramonti J, Wittmann T, Bueno L (2007) A pilot study of fecal serine-protease activity: a pathophysiologic factor in diarrhea-predominant irritable bowel syndrome. *Clin Gastroenterol Hepatol* 5: 550-555

Salonen A, de Vos WM, Palva A (2010) Gastrointestinal microbiota in irritable bowel syndrome: present state and perspectives. *Microbiology* 156: 3205-3215

Saulnier DM, Riehle K, Mistretta TA, Diaz MA, Mandal D, Raza S, Weidler EM, Qin X, Coarfa C, Milosavljevic A, Petrosino JF, Highlander S, Gibbs R, Lynch SV, Shulman RJ, Versalovic J (2011) Gastrointestinal Microbiome Signatures Of Pediatric Patients With Irritable Bowel Syndrome. *Gastroenterology*

Schmulson M, Chang L (2011) Review article: the treatment of functional abdominal bloating and distension. *Aliment Pharmacol Ther* 33: 1071-1086

Schoepfer AM, Schaffer T, Seibold-Schmid B, Muller S, Seibold F (2008) Antibodies to flagellin indicate reactivity to bacterial antigens in IBS patients. *Neurogastroenterol Motil* 20: 1110-1118

Sekirov I, Russell SL, Antunes LC, Finlay BB (2010) Gut microbiota in health and disease. *Physiol Rev* 90: 859-904

Si JM, Yu YC, Fan YJ, Chen SJ (2004) Intestinal microecology and quality of life in irritable bowel syndrome patients. *World J Gastroenterol* 10: 1802-1805

Sokol H, Seksik P, Furet JP, Firmesse O, Nion-Larmurier I, Beaugerie L, Cosnes J, Corthier G, Marteau P, Dore J (2009) Low counts of Faecalibacterium prausnitzii in colitis microbiota. *Inflamm Bowel Dis* 15: 1183-1189

Spiller RC (2007) Role of infection in irritable bowel syndrome. *J Gastroenterol* 42 Suppl 17: 41-47

Spiller RC, Jenkins D, Thornley JP, Hebden JM, Wright T, Skinner M, Neal KR (2000) Increased rectal mucosal enteroendocrine cells, T lymphocytes, and increased gut permeability following acute Campylobacter enteritis and in post-dysenteric irritable bowel syndrome. *Gut* 47: 804-811

Swidsinski A, Weber J, Loening-Baucke V, Hale LP, Lochs H (2005) Spatial organization and composition of the mucosal flora in patients with inflammatory bowel disease. *J Clin Microbiol* 43: 3380-3389

Tana C, Umesaki Y, Imaoka A, Handa T, Kanazawa M, Fukudo S (2010) Altered profiles of intestinal microbiota and organic acids may be the origin of symptoms in irritable bowel syndrome. *Neurogastroenterol Motil* 22: 512-519, e114-515

Treem WR, Ahsan N, Kastoff G, Hyams JS (1996) Fecal short-chain fatty acids in patients with diarrhea-predominant irritable bowel syndrome: in vitro studies of carbohydrate fermentation. *J Pediatr Gastroenterol Nutr* 23: 280-286

Zaura E, Keijser BJ, Huse SM, Crielaard W (2009) Defining the healthy "core microbiome" of oral microbial communities. *BMC Microbiol* 9: 259

Zoetendal EG, Akkermans AD, De Vos WM (1998) Temperature gradient gel electrophoresis analysis of 16S rRNA from human fecal samples reveals stable and host-specific communities of active bacteria. *Appl Environ Microbiol* 64: 3854-3859

Zoetendal EG, Vaughan EE, de Vos WM (2006) A microbial world within us. *Mol Microbiol* 59: 1639-1650

Zoetendal EG, von Wright A, Vilpponen-Salmela T, Ben-Amor K, Akkermans AD, de Vos WM (2002) Mucosa-associated bacteria in the human gastrointestinal tract are uniformly distributed along the colon and differ from the community recovered from feces. *Appl Environ Microbiol* 68: 3401-340